THE SILENT EPIDEMIC:

THE SILENT EPIDEMIC:

**What Everyone Should Know
About Brain Injury**

MARK JOHN CONDON

To order additional copies of this book, contact:
Xlibris
844-714-8691
www.Xlibris.com
Orders@Xlibris.com
755091

CONTENTS

DEDICATION

I dedicate this book and all the effort involved in writing it to my daughter Lia Salome' who is the best person in my life: May it help Lia better understand her father's inconsistencies and put my few accomplishments in perspective. Also, I dedicate this book to my amazing parents and family who have sacrificed and worked on my behalf, for so many years, making my post- brain injury life a life that I am happily and gratefully living to the fullest. Thanks be to all of you.

ABOUT THE AUTHOR

Mark John Condon's life as a child was unremarkable and average in every way. Born in 1958 in Ontonagon, Michigan, he was the middle child of five kids in a middle-class family. He was a no-nonsense kind of guy with a great sense of humor, who loved the outdoors, athletic sports, and his friends. When Mark John suffered a severe traumatic brain injury as a collage student, his world and his family's world, was turned upside down. Being abruptly and gravely compromised by the most complicated disease known, lost in a maze of medical misinformation, insurance policy denials, and offered only inadequate options for rehabilitation—he found life to be a struggle more difficult than anyone can imagine. Now, more than forty years forty years later, he has shown an uncanny ability to maintain and achieve goals in the face of the strictest adversity. No one can understand Mark John without knowing the source of his remarkable grit—his close-knit, resilient family. With his family's love and support, today this independent brain injury survivor embraces life in the moment and looks forward to tomorrow. His approach to problems, a combination of compassion and pragmaticism, has worked again and again not only to his own benefit and but also to the benefit of other survivors. Mark John hopes this book will help reframe any reader's confusion and concerns regarding post-traumatic life with a brain injury or with a brain injury survivor—in such a way as to help him or her gain insights that lead to breakthrough experiences.

ABOUT THE BOOK

Every year over 50,000 people will die from brain injury. Annually, one million more brain injury survivors will suffer long-term disability. Yet those closest to neurological research aimed at "understanding the brain" say that to date researchers have only scratched the surface. There is an urgent need for rehabilitation professionals to be much better informed about the personal consequences of brain injury. The dysfunctions associated with brain injury can be subtle, complex, and wide ranging in their effects on quality of life for both survivors and their families. Doctors attest that what Mark John Condon has learned through his brain injury experience and shared in The Silent Epidemic: What Everyone Should Know about Brain Injury is something they could never have learned in all their years of studies. This book could not be published at a better time, since education is recognized as the greatest preventive measure against future brain injuries. Severe brain injury will cost a survivor, his or her family and the community millions of dollars over the survivor's lifetime; it is costing trillions of dollars to the nation as a whole: That is with the most commonly prescribed medical approaches. Mark Condon, however, has searched out, put together, and followed an effective protocol for recovery and rehabilitation that is much less expensive and with which he has broken and dramatically surpassed conventional medical rehabilitation records.

DISCLAIMER

This book relates the story of the author and an approach to rehabilitation that he developed and has personally found to be effective. He is not a medical professional, and this book does not constitute medical advice.

INTRODUCTION

When I was twenty-two years old, driving a couple of blocks in front of the State Capitol Building in Downtown Lansing, Michigan, a drunk driver in a pickup truck ran a red light and crashed—going an estimated 50 miles per hour—into the passenger door of my automobile. The impact swung me around, the right side of my head smashed into the dashboard, and I was knocked unconscious. The stick shift broke six ribs as it ripped open my chest, collapsed my lung, and together with the brain damage stopped my breathing. The drunk driver's truck plowed my car into a parking lot, and I was thrown under the passenger-side dashboard as it crushed in around me, trapping me and making it impossible for me to be removed. Had the bleeding not been stopped and my breathing resuscitated within ten minutes, I would have been completely dead. (I say "completely," for much of me was already dead as a result of *extensive brain damage*). That would have been the end of me had Providence not manifested itself.

At just that moment, there happened to be an ambulance at the same intersection, waiting between calls for the next green light. The paramedics saw the two vehicles crash right in front of them. Somehow they resuscitated my breathing and kept me alive while they waited for the fire department to arrive and extract me from the car. That was when I became a *survivor*—a term used by those in the rehabilitation field to describe a person who experiences disability because of a brain injury (BI).

Traumatic brain injury (TBI) is called the "Silent Epidemic" because the uninformed public is being ravaged on a large scale by its devastating repercussions. According to the National Center for Health Statistics, the total number of injuries to the head (of all types) in the United States is estimated to be over eight million per year. Put another way, every four seconds, someone in the United States may suffer a degree of brain damage. Most of those who are subjected to head injuries will not experience life-changing consequences because their injuries do not result in brain damage. However, every ten minutes, one of those eight million will die; and every minute, two others will suffer with long-term disability from a brain injury that is truly traumatic.

In 2015, the Centers for Disease Control and Prevention (CDC) estimated that annually in the United States, TBIs result in 53,000 deaths, 300,000 hospitalizations, 2.1 million emergency department visits, 1.1 million physician office visits, and 84,000 other outpatient department visits. The CDC reports at least 3.2 million people in the United States currently live with long-term disability resulting from TBI. Yet according to a 2015 survey by Whiteneck et al.,[1] "Prevalence of Self-Reported Lifetime History of Traumatic Brain Injury and Associated Disability: A Statewide Population-Based Survey," the CDC's estimate is based entirely on the number of people hospitalized with TBI, and only 1 in 10 people who sustain a TBI of any severity in the United States is hospitalized. Further, about one-third of these nonhospitalized people will have long-term disability, putting the true estimate of US citizens living with long-term disability resulting from TBI closer to 10 million.

According to Faul and Wald[2] (2010), the leading causes of TBI are falls (35.2 percent), motor vehicle accidents (17.3 percent), being struck by/against an object (16.5 percent), assaults (10.0 percent), and unknown/other (21.0 percent). Blasts are a leading cause of TBI for active-duty military personnel in war zones. Before the age of 65, 2 out of every 3 Americans (66 percent) will have suffered a form of brain injury ranging from mild to severe. The people who endure the ravages of TBI each year are primarily children 0 to 4 years old, teenagers 15 to 19 years old, and adults 65 years old and older. Commonly, children are injured playing or riding bicycles, teenagers in car accidents or sports, and the elderly by falling. Although BI can happen to anyone, statistics show that almost twice as many young men as young women suffer head trauma in large part because young men take greater "recreational" risks, participating in contact sports and driving cars aggressively. Your sons and daughters and elderly parents are in the age groups most at risk of becoming one of the more than 3,637,000 annual BI survivors in the United States.

Typical survivors, before they were injured, were excited about life, full of promise and possibility, growing more comfortable with their identities, engaged in education or employment, and moving through life with carefree ease. Then interrupting everything just like an unexpected phone call, a car crashed into them when they were driving around town, not wearing a helmet they accidentally fell off a bike on the way to a friend's house, or they slipped and fell while showering in the bathtub—and they became incapacitated social welfare recipients. Every twenty minutes, that phone call comes for someone in the United States. The message "life as the survivor knew it," *"life as the family knew it"*—is over.

The survivor now has to relearn how to walk, how to talk, how to chew food without offending others, how to put clothes on in the proper order, and how to be a friend, a son or daughter, a mother or father, a grandma or grandpa, or an employee. He or she has to learn all over again how to read, how to count change when making a purchase, how to follow a schedule or recipe, and on and on. In essence, BI survivors have to relearn the activities of daily living (ADLs) and how to behave all over again—from scratch. Everyone knows about growing pains, but few can imagine how difficult it is to have to resocialize, reintegrate, recoordinate, and relearn nearly everything when it is no longer age appropriate and this time around with a fatigued, overwhelmed, damaged brain that does not work correctly.

Often no immediately noticeable signs show that a person has been brain-injured. It is, by and large, an invisible disability. Yet more than other acquired disabilities, BI will cause some survivors to seem "less human" because it paints its victims with a *mysterious otherness* that is difficult to understand. The Silent Epidemic, as its name implies, finds millions of people oblivious of its devastating consequences. Once severely afflicted with life out of control, survivors may never again enjoy personal satisfaction, and their self-esteem may be only a memory of the past, if they can even remember having had self-esteem. Surprisingly, the life-changing consequences of brain injury are met with less sympathy, empathy, and understanding from other people than those of almost any other disability.

I entered the *other world* of the brain damaged as a young man. Since that time, I have undergone nearly every form of rehabilitation recommended for brain injury. I have an unenviable wealth of experience with life post-BI, and I have personal knowledge of what does and does not work therapeutically. I believe, therefore, that I am in a position to offer a helpful perspective for the survivor, the spouse, the family, the friend, the employer, and the professional who deal with the ramifications of brain injury. Nearly every article on BI mentions the need for further education of rehabilitation professionals regarding the personal consequences of brain injury[1]. For such professionals, the perspective I offer may be especially helpful. However, the recognized need to educate professionals, who may only see a survivor for an hour each week over several months, only underscores the need for both the survivor and the supporting family to become knowledgeable about life with a brain injury because they will have to deal with it, and keep on dealing with it, each day for the rest of their lives.

Education can provide a bridge of understanding to help family members and friends relate to a survivor in the most beneficial ways. Education is also the greatest preventive measure against future brain injuries. The more people who know the high risks and the life-changing consequences of BI, the more they will employ effective precautionary measures—and fewer will be those so injured.

The Individuals with Disabilities Education Improvement Act of 2004 is a law that makes available a free appropriate public education

---

[1]   According to Brent E. Masel, MD, medical schools are not teaching brain injury. "Most medical professionals have very little knowledge and training in brain injury. Therefore, it is the educated patient and family who become the manager of the disease" (www.brainline.org/article/ brain-injury-chronic-disease-interview-brent-masel-md).

to eligible children with disabilities throughout the nation and ensures special education and related services to those children. The IDEA defines *TBI* as "an acquired injury to the brain caused by an external physical force, resulting in total or partial functional disability or psychosocial impairment, or both, that adversely affects a child's educational performance." Traumatic brain injury applies to open or closed head injuries resulting in impairments in one or more areas, such as cognition; language; memory; attention; reasoning; abstract thinking; judgment; problem-solving; sensory, perceptual, and motor abilities; psychosocial behavior; physical functions; information processing; and speech.

While this book is based on my experience with TBI, it incorporates essentially all the elements of other types of brain damage. Much of what is said about the person with TBI—whether that injury is the result of a car crash, a blast injury in Iraq or Afghanistan, or a chronic traumatic encephalopathy (CTE) from contact sports—will also apply to people with other types of BI, such as those resulting from aneurysms, anoxia (loss of oxygen), arteriovenous malformations (AVMs), brain infection (encephalitis, meningitis), metabolic disorders (diabetic coma, insulin shock), stroke, toxic exposure (substance abuse, toxic agent inhalation), tumors, and viral illness. This book's relevance in so many different circumstances of brain injury has led me to take *Traumatic* out of the title and name it *The Silent Epidemic: What Everyone Should Know about Brain Injury*.

I invite you to read my book as an introduction to living with brain injury. Although it is by no means comprehensive, this book may help you better understand yourself as a survivor or—not being personally injured—understand people with brain injuries, suggest how to develop a more effective rehabilitation protocol for yourself or the survivor in your life, and persuade you to take simple steps to prevent yourself or your family member from being brain-injured again or for the first time. I also want my book to encourage each survivor to hope for a better future for him- or herself.

1   G. Whiteneck et al., "Prevalence of Self-Reported Lifetime History of Traumatic Brain Injury and Associated Disability: A Statewide Population-Based Survey," *Journal of Head Trauma Rehabilitation* (April 29, 2015), http://journals.lww. com/headtraumarehab/pages/results.aspx?txtkeywords=Prevalence+of+Self-Re ported+Lifetime+History+of+Traumatic+Brain+Injury+and+Associated+Disabi lity%3a+A+Statewide+Population-Based+Survey

2   M. Faul et al., *Traumatic Brain Injury in the United States: Emergency Department Visits, Hospitalizations and Deaths, 2002–2006* (Atlanta, GA: Centers for Disease Control and Prevention, National Center for Injury Prevention and Control, 2010).

1

A DEGREE OF MY EXPERIENCE

If you visualize a circle, a degree is barely a pinpoint on its circumference. What I am about to describe shows you, and can only show you, about that much of what I experienced in the days, weeks, months, and the first years after those paramedics saved my life.

To begin with, for thirty-two days, I was in a coma. I remained in a torpor (a state of lifeless inactivity) of gradually lessening severity for another month after that. At least that is what the hospital report says, for I have anterograde amnesia; I cannot remember the months after the accident. I also have retrograde amnesia; I cannot remember the months before the brain injury. While I lay in a coma, they performed brain surgery to monitor my intracranial pressure, which was 9.75 mmH_2O on the medical scale. Health records show that when the pressure exceeds 8.0 mmH_2O, the patient "always dies." The doctors were certain 9.75 mmH_2O would kill me, so they worked as quickly as they could to reduce the inflammation.

I was fortunate the medical team was able to lower the inner-cranial pressure with a Nembutal drip that kept my brain asleep by slowing its activity and turning down the nervous system. There are inherent complications with a Nembutal drip, however, and for that reason, doctors always want to get a patient off it as soon as possible. In my case, each time they tried to remove the Nembutal drip, my brain pressure went up again. My body temperature was dangerously high as well, so they put me naked, except for a loincloth, on an ice mattress, where I would lie shivering and shaking all night. I cannot remember any of this, but my mother said she could not bear walking in the room and seeing me like that. For a considerable time, I could not eat and had to be fed through a nasogastric tube inserted into my stomach. My muscles were quickly wasting away, and I dropped down to 120 pounds.

When I began having great difficulty breathing, they performed a tracheotomy—that is, a surgical procedure of cutting into the throat to attach an artificial breathing machine. On the respirator, I caught two different strains of lethal pneumonia (staph and anaerobic), both resistant to antibiotics. People on assisted breathing with a single strain of lethal pneumonia usually do not survive because they cannot cough to emit the disease, and the disease kills them.

The neurologist Dr. Posada (a neurologist is a doctor with specialized training in diagnosing, treating and managing disorders of the brain and nervous system such as TBI, Alzheimer's disease, stroke, Parkinson's disease and epilepsy) and the pulmonologist Dr. Allen Nieberg (a pulmonologist, or pulmonary disease specialist, is a physician who possesses specialized knowledge and skill in the diagnosis and treatment of lung conditions and diseases) at Sparrow Hospital in Lansing, Michigan, told my parents they were certain I would not survive. The only option they could recommend was an unconventional treatment that sprays antibiotics directly into the lungs through the respirator. Both doctors soberly said, "This treatment will either make Mark better or kill him." In comparison with certain death, the fifty-fifty unconventional treatment seemed to my parents to be the right thing to do, so they signed the hospital liability release waiver and authorized the procedure.

After the treatment, my condition began to improve, but my neck was swollen grotesquely huge as a result of air leakage from my lungs. This naturally scared my family. My nurses followed a simple procedure to aspirate/deflate my neck, however, and that took care of that.

Before the unconventional antibiotic spray procedure turned things around, the hospital staff and doctors were trying to prepare my family as best they could for my death. When my condition improved, the unprepared doctors—who had both thought I would certainly die—told my family what then seemed to be *inevitable.* "Mark's brain injury is so severe he will be institutionalized for life." The fact is, since being released from the hospital more than forty years ago, I have not been in a single institution. What I *have* done is continue to gradually improve as I practice my rehabilitation program every day since then.

I am told that after coming out of my coma in the hospital, I would open my right eye and track/follow people around the room with just that eye. I also started moving my right hand. The brain injury caused hemiparesis (unilateral weakness affecting one entire side of the body) on my left side. My left eye was always closed, and my left arm and hand were always inactive, curled up and constricted against my chest. My left leg was also curled up and could not straighten out. One of my college buddies came to visit me in the hospital, and when he saw me in that condition for the first time after my accident, he immediately fainted, fell and hit his head on the floor. I was told they rushed him to the ER and examined *his* head. Thankfully, Kelvin was okay. He was a fellow athlete and one of my toughest friends.

The first thing the hospital staff worked on was teaching me to sit up in bed because with most muscle control lost, especially on the left side, I could not do that. Once when my younger brother Jeff and my mother were visiting me while I was in that condition, I coughed so hard that the bloody tracheotomy tube blew out of my neck and flew all the way across the room, hitting a poster on the wall. It scared them both, but my mother, a former nurse, remembered that tracheotomies have an inner tube, so a patient can keep breathing even if the outer tube is dislodged. Later when I could sit up, I would become agitated and flop around in bed. One time I fell out on the floor, so for safety reasons, the hospital restrained me (tied straps around my waist, wrists, and ankles) for two months until the day I was discharged. When they finally started getting me out of bed, they would strap me in a chair, and I would just sit there, rocking up and down for hours at a time.

My mother would help me in physical therapy. Once when she was doing that, a visitor asked her, "Was he ever normal?"

She replied, "Yes, Mark was a senior at Michigan State University a month ago." The visitor could hardly believe it.

Something hard for even my mother to believe was my inability to put together a simple eight-piece puzzle when I was in cognitive therapy. My left eye was closed for a long time and then barely halfway open. My family told me that on one occasion, when my father was pushing me in a wheelchair past a mirror, I said, "I must look gruesome with that eye closed."

When I began talking, it was hard to understand my pronunciation. I would also, at times, say crazy things like, "I want you to go and get a blue Sphinx. Kathy has one in her tank." Kathy is my sister, but she didn't have a tank, and I do not know what a blue Sphinx is. When my younger brother Tom came to visit, he sadly asked my mom if I would always talk that way.

I have no recollection of those events during the critical phase of my recovery nor of the first time I was able to stand up. My first memory post-coma is of my elder brother, Dan, holding me up as I used the urinal in a bathroom. I had no idea what had happened to me or what my condition was, but somehow I knew that I needed Dan's help, and somehow I understood that all that mattered at that moment was to keep my balance as I relieved myself. My memory and awareness did not return all at once like a light turning on at the flip of a switch. It was more like the slow clearing of a northeastern inclement weather pattern or, even more accurately, like the digging of a copper mine—and all the years it takes to do that.

The next thing I remember is that I had to learn to walk between parallel bars. Then I had to learn to walk without assistance. Once I could do that, I had to learn to walk *better* because my left foot was inverted and drooped down from the heel. My toes would hit the ground before the heel and drag on the floor instead of picking up, and my left knee would hyperextend backward in a snaplike fashion before the next step. I had to think about every aspect of walking with each step and have continued doing so ever since.

From those early days in the hospital and for the next ten years, every time I walked, I felt like a freak because even with the greatest effort, I was unable to correct my gait—all I could do was try to compensate for it, and I could barely do that. I had never realized how difficult graceful walking can be, but it is indeed a complicated series of actions/inactions that involves the whole body.

Dr. David Ludden, who received a PhD in cognitive psychology from the University of Iowa and authored the book *The Psychology of Language: An Integrated Approach*[3], explains that many muscles must coordinate—contracting and relaxing in harmony with or in opposition to adjacent/opposing muscles—for us to walk. A part of the body on one side moves in one way while a different part on the other side must move in the opposite way. As the right foot is lifting and moving forward, the right arm is swinging backward. Then as the right arm swings forward, the left foot must rhythmically lift and step ahead as the left arm swings backward. All the while, the hips are rotating left and right, and the spine is slightly dipping back and forth. At a normal pace, the whole amazing process repeats up to fifty times per minute—all in perfect timing and seemingly without effort, like a well-rehearsed symphony. Unlike the beautiful cadence of a normal stride, the "gait music" coming out of my damaged brain was an awful syncopation (which involves a variety of rhythms that are in some way unexpected, causing part or all of a tune or piece of music to be offbeat) with a variety of unpredictable rhythms played on the ligaments, sinews, and anatomy of my normal-looking neurologically compromised body, producing a terribly offbeat "tune."

In the hospital, I tried my very hardest in therapy. Everyone commented to my family that I gave it my all. One time, I am told, I insisted that my mother walk me around the hospital by herself and told her, "You will do good, Mom." She wanted to encourage me, so she walked me the whole length of the hall and around the floor. She told me I did great. Another time later on, when I insisted on pushing her in the wheelchair, I terrified her because I kept going faster and faster, laughing and laughing all the while. (Fortunately, neither of us was hurt during those *ill-advised, dangerous activities.* Over forty years ago when I was injured, so little was known about brain injury that good advice was hard to come by. Today people are warned against doing such reckless things because they often cause secondary injuries to the survivor and serious primary injuries—back injuries especially—to the family member/friend, injuries that can prevent those others from continuing to physically assist survivors or from moving freely themselves. Naturally, survivors want to do what they did before being injured; but all too often, they want to before they are able to do so safely, and their attempt to undertake certain activities is a recipe for disaster.)

After my discharge, followed by four months of outpatient therapy, the doctors told my family, "Don't expect Mark ever to be able to get a job again. He won't make much progress from this point forward. Mark has reached his maximum medical improvement (MMI)." I was already back in college, however, working to finish the packaging design engineering courses I had been enrolled in at the time of my accident—the ones that had, meanwhile, been recorded as "incomplete"—and I was doing a good job of it. My family was hopeful that I would graduate and be employed as an engineer someday.

Besides learning how to walk again, I had to learn to speak intelligibly. I would say something, and my sister, Kathy, would ask what I had said. I, of course, knew what I had said, so I would repeat it, but she would ask me again what I had said. So I would say it again very slowly, but I could not pronounce the consonants properly and often left off the ends of words. My family became so used to this that they began to understand me regardless of the dissonance. Still, they would insist I repeat my words until I spoke them more clearly. I would get frustrated because, to me I sounded like I was saying everything correctly (I could not hear my mispronunciation), so why repeat myself—again and again? At times, my frustration was expressed as anger toward Kathy, whom I typically singled out. Fortunately, neither she nor the rest of my family gave up on me, nor did my circle of support, which in hindsight is quite remarkable.

In addition to rehabilitating my gait and speech, I had to relearn how to maintain personal hygiene, how to groom and dress myself, how to follow social etiquette around the dinner table, how to organize and clean my bedroom, and on and on—all the many things of that kind. The ADLs (*Activities of Daily Living*)—are what I call the *tangibles*, obvious things that can be observed and measured, things people normally do by and for themselves—such as feeding, bathing, dressing, grooming, homemaking, and leisure activity. With a severe traumatic brain injury, relearning the tangibles is a lot of hard, hard work, but it is nothing compared with the job of trying to get a grasp again of the intangibles—*the elusive, vague aspects of life*, the thousands of relational, social, and executive skills that survivors learned over the years before their brain injury, skills such as how to be with other people without embarrassing or offending them, how to communicate eloquently and pick up on nonverbal nuance, how to be true to oneself and one's values, how to appropriately reciprocate a favor given, what the comfortable personal space is in public encounters, how to be sexually intimate with your spouse, how to make decisions in different contexts, and on and on. (Years after a brain injury, intangibles can even come to involve matters such as how to maintain business correspondence, how to consistently be on time for vocational commitments, or how to initiate and monitor work and recreational activities; nonetheless, they remain just as difficult.)

The intangibles are all situational, so I could not apply an exercise program to them. It was doubly hard for me to get a handle on the intangibles because my thoughts were no longer consistent. It was like trying to hit a moving target using a gun with sights that kept changing. I would think I had it figured out as I looked through my scope, and then for no reason I could understand, I would have to refocus through new peep sights; but by then, the target would have moved somewhere else. Consequently, I could never hit it. I did not know what to do about the intangibles, and the stress of that made it all the more difficult to focus on the hours and hours of therapies for the tangibles.

After several years, the full ramifications of my severe brain injury became evident both to my family and to me. At times, I wished that ambulance had not been waiting at the intersection when my car crashed. I wished I had died then and there because I hated the life those paramedics saved. Dying would have been so much more convenient. People would have remembered me for what I was before the accident—a fun, popular guy in high school, an engineering student at college, an active participant in sports, a loyal fraternity member, an effective counselor for a university outreach effort, and other good *normal things* like that. After the accident, I became the guy who was awkward with relationships, the guy who could not keep a job, the guy who could not compete in sports, the guy who could not walk or talk right, the guy who *always* tried to be funny *but wasn't*, or the guy who had a hard time managing and understanding himself, let alone other people. I can fill pages with what I could not do right.

3   David Ludden, *The Psychology of Language: An Integrated Approach* (Thousand Oaks, California: SAGE Publications, Inc., 2016), https://www.amazon.com/Psychology-Language-Integrated-Approach/dp/1452288801

2

THE FIRST DECADE OF MY BRAIN-INJURED LIFE

At my one-year checkup, my neurologist, Dr. Posada, examined and tested me, turned away to review my hospital records for a good while, looked at my post-injury college course record, and murmured to himself in his thick Jewish accent, "It is a miracle."

He then turned back to me and said in a loud, clear voice, "It is remarkable that you are doing so well!"

At the time, I was encouraged. I thought, *Great, I will keep making "miraculous" progress, getting better and better, until I am just like I was before the accident.* That all changed when I hit the "two-year plateau" no one had told me about. After two years, the American Medical Association (AMA) maintains that survivors reach their maximum medical improvement and will not significantly progress beyond that. Consequently, insurance companies declare that therapy beyond that point is unnecessary. Sure enough, in my third and fourth years after brain injury, I was clearly not making the consistent improvements I had made during the first twenty-four months. If Dr. Posada had "examined" a whole day of my life five years post-injury—with all the problems I was having then, both physically and psychosocially—I do not think he would have called it a miracle.

Although I had "successfully" completed an initial therapy program, the never-ending struggle to be normal still awaited me each and every day. Recovery from brain injury is often accompanied by intense headaches, seizures, and spastic (jerky, epileptic-like) muscle contractions. I was fortunate not to experience any such physical pain or convulsions, but I did suffer many emotionally painful moments and frightful, hopeless thoughts. Moreover, I faced a constant challenge to improve, to be *normal*, to be "myself"—my *former* self. As my self-awareness began to resurface, it felt as though I were imprisoned because, while I could do some things, I could not do everything I used to do.

Other people could not see my "prison bars," of course; my disability was and is invisible. I was not an amputee, and I was not in a wheelchair. People had no way of knowing, just by looking at me, that I was severely disabled. I wanted everyone to see my tracheotomy and brain surgery scars; I thought those ugly marks would help explain things. However, even my scars were not obvious. If I were not walking or talking, no one could tell there was anything wrong with me.

What was wrong was my damaged brain—not me. How could I understand this? How could my family and friends understand it? How could people separate my physically damaged brain from my personal self? It had to be me that was wrong. Was it not *me* who was socially inappropriate? Was it not *me* who would get stuck in procrastination? It was *me* who—to defend myself in a relational conflict—would not tell the whole truth, wasn't it? When you have a broken leg, your friends say, "I hope your leg gets better soon." When you have a damaged brain, they do not say, "I hope your brain gets better soon." It is *you* they expect to get better. If you stop to think about it, our brains *are* us; I *am* basically my brain—for nothing defines me or you more than the manifestation of our brain's abilities/disabilities.

My family and friends were torn. They saw the same me on the outside. I looked pretty good; they said I looked great. They thought I was the same, they wanted me to be the same, and they tried to relate to me the same. But I was not the same. I did try to do the same things, be the same way, and tell the same kinds of jokes. (I often hid behind humor—laughing and making people laugh.) I wanted to be the same me I had been. My "new style" did not work so well, however, and it kept getting in the way. I was the same me, yet somehow I was a different me with a different style. It was confusing, and I was confused.

People did not understand brain injury (how could they?), so when I would blurt an opinion out of turn, they naturally thought *I* was rude.

There was a time during my early recovery when I thought that every attractive, healthy woman who was nice to me should certainly be my girlfriend and that maybe we would even get married someday. I have been reminded that it was also common for me to get stuck for hours and hours on certain "tasks" like copying recipes, organizing storage items that I had not used and would not use for years, or learning about something I had heard on the radio regardless of how irrelevant it might be to me and my life. Such odd behavior would make my mother feel terrible. Here was her son, a grown man, having to be treated like an adolescent. She remarked to my father how sad it was that I had to "grow up again"—how many other people, she wondered, have to go through their adolescent years twice?

I tried and tried to be normal. I was willing to work hard at being normal, and I did work hard—I worked my hardest. After ten years, I had tried every therapy and every program we knew of—and anything else that might help—but I was still not my normal self. Even as I worked at being normal, I repeatedly rubbed people the wrong way. I could not coordinate my body, maintain a healthy friendship or an intimate relationship, or secure long-term employment. My balance was compromised, and I would often stumble, even "bounce" off walls. Mercifully, I was always able to keep from outright falling or hitting my head. For several years, I struggled with short-term memory loss. I forgot appointments, lost clothes, forgot where I put the keys, lost checks my parents had sent, and repeatedly forgot what I was doing. It was not working. What was *it*? *I* was *it*, and I wasn't working. Why? Why? Why? Maybe I just had to work at it harder?

I was fired from several jobs before I successfully completed a packaging design engineering contract with General Motors. However, GM did not hire me permanently or offer me another contract. My next job was with a packaging company outside Lansing, Michigan, but I only worked there for two months. Because of my poor balance and only partial use of my left arm/hand, the manager was afraid I might get hurt on the large stamping equipment. My mom told me recently that she thought it must have been demoralizing for me, a Michigan State University (MSU) graduate, to be dismissed from his career job because he couldn't walk right. In hindsight, we are both thankful the manager was as perceptive as he was. I probably would have injured myself seriously—if not fatally—in that factory.

Initially, employers could not see any visible signs of my injury beyond the left hemiparesis, so they thought I should be *acting* normally. Most would get frustrated with my "different" behaviors and, in time, let me go. I did not seem to have a full understanding of what I was doing wrong on the job. Consequently, I would be terminated again and again, and life was a continual struggle. It would have helped if I had had a job coach or a brain injury specialist to work with the employer *and help me with my vocational problems*, but no one told my family that such a service was available or important.

The connections in my brain were broken or scrambled, and the fatigue I experienced on top of that made an eight-hour job very difficult for me—it still is. I did not learn until fifteen years after my injury that when survivors of a moderate or severe brain injury try to do *too much* in the first months or year(s) after being injured, it complicates their recovery and reduces their overall rehabilitation success.

My family and I could have done a better job of managing the balance between rest and activity during the early years of my recovery had we had access to the REAP Project.[2] That said, I remained significantly slower in my physical movements, had problems relating to people, made poor judgments, and like many survivors was easily taken in by salespeople. (More than once, I got talked into selling multilevel-marketing products.) I would sometimes have laugh attacks and be unable to stop laughing for five minutes or longer—which, of course, made people look at me strangely. Naturally, no one without

---

[2] www.concussiontreatment.com/images/REAP_Program.pdf.

knowledge of my post-brain-injury status could possibly understand where my inappropriate behaviors were coming from—behaviors such as taking food off other people's plates when dining out or eating the whole plate of cookies all by myself at a friend's house. I would get tired in the afternoon while visiting a friend and simply go take a nap anywhere in that friend's house without even asking. Sometimes I would just sit and stare.

After a while, some of my friends couldn't handle the *new Mark*. They dismissed me as weird and abandoned me. The sad part was, for me as it is for many survivors, because my brain was broken, I simply couldn't figure out that some of the things I was doing were peculiar, "off key," or socially awkward. My family shed many tears for me, the son and brother they loved so much, because I had to struggle with practically everything, suffered such rejection, and had to face so many disappointments.

The consequence of my injury was that much of my life had been taken out of my control, and I, in no way, understood what was happening. If anyone did understand, no one told my family or me. We were led by the professionals to believe that if I would just work harder at it, I would get better. The fact was they really didn't know. How could they? Sure, I wanted to be *better*, I wanted to be the same me I had been, the me that almost everyone liked, but I *couldn't* be that me. I didn't want to think *can't*, so I thought *can* and kept at it, working harder and harder, day after day, year after year, into the next decade. But with what results?

I could walk a little bit better, but my gait was still a huge problem and far from normal. I could talk a little better, but I could not speak the way I used to, and when I was fatigued, it was so much harder to understand me. I could move my left fingers a little bit better for a certain amount of time, but they were still severely disabled. If I moved them fast, they would hyperextend, lock, and get even weaker—it still took a sizable effort to tie my shoes. I was easier to get along with, but I was still not as socially polished as I had once been. What was all my effort worth? I still had to think about everything I said, how I said it, when I said it, why I said it, and whom I said it to before I said it. I had to examine and reexamine every movement I made was it straight enough, was it far enough, was it strong enough, was it relaxed enough, was it coordinated properly, was it timed precisely, was it in balance proportionally with everything else? Too many choices had to be made all the time, and my very best efforts were not enough. Try as I would with my depleted ego, I could not be normal.

My brain injury was just too much for me. I wanted my life to be over. I was ashamed of myself. I—who used to be one of the best hockey players in my high school, deft at handling a puck—could no longer eat properly with a fork. I was ashamed for my family. I, who used to teach and bring understanding to other college students, no longer understood myself. Should the *new me* really have a right to exist in this world? It seemed to me that, for everyone's sake, I would be better off dead. I wished I were dead, and several times, I thought of ways to kill myself. I am thankful that with the resilience my family's love and support gave me, along with my faith in God, I was able to self-regulate that awful impulse and never attempt suicide. Still, I was very tired of trying to do *everything right*. It was too much. Why couldn't I just *be* right? I had never been so frustrated, so ashamed, so uncertain, and so discouraged in my life.

That was how it was with me for the first ten years of my life post-TBI. In Steven Spielberg's movie *AI: Artificial Intelligence*,[3] Haley Joel Osment stars as the prototype child-robot named David Swinton. At one point in the film, David—who is lifelike—pleads with its scientific creator, Prof. Allen Hobby, "Make me a real boy." That scene portrays what I felt. I wanted to be a real man, the real Mark Condon and not the impostor standing in his place.

The feeling that you are not who you are after brain injury is very common for survivors. (Their families see them as somehow not the

---

[3]   https://en.wikipedia.org/wiki/A.I._Artificial_Intelligence

same person too). In fact, if you have recently been brain-injured, you
should expect such feelings and prepare yourself to be able to deal with
them better than I did. There came a time when I insisted that everyone
no longer call me Mark because I was not the same person, not the same
Mark; instead, they were all to call me by my first *and* middle name—
Mark John. I began introducing myself to everyone as Mark John,
and I continued to do that for more than ten years. I have learned it is
not uncommon for survivors to change their names, and I understand
why—a name change can symbolize the all-encompassing life change
associated with a brain injury. Have no doubt, after a brain injury, there
is a good chance that you will never feel like yourself again. You too may
change your name. The brain is a central part of our personhood, the
pinnacle of who we are apart from our soul. When the brain is injured,
we often express ourselves in confusing ways.

At that point in my rehabilitation journey, I was nowhere near
accepting my brain-injured self. I did not, or could not, really grieve my
loss (which is an important part of acceptance) until I had lived with
my disability for many years. That was a major reason why I could not
accept the new me. One night after ten years had passed, however, I was
with my family in my parents' living room when at last I *fully* realized
that no matter how hard I worked at rehabilitation, I would never again
be able to do a great many of the things I had done before my brain
injury—I simply would not ever be the "normal Mark" again. Fully
grasping that reality, I broke down and cried—I cried so hard for so long
(more accurately, wailed) that for more than forty minutes, I couldn't
catch my breath. Everyone else in the room was crying with me.

Carl Jung—the founder of analytical psychology, whose work
has been influential not only in psychiatry but also in anthropology,
archaeology, literature, philosophy, and religious studies—has said,
"There is no coming to consciousness without pain." That was never
truer for me than with my family that night, when I became more
conscious of the full ramifications of my brain injury—and felt the
pain. Beyond being truly painful, it was a profound moment in my

life and in my family's life post-injury, for it allowed me and us to more fully *accept* my disability and begin to grow past it. I did not quit my rehabilitation programs after that night, but I did begin to approach them with a different attitude. Later, on the referral of Dr. Gerald McIntosh (see "My Progressing Brain-Injured Life," chapter 7), I was able to dramatically improve the effectiveness of my rehab programs with the help of Dr. Bernard S. Brucker's biofeedback center (see "Remarkable Professionals and Their Therapies," chapter 10).

3

BRAIN INJURY CONSEQUENCES YOU COULD EXPERIENCE

The medical profession has learned so much about the human brain since I was injured in 1981 that it is remarkable. However, those closest to neurological research say they have only scratched the surface. Paradoxically, impressive scientific breakthroughs made over the last forty years have only highlighted the huge deficits in our neurological knowledge and understanding.

We do know the skull, made up of twenty-two bones, holds and protects the brain along with three internal membrane envelopes: the dura mater, arachnoid, and pia mater. Cerebrospinal fluid flows around the brain, between the membranes, and down into the spinal column. The primary function of the three membranes and of the cerebrospinal fluid is to protect the central nervous system. According to a wonderful *National Geographic* 2018 special publication – *Your Brain A User's Guide: 100 things you never knew*,[4] the brain is built on the brain stem, where unconscious survival functions such as heartbeat and breathing originate. On top of the brain stem is the cerebellum, which coordinates such voluntary movements as balance, posture, speech, and precise, fine finger movements. The four key parts of the brain are as follows:

1. Frontal lobe – responsible for organizing incoming information and planning as well as controlling behavior and emotions
2. Parietal lobe – crucial for integrating sensory and visual information
3. Temporal lobe – used for processing language and storing information in long-term memory

4. Occipital lobe – dedicated to vision

In *Your Brain A User's Guide* Patricia S. Daniels explains further that the cerebral cortex—the outermost brain layer—is where higher and executive functions originate, including reason and problem-solving, creative thinking and organizing, and language and self-knowledge. The cerebral cortex—most susceptible to damage from traumatic injuries—is, when injured, directly associated with the four classic brain injury aftereffects listed below, as well as with lack of self-knowledge, emotional lability, and behavioral/cognitive dissonance. The prefrontal cortex, right behind the forehead, is widely considered responsible for most of the neural processes associated with general intelligence. General intelligence, also known as *g factor*, refers to the existence of a broad mental capacity that influences performance on cognitive ability tests or measures. When the prefrontal cortex is injured or compromised, abstract reasoning is proportionally affected.

To better grasp the marvelous aspects of the human brain, read *National Geographic's* entire *Your Brain A User's Guide* magazine and Daniels's book *National Geographic Mind: A Scientific Guide to Who You Are, How You Got That Way, and How to Make the Most of It*. A healthy brain orchestrates the magnificent symphony performance of all members of the body and of the four key brain parts with their more than one hundred billion nerve cells that enable every human being to live, learn, experience, and express him- or herself in this world. Correspondingly, the brain dysfunction associated with a brain injury can be subtle, complex, and wide ranging in its consequences for survivors' quality of life.

Classic Aftereffects of Brain Injury

It has been said that if you see one brain injury, you have seen one brain injury (in that each one is vastly different from the next). Degrees of disability from brain injury vary widely depending on what a person's inherent and learned physical, emotional, and cognitive attributes were before being injured; on what his or her characteristic ways of relating to other people were; on the manner and severity of the injury; on what part of the brain was affected; on the level of care received immediately after the injury; on his or her level of resilience both pre- and post-injury; on what kind of insurance or financial resources were/ are available for ongoing rehabilitation/health care; on the availability of competent therapists with effective neurological/physical/cognitive/ speech programs for appropriate long-term rehabilitation; and on what kind of family support system there was and is in place. With some severe survivors exhibiting impressive recovery while other moderate/ mild survivors are vexed with long-term significant disability (Thornhill et al., 2000), the heterogeneous (varied, diverse) evolution of outcomes with BI over time remains unexplained (Betz et al., 2012; Corrigan et al., 2015; Davis et al., 2012; Forslund et al., 2013). However, in this Rubik's Cube of injury/outcome possibilities, there are four classic post-injury traits consistently found in survivors of moderate/severe injuries: perplexity, distractibility, fatigue, and short-term memory loss.

Understanding these recognizable effects of organic brain injury is crucial for a positive adjustment to the "new life" by both survivor and family.

1. *Perplexity* prevents some survivors from applying their knowledge outside the context where they learned it. Many times, survivors are able to perform the same vocational routine or functional duty they performed pre-injury, but often they cannot learn a new routine or even apply the old one in a new situation. They lose the ability to infer from their knowledge. Every season of life requires a different set of skills—as we grow, we mature gracefully by incorporating what we have learned socially, academically, vocationally and spiritually from prior seasons. Perplexity is especially confounding for some young survivors who become completely lost when they enter the next season of life. In fact, for many survivors it is as if he or she

remains stuck in childhood or adolescence—the "season" when they were injured—for the rest of his or her life.

2. *Distractibility* involves the tendency to pay attention to things that are not related to the activity at hand. In the case of some survivors, it is as if all their thoughts are loose in their heads at the same time. Whichever one is clearest or loudest at any given moment gets their attention. Things like eating or watching TV can totally eclipse situational awareness and the norms of social etiquette. Fluorescent lights in the ceiling, pictures on the walls, or any number of things in a young survivor's classroom can distract and obstruct his or her ability to focus and learn. Because of distractibility, driving is much more difficult and riskier for many survivors or altogether impossible—especially if fatigued or during rush hour.

3. *Fatigue* may curtail a survivor's ability to follow a procedure for any meaningful period. When the brain-injured person gets tired, which happens more often than before the injury, the hemiparesis-affected side of his or her face may sag, his or her compromised/diminished social skills become even more difficult to endure by others, and his or her already limited physical/mental agility regresses even further. Fatigue can significantly limit the application of a survivor's vocational abilities. The medical profession has long recognized that a good night's sleep is necessary for the brain to organize memories into retrievable files for future reference, an activity that is the foundation of learning. Further, without quality sleep, people have difficulty retaining memories, may become emotionally and behaviorally untoward, and are greatly disadvantaged when it comes to making decisions or solving problems. I, along with millions of other survivors, have not gotten a good night's sleep since being brain-injured, and I have to battle with fatigue every day. The results of twenty-one studies found that 50 percent of survivors suffer with some form of sleep disturbance after TBI, and between 25 and 29 percent have either insomnia, hypersomnia, or apnea (Mathias and Alvaro, 2012). I along

with other survivors am often overcome by lassitude and have to withdraw for a time from both social interactions and vocational responsibilities.

4. *Short-term and other forms of memory loss* are a wicked hindrance to daily life. A survivor may walk into a supermarket and not remember the way out, or he may make a commitment he intends to keep but then forgets it in two minutes, or she may keep circling a block five blocks away from her own home, which she somehow cannot find. Memory loss is another obstacle that interferes with many forms of employment and complicates social relationships. When working memory[4] is compromised, survivors are more prone to distraction, finding it all the harder to fulfill job requirements and maintain personal relationships.

Memory issues may, in fact, be the most vexing aspect of living with a brain injury. Think for a moment how critically important memory is. According to *Your Brain A User's Guide,*[4] the foundation of memories is what each person uses to build and communicate his or her personal, social, and professional identity. Memories are located all over the brain in various neural circuits that are interconnected with many other neural circuits/memories. (One memory often triggers the recall of another.) *Motor memory* provides the precise controls over every muscle, including those that, for example, help a person maintain balance while walking up or down the stairs, use the fingers properly for penmanship or typing on a computer, or activate the tiny vocal cord muscles imperative for speaking. When someone loses vocal motor memory, that person's

---

[4] *Working memory* is a short short-term capacity that retains information or sensations for just a few seconds. (You remember *briefly* what your boss just said, what you said in reply; or you remember *briefly* some sensory data from an experience—the smell of Grandma's chicken, for example—but then working memory has done its job and bows out.) *Long-term memory*, on the other hand, analyzes the working memory's "ticker tape," organizes what is necessary for the future, and places those memories into "filing cabinets." Temporary or permanent (short-term or long-term) filing cabinets can be called upon throughout a day and even over the years into the future—allowing us to correctly perform a job task at the end of the day or throughout a career.

speech is greatly compromised—becoming difficult, if not impossible, to understand—and leads to negative social consequences.

Sensory memory involves the five senses, with sight claiming the crown since it occupies the most brain matter and is universally held to be the most cherished sense. All the experiential information flowing from the five senses and being analyzed by the brain dynamically affects thoughts, emotions, memories, and personality. Stimulation thresholds are often altered by a brain injury. Either higher or lower minimum levels may be required before the brain perceives a sensation. A brain injury may therefore greatly alter (heighten or reduce) what a person can see, hear, taste, smell, and touch. It can also affect physical coordination, personality, communication skills, and relationships. *Face recognition memory* is especially important for relationships—not only to remember a person and his or her name, but also to recognize feelings and intentions. A healthy brain is superbly hardwired to perceive all the different nonverbal cues and emotions a face can communicate.

According to David McRaney, who wrote the book *You Are Now Less Dumb: How to Conquer Mob Mentality, How to Buy Happiness, and All the Other Ways to Outsmart Yourself*,[5] "You have an origin story and a sense that you've traveled from youth to now—along a linear path, with ups and downs that ultimately made you who you are today. That sense is built around events that you can recall and place in time. . . . Without episodic memories, there is no narrative; and without any narrative, there is no self" (p. 42). Our memories are far more than what we have or have not accomplished; they include everything we have felt, learned, believed, thought, admired, and detested. Some severe brain injuries can altogether rob the brain of its ability to refer to the past, generate and keep new memories or possess an awareness of self.

Language Issues

Language memory is responsible for connecting words with objects, emotions, beliefs, and everything else. It is the paramount underpinning of communication. It is not unusual for survivors to lose the ability to understand spoken language unless it is said slowly with clear enunciation. A brain injury can rob survivors of learned and well-developed "verbal pattern recognition" ability, without which they struggle over and over again to understand what is being said or how to say something. It can be as if, repeatedly, it is the first time they have ever formulated and spoke a sentence—or heard one. Some survivors may altogether lose the ability to speak and be understood. Communication is so important to human existence that a vast amount of brain matter is dedicated to this skill.

Daniels[4] quotes Derek Bickerton, an expert on Creole languages. "Although some scientists believe the mind can exist without language, others argue that language produces mind. Without language, I wouldn't say that it is impossible to have a mental experience, but I'd say the mental experiences would not be very coherent" (p. 45). (If you, as a reader of this book, are a survivor who has memory issues [or a family member of a survivor], I strongly recommend that you obtain the special edition of *National Geographic* referred to in reference 4 of this book and better inform yourself. Your local librarian can help you locate a copy.)

The renowned author Gertrude Stein, who created a unique place for herself in the world of wonderful letters, famously said, "Why should a sequence of words be anything but a pleasure?" Unfortunately for many survivors, hearing a sequence of words is the farthest thing from a pleasure. Instead, it is a painful reminder of how awkward and foreign life has become post-injury. A simple, coherent sentence can be for them, when it is their turn to speak, a very difficult thing to produce. Damage to the Broca's area of a person's brain renders him or her unable to articulate language—and speak intelligibly—yet such damage may not affect his or her ability to *understand* both spoken and written language. Conversely, if the Wernicke's area of a person's brain is damaged or if brain cells in the Wernicke circuit are damaged, that damage disables his or her ability to understand spoken and written language and severely compromises the ability to write yet does not affect the ability to speak.

Dr. Ludden explains in his 2016 book, *The Psychology of Language: An Integrated Approach*,[3] that in the same way we ambulate—walking with parallel but opposite left and right steps to cover ground—we speak with parallel but opposite consonant and vowel sounds to produce the syllables that form words. The balance required to walk straight is reflective of the coordination required to talk "straight." According to Ludden, speech employs a multitude of delicate contract/relax muscle responses throughout and around the mouth—in the lips, tongue, jaws, and neck—to establish the necessary and complementary positions between each to produce the desired sounds, to communicate the intended words. Ludden illustrates that on a map of the brain, many of the geographical brain structures that are responsible for locomotion are the same brain structures responsible for speech.

Difficulty speaking or understanding spoken words has far-reaching consequences in the lives of survivors. You may not have sufficiently appreciated up to now just how valuable and necessary your ability to communicate is. According to Richard Knox—who discussed his 2007 "Study: Men Talk Just as Much as Women"[5] on National Public Radio—people speak on average sixteen thousand words per day. Take away a person's ability to converse or greatly diminish it, and you automatically take away or diminish his or her ability to stay socially connected. Even when a survivor is able to speak, if his or her level of speech is greatly compromised, it will have far-reaching negative consequences.

Matthias R. Mehl, Simine Vazire, Shannon E. Holleran, and C. Shelby Clark conducted a study at the University of Arizona titled "Eavesdropping on Happiness: Well-being Is Related to Having Less Small Talk and More Substantive Conversation."[6] Aligning with past studies they found, "Higher well-being was associated with spending

---

[5]   https://www.npr.org/templates/story/story.php?storyId=11762186

less time alone, and more time talking to others. Further, higher well-being was associated with having less small talk and more substantive conversations." The happiest participants spent 25 percent less time alone and 70 percent more time talking—with twice the number of substantive conversations (p. 2). The research stated, "A happy life is social rather than solitary and conversationally deep rather than superficial. . . . Deep conversations may actually make people happier. Just like self-disclosure can instill a sense of intimacy in a relationship, deep conversations may instill a sense of meaning in the interaction partners." This deduction made them entertain the possibility that "happiness can be increased by facilitating substantive conversations" (p. 3).

Conversely, diminished speech ability is one of the major negative consequences of a brain injury that can detract from happiness, diminish the quality of relationships, and depress satisfaction with life.

To help you begin to appreciate better the loss of brain function, count every *F* in the following text:

> FINISHED FILES ARE THE RESULT OF
> YEARS OF SCIENTIFIC STUDY COMBINED
> WITH THE EXPERIENCE OF YEARS

How many *F*s are there? Count them again. How many *F*s?

There are six. Go back and read it again from left to right and try to find the six *F*s before you read any further.

I saw this on the Internet and learned that the reason most people count only three *F*s the first time they read it from left to right is that the brain cannot process the *F* in *of.*

FINISHED FILES ARE THE RESULT OF
YEARS OF SCIENTIFIC STUDY COMBINED
WITH THE EXPERIENCE OF YEARS

Every normal brain has several "blind spots" in addition to not processing the *F* in *of.* After even a mild brain injury, however, there are a thousand times *more* physical, mental, and emotional matters a damaged brain simply cannot process. Being aware of being aware is what makes us human, seperates us from animals, and is implied with the name *Homo sapiens*, "wise man." A brain injury clearly can devastate our wisdom if it steals our self-awareness, our ability to process and interpret sensations or to create the sounds of speech. Some will argue that a brain injury can make us less human than other acquired disabilities. Dutch philosopher Baruch Spinoza (1632–1677) said that people who lack the power to be in charge of or in control of their emotions are subject to what he called "enslavement." Depending on the location and severity of their injuries, people with BI likewise may be enslaved to the degree that they lose control of their emotions or remain unaware of the nature of their limitations and losses. Under such "bondage" they do not know that they do not know.

The CNS (Central Nervous System) Medical Group affiliated with Craig Hospital[6] in Denver, Colorado, told me that neuropsychologists

---

6   Craig Hospital is an institution exclusively dedicated to spinal cord injury, traumatic brain injury, and research. They have treated more than 27,500 patients since 1956 and have been ranked in the top ten rehabilitation hospitals for twenty-one consecutive years (Craig Hospital, 3425 S. Clarkson St., Englewood, CO 80113, 303-789-8000, www.CraigHospital.org).

call "not knowing that you do not know" *anosognosia*.[7] A degree of anosognosia manifests in most survivors, whereas pervasive anosognosia manifests in only a few. It is not uncommon for survivors with anosognosia to also exhibit *insouciance*; that is, detachment from concern, worry, and anxiety. They are basically carefree—oblivious of their limitations and to the full ramification of their brain injury. Other survivors, though they may be aware of their post-brain-injury negative behaviors (disinhibition, lack of executive function, inability to control anger, short-term memory problems, etc.) and even though they may know effective strategies to accommodate for such faux pas, simply fail to employ those compensation strategies. Such nonproductive behaviors can "enslave" them just as if they suffered from full-blown anosognosia.

Reduced Self-Awareness and Situational Comprehension

Highlighting degrees of anosognosia in respect to self-awareness I refer to what Maimonides said, "We naturally like what we have been accustomed to, and are attracted towards it." Some survivors never like or become accustomed to any aspect of their lives. He or she lose the awareness of his or her associated "attraction compass," and end up directionless—indefinitely. Workers with moderate brain injury are often puzzled about, or refuse to believe, the changes in their personality and functional ability. Ensuing abandonment by family, "friends," and coworkers—along with imprecise psychological/medical diagnoses by professionals who treat mild/moderate brain

---

7   *Anosognosia* is a deficit of self-awareness where one is oblivious to their mental health condition or cannot grasp the full extent of it. Anosognosia, from the Greek language, means "to not know a disease" and is a common symptom of certain mental illnesses. Degrees of anosognosia can vary over time, with a person fully cognizant of their mental illness one day and altogether denying it the next. Variations in awareness are typical with anosognosia and should not be attributed to personal choice or stubbornness (https://www.nami.org/learn-more/mental-health-conditions/related-conditions/anosognosia).

injury—amplifies the stress, fear, and anxiety of these survivors. The stress they feel certainly magnifies the negative consequences of their brain injury and, more often than not, short-circuits their compensation strategies. Some survivors hold far-fetched vocational expectations because of their reduced self-awareness and diminished ability to correctly assess the world around them. They may continue on their chosen course full of anger, assigning to others the responsibility for their problems. Other survivors may withdraw completely to reduce the overwhelming frustration and depression they experience.

Psychologists have compiled an extensive body of research with the normal population on what is called "locus of control." To the degree that you feel life is under your control (i.e., you believe that your actions can change the circumstances of your life), you have an internal locus of control and a positive and passionate feeling about life. Conversely, to the degree you feel life is out of your control (i.e., you believe that there is nothing you can do to change the circumstances of your life— everything just happens to you), you have an external locus of control that generates a negative and apathetic feeling about life. Brain injury always results in a shift toward an external locus of control. *To the extent that survivors of moderate/severe brain injury cannot manage themselves or their lives, remain unaware or unaccepting of the injury's control-robbing consequences, and adopt an external locus of control, they are inconsolable and bewildered to a degree far beyond that felt by the normal population.*

Nancy Gibbs[7] reports that Antonio Damasio,[8] professor and head of the Neurology Office at Iowa University and author of *Descartes' Error: Emotion, Reason and the Human Brain*, learned from working with survivors how necessary the invisible neurological pathways are for a normal life. Although people who have lost those pathways may be just as intelligent and able to perform their jobs, their lives commonly become unmanageable. Such survivors cannot make decisions because they cannot foresee consequences and are confused or uncertain about their feelings related to their choices. Some survivors have to be satisfied instantly and cannot delay gratification; others may lose the ability to read the emotional cues so easily understood and displayed by others. (As much as 90 percent of emotional communication is nonverbal.) If some survivors make a social mistake, they are likely to repeat the same mistake again and again because they feel no regret or shame. It is not their audacity or arrogance that emboldens them to feel no shame but the fact they have lost their social awareness capacity or the grounded self-consciousness that will allow them to avoid social blunders in the first place.

Families often report they wish their survivor were *normal*. Not being normal is the mysterious "otherness" that vexes survivors who lack self-awareness and do not know they are "off the mark." Gibbs reports,

> If there is a cornerstone to emotional intelligence on which most other emotional skills depend, it is a sense of self-awareness, of being smart about what we feel. . . . Self-awareness is perhaps the most crucial ability because it allows us to exercise some self-control. The idea is not to repress feelings but rather to do what Aristotle considered the hard work of the will. "Anyone can become angry—that is easy," he wrote in the *Nicomachean Ethics*. "But to be angry with the right person, to the right degree, at the right time, for the right purpose, and in the right way, this is not easy."

Today's radio psychologist David Visgot maintains, "Not to be aware of one's feelings, not to understand them or know how to use or express them, is worse than being blind, deaf, or paralyzed. Not to feel is not to be alive. More than anything else, feelings make us human."

Benjamin Franklin said, "To cease to think creatively is but little different from ceasing to live."

The following exercise is an attempt to give you "experience" of just one dimension of what it can feel like to live with a brain injury.

(I normally only give this "exercise" aloud when I speak publicly, but I want to include it for you here in print since it is so effective for my audiences.) You will have to allow yourself to feel what it is like to "hear" a short text without the schema required to make sense of it. If you are wondering what a schema is, it's an unconscious organization of experiences in your brain, a reference in your mind that helps you interpret the intent or meaning of what's going on around you. Most of you will immediately know what I am referring to, but those who do not should pay attention to how difficult it is to understand the written text, even though all the words are easy. (If the meaning of what follows escapes you, please let yourself feel the feeling of not knowing what I am talking about—when you should—and then multiply that awkward feeling by a million, and you will begin to appreciate what it is like for many survivors of brain injury to live life without the references their minds used in the past, and currently need, to interpret/understand ordinary life.) Here is the text:

> This is an easy thing to do. If possible you will do it at home, but you can always go somewhere else if it is necessary. Beware of overdoing it. This is a major mistake and may cost you quite a bit of money. It is far better to do too little than attempt to do too much. Make sure everything is properly placed. Now you are ready to proceed. The next step is to put things into another convenient arrangement. Once done, you'll probably have to start again real soon. Most likely, you will be doing this for the rest of your life.

What is this about? Do you know? Are you certain you know what the text is referring to? How hard is your mind working to figure this out? Some scratch their heads, thinking that it does not make much sense. There is a good reason it does not make sense. The schema or clues that your brain normally will use to understand the text have been omitted. When the schema is in place, it all makes sense. Watch the clarity you get instantly with the schema included. "*Laundry* is an easy thing to do. If possible, you will do it at home, but you can always go somewhere else if it is necessary..." Laundry is the schema. With the schema in place, it all makes sense; there's no problem.

If you put yourself into this exercise wholeheartedly, you may have been doubly frustrated because you thought, *Most people will know what it means.* And you want to be among those people—among the most, among the normal. *The truth is the majority of us cannot easily make sense of this text without knowing its schema, and that is actually* normal. What is missing from many survivors' awareness is the schema needed to place social, vocational, or personal situations in their proper context. The amount of work these people have to go through to understand things that, pre-injury, they would have understood with no effort at all is exhausting. Under post-injury circumstances, however, their need to make such effort is *truly normal.* Not realizing that having to put forth considerable effort is the new normal, some survivors choose one of the first interpretations to cross their minds—instead of struggling or relying on/deferring to others for the correct understanding. When it turns out that their interpretation is wrong, they may become defensive or aggressive in an attempt to justify their position. Other survivors, as was mentioned earlier, may choose to socially withdraw. They feel overwhelmed and may blame themselves for their awkwardness and lack of comprehension when, in fact, their bafflement is not due to themselves personally—but rather to organic brain damage.

Emotional Bankruptcy

All throughout life and even in a mother's womb, people experience emotions. Emotions are critically important to understand and manage life well, develop significant relationships, plan/prepare for a satisfying future, and make sense of our experience. Being able to express and perceive a full range of emotions is foundational—twenty-seven emotions have been identified to date, and I am sure more will be added.

Emotions are complex. The theory of constructive emotion promoted by Lisa Feldman Barrett, a neuroscientist at Northeastern University, holds that emotions do not *happen to* you, nor do they have a universal look; but rather, they are individually generated and expressed by several brain regions and innumerable neural connections simultaneously interfacing with one another. Emotions are something that our brains construct, and a healthy brain is very much in control of emotions. Conversely, a damaged brain often can no longer feel, recognize, or control emotions.

The hippocampus, which has a significant role in memory—receiving information and impressions from the whole brain to integrate them into a single experience—may play a supporting role in emotions. The prefrontal cortex (the primary brain region injured with TBI and a major part of the "empathy network") is responsible for regulating the escalation of emotions. When the prefrontal cortex is damaged, we can have great difficulty being empathetic and fostering meaningful relationships. Empathy is the ability to imagine and feel other people's emotions—the ability to put yourself in their shoes and to feel their feelings. However, when you cannot feel your own feelings and cannot recognize the body language/vocal expression of another's emotional state, you are at a great disadvantage. Some people are innately better at controlling their emotions and we naturally feel both welcomed and peaceful in their presence. Almost everyone can learn to be more skilled at emotional regulation and the efforts in this direction are well worth it. (The exception may be survivors with prefrontal cortex, hippocampus, or pervasive brain damage.)

Involuntary Emotion

In contrast to the four already mentioned common post-injury traits—perplexity, distractibility, fatigue, and short-term memory loss—if ever there is a disconnection between the parts of your brain that express emotion and those that control emotion, you will experience frequent outbursts of involuntary crying or laughing known as *pseudobulbar affect* (PBA). The impact of PBA is substantial, resulting in embarrassment for the patient, family, and caregivers as well as upsetting the people around them, all of which may then lead to restriction of social interactions and a lower quality of life. According to Avanir Pharmaceuticals, Inc. (www.pbafacts.com), PBA can occur when brain injuries or certain neurologic diseases damage the *bulb* area of the brain stem that controls normal expression of emotions (*affect*). Injury to this area of the brain can disrupt brain signaling, causing a "short circuit" that activates involuntary (false or *pseudo*) episodes of crying or laughing. A telltale sign is that the uncontrollable crying or laughing episodes are inappropriate to the situation in which they occur. Many PBA patients describe occasions where they laughed when they were actually feeling sad or cried when they really felt happy. Although PBA is uncommon, for those afflicted with it, it is not uncommon enough.

Hydrocephalus

Yet another complication that can follow brain injury is hydrocephalus, which comes from the Greek words *hydro*, meaning "water," and *cephalus*, meaning "head." Translated, *hydrocephalus* means "water on the brain." According to the Hydrocephalus Association (www.hydroaasoc.org), hydrocephalus is an atypical buildup of cerebrospinal fluid (CSF) within the brain's ventricles. Cerebrospinal fluid is produced in the brain's cavities and choroid plexus and then circulated, surrounding the entire brain and spinal cord, delivering the necessary nutrients and proteins, removing accumulated wastes and toxins, and providing an absorptive liquid cushion to prevent injury— before it exits into the bloodstream via tissues at the base of the brain. Normally, CSF is absorbed into the bloodstream at a coequal rate to its production. When absorption is deficient, CSF builds up, and hydrocephalus develops with enlarged ventricles and increased pressure inside the head.

I had never heard of hydrocephalus or of its connection with head injury until more than thirty years after my own TBI when a friend in Florida developed it. A year after his brain injury, he was still unable to work, had balance issues, had become very forgetful, and suffered from loss of bladder control (incontinence). I was helping him as best as I could with rehabilitation recommendations and counseling over the phone from Colorado, but he was making little improvement. He went to the best doctors. He brought an MRI of his brain with him when he saw one of the top five neurosurgeons in the United States. Even looking at the image, however, this well-known neurosurgeon did not recognize my friend's enlarged ventricles as atypical, nor did he properly diagnose his symptoms. He said, in fact, that he saw no sign of a brain injury in the MRI, and he totally failed to mention any possibility of hydrocephalus. Serendipitously then, just when my friend was terribly frustrated and losing hope, he was introduced to Dr. Aizik Wolf, the director and founder of the Miami Neuroscience Center at Larkin Hospital in Miami, Florida, who immediately diagnosed hydrocephalus.

The Hydrocephalus Association[8] explains that the actual cause of hydrocephalus is not always clear, and it differs with age and circumstances. More than 70 percent of all hydrocephalus cases are congenital (present at birth). However, a head injury can damage the brain's tissues, nerves, or blood vessels and cause acquired hydrocephalus. Blood from ruptured vessels may flood the CSF pathways with scarred membranes or meninges, causing inflammation that blocks CSF absorption sites. (Alternatively, a tumor in the brain may fill or compress a local ventricle and block the flow of CSF to cause acquired hydrocephalus [www.ninds.nih.gov].) Finally, normal pressure hydrocephalus (NPH) may occur in older adults when the ventricles of the brain are enlarged, but there is little or no increase in the pressure within the ventricles. Sometimes the cause of NPH is known, but most often it is idiopathic (unknown).

---

[8]   www.hydroassoc.org/symptoms-and-diagnosis-nph.

Symptoms of NPH include the following:

- *Mild dementia* is described as a loss of interest in daily activities, forgetfulness, difficulty dealing with routine tasks, and short-term memory loss. NPH is one of the few treatable forms of dementia.
- *Impairment in bladder control* in mild cases is typically characterized by urinary frequency and urgency and in severe cases is a complete loss of bladder control or urinary incontinence. Some people with NPH never display signs of bladder problems.
- *Gait disturbances* range in severity from mild imbalance to the inability to stand or walk at all. Gait is often wide based, short stepped, slow, and shuffling. Gait disturbance is often the most pronounced symptom and the first to become apparent.

That friend in Florida was Bodhi Kocica, director of the Hoshino Therapy Clinic, who suffered a TBI after falling down a flight of stone stairs back in his homeland of Prague when he was visiting family in 2015. Bodhi's TBI resulted in hydrocephalus and has rendered him unable to perform his amazing Hoshino Therapy (see "Remarkable Professionals and Their Therapies," chapter 10) for more than an hour in a day, if at all, ever since.

◆

Brain damage may cause you, if you have been so injured, to be unaware, inflexible, inappropriate, incontinent, irritable, socially awkward, imbalanced, chronically fatigued, impulsive, devoid of self-awareness, ragingly aggressive, socially isolated, extremely forgetful, unable to speak or read a simple sequence of words, unable to pick up on emotional facial expressions and body language, or unexplainably slothful. Then you, like many survivors, will be mistakenly blamed for these neuropathological conditions, and your upset family will request again and again that you be your normal self. Usually, it will be your injured brain, not your personal choice, that is the cause of such problems. The brain is a physical organ, and brain injury (a neurophysical injury) simply brings about these kinds of psychological/behavioral/physical abnormalities.

"TBI remains a tremendous public health problem. The brain is arguably the most complicated organ we've got, and brain trauma is the most complicated form of disease. What society thinks of as a treatment though is 'cure,' and it is difficult to put the concept of cure into the brain,"[9] said David Hovda, PhD, director of UCLA Brain Injury Research Center, US Defense Health Board adviser, who in 2011 received the US Army's Strength of the Nation Award (the highest civilian award given by the army). That a survivor's abnormal behavior is the result of a complicated brain injury—that it is caused, in other words, by the most complicated neurophysiological condition known to man and is not just a matter of his or her personal choice—is a fact commonly beyond the ability of family, friends, teachers, and health-care providers to grasp (not because of any deficiency on their part but simply because *brain injury* education is lacking).

A survivor often hears, "Why don't you stop doing that? You never did that before." But his or her damaged brain is afflicted with the most complicated, misunderstood disease—how could he or she stop. The *disease* will not *let* him or her stop. Being the target of undeserved blame may add to a survivor's depression, stress, and defensiveness, which impair stable identity and compromise healthy self-esteem. Self-esteem amounts to how much you like and respect yourself, yet it can be greatly influenced by how much you are liked and respected by others. When your family, friends, and spouse have deserted you; when you are no longer able to do what you did; and when you have not yet become aware of the consequences of your brain injury, healthy self-esteem is practically impossible. The belief of some psychologists that self-esteem is the core component of a sound personality underscores the *disadvantage* that you,

---

9   https://www.brainline.org/video/dr-david-hovda-talks-about-progress-field-tbi.

as a survivor, are under if, as so many survivors do, you lose your self-respect, your self-esteem.

Normalcy Bias

The term for a certain dynamic that can occur in our human psyche, namely, *normalcy bias* or *normality bias*, refers to the mental state people can enter when they are facing a disaster. It causes them to underestimate both the likelihood that a disaster will occur and its possible effects if it does occur. Normalcy bias assumes that, since a disaster never has occurred in one's life, a disaster never will occur. People with normalcy bias also have difficulty *responding* to something they have not experienced before.

It is no surprise that normalcy bias often manifests both in survivors and in the people surrounding them. For one thing, scarcely anyone without special experience or education can accurately "estimate" the very real likelihood of becoming brain-injured; still less, deal competently with the consequences. Additionally, it is always the obstacles that we do not see coming that are the biggest challenges in life. I have never met anyone who saw in advance and was adequately prepared for a brain injury disaster nor anyone who understood its far-reaching consequences or knew how to best accommodate/rehabilitate BI. People with normalcy bias also tend to interpret warnings in the most optimistic way possible, seizing on any ambiguities to infer a less serious situation. They are apt to underestimate survivors' need for accommodations and for ongoing therapy.

Yet another manifestation of normalcy bias in mild and moderate survivors (and more importantly in their family and friends) is a tendency to regard the problems associated with a brain injury as temporary or of no great consequence. In the aftermath of a brain injury disaster, it is only natural to have a degree of normalcy bias. Normalcy bias lies behind the advice of family and friends for the survivor to "get over his/her brain injury and get on with life" or "just stop doing X" or that "Y shouldn't be a problem." (*X* and *Y* could stand for a hundred different things.) Getting over a brain injury or stopping a negative behavior, however, has never been that simple for any of the survivors I know or have worked with (including myself). Everyone involved would be best served by dropping all normalcy bias when it comes to brain injury.

Psychosocial Deprivation

Paul Aravich, PhD, is a professor at Eastern Virginia Medical School who teaches a course on medical neuroscience and who has won several awards, one being the AOA Glaser Distinguished Teacher Award[10] for "significant contributions to medical education" from the medical school faculties in the United States and Canada. According to Aravich, the effect of brain injury on successful aging, on longevity, and on the ability to resist the diseases of aging is remarkably understudied. He thinks part of the reason is we do not focus on the "whole person who has a brain injury as much as we should." Aravich maintains that the question of what effect brain injury has on successful aging is a very important one because, according to the United Nations, the largest single minority group on the earth is people with disabilities. Dr. Aravich says further that, regardless of where you go, disabled people are marginalized, disenfranchised, socially isolated and face barriers to good care.

According to Aravich as reported in his PBS original series, *The Secret Life of the Brain*, "One of the things we know is that successful aging is very much a 'brain thing.'" It has been said that the human brain is a "social brain," and one of the common denominators for people with any form of disability is psychosocial deprivation.

---

[10]   Alpha Omega Alpha (AOA) Robert J. Glaser Distinguished Teacher Awards are presented annually at the awards dinner of the Association of American Medical Colleges (AAMC) by the president of Alpha Omega Alpha that funds the program. This award recognizes outstanding contributions to the education of medical students by four faculty at LCME-approved schools of medicine.

Psychosocial deprivation injures a specific part of the brain known as the hippocampal formation, which has adult stem cells in it. (Studies have shown that in psychosocially enriched environments, neurons in the hippocampal formation can continue to divide long after maturity occurs.) Observing that hippocampal function plays a primary role in both short-term memory and the formation of long-term memory and that as we grow older cognitive impairments sometimes occur, Dr. Aravich concludes:

> So to the extent you have impairment in hippocampal function from a brain injury to begin with, psychosocial deprivation will necessarily damage it further, putting you at greater risk for mild cognitive impairment later on. That does not mean you are going to get mild cognitive impairment, nor does it mean you are going to get Alzheimer's disease or the chronic traumatic encephalopathy that has already been mentioned, but we do know your risk is going to be greater than average, depending on the severity of the injury.[11]

In 2005, the researchers Jean M. Twenge, Roy F. Baumeister, C. Nathan DeWall, Natalie J. Ciarocco, and J. Michael Bartels[9] conducted a study that revealed that social exclusion impairs self-regulation in part because of something called ego depletion (more on ego depletion below). The effort required to self-regulate is an important part of being a person. Self-regulation is critically important when it comes to maintaining relationships. Failure to self-regulate always increases social isolation and vice versa. At some point after a person has been rejected by friends and family because of socially inappropriate speech or behaviors and by society in general for the same or different reasons, it is easy for the rejected one to believe that it is not worth the effort required to get along with others, to self-regulate, because "No one pays attention or cares about me anyway."

---

11   https://www.brainline.org/video/why-brain-injury-and-aging-so-understudied.

We humans survive and thrive because we stick together in one or several groups by respecting all those unspoken but clearly understood (by normal people) social variables—such as professional level and personal standing, character and ability, political coalition and sexual predisposition, spiritual outlook and worldview—all to prevent being ostracized. The effort involved in this social dance is worth it. Most everyone does his or her part without a second thought because that is how we stay connected. Staying connected is how we develop in healthy and vigorous ways. Most of us grow up with an inborn ability to recognize what will cause people to push us away.

The key denominator in the "socially unacceptable equation," besides obscenities and vulgarities, is selfish behaviors. Narcissistic people who fail to do their part in a group activity, who are selfish and cannot be relied on to contribute, or who are oblivious to others' feelings when they talk and relate are naturally excluded from social circles. Unfortunately, that kind of behavior is just exactly what is displayed by many survivors who, with low self-esteem, lack the social awareness required to self-regulate and maintain intimate relationships or close friendships. With the loss of friends and an increased dependence on family, the size of a survivor's social network grows smaller and may lead to psychosocial maladjustment—which inherently perpetuates social isolation.

Once a survivor has been pushed to the social fringe, any attempt to help that person undo the relationship damage already done—to help him or her move toward healthier, reciprocal relationships—requires working with *both* the survivor *and* his or her social circle. That, as a rule, is very hard to bring about. According to McRaney[5] (p. 112), Baumeister along with his coauthors wrote in their social exclusion paper that members of society enter an unspoken agreement with one another. The expectation is for each to self-regulate, at times cooperate and support, and not to selfishly isolate him- or herself from the whole. When a person does these things, he or she is part of a group (society has many groups whose members know and acknowledge one another) that gets "picked up" when down, that picks up others when they are down, that is "one of us"; and his or her personhood is reciprocally nourished and strengthened by family, friends, and the greater community. However, if someone fails to self-regulate or continues breaking some other aspect of the agreement, that person will be excluded and "kicked out" of the group, out of the community. After being rejected, that person will not be included in social outings or backyard parties, and his or her phone calls or text messages will not be returned.

According to the World Health Organization (WHO), the quality and quantity of social relationships is one of the primary factors that combine to affect the health of individuals and communities. "Whether people are healthy or not is determined by their circumstances and environment. To a large extent, factors such as where we live, the state of our environment, our genetics, our income and education level, and *our relationships with friends and family* all have considerable impacts on our health" (italics added).[12] WHO's key determinants of health include social and economic environment, physical environment, and individual characteristics and behaviors. According to WHO, social status and finances combined is the first key to overall health. Said another way, the better a person's social environment—his or her family, friends, and community—the better that person's health. Lack of social support or opposition from family and friends is directly linked to unfavorable health outcomes. The importance of quality social relationships for survivors and their families cannot be overemphasized in the rehabilitation process; literally everyone needs to work on it. Of equal importance is financial well-being—the greater the gap between the richest and poorest people, the greater the disparities in health. Nearly every brain injury survivor has difficulty managing money, and nearly every involved family suffers financial loss. That is beyond the scope of my book, but I strongly encourage survivors to learn how to better manage their money by following experts and authors who know how to do that.

---

[12]   https://www.who.int/hia/evidence/doh/en/.

So much is at stake in "working on the quality of our social relationships" that it is imperative to understand what makes for a quality relationship. Debra Umberson and Jennifer Karas Montez in "Social Relationships and Health: A Flashpoint for Health Policy," as published in the *Journal of Health and Social Behavior,*[10] explain that social support refers to the *emotionally sustaining qualities* of relationships (e.g., the sense that one is loved, cared for, and listened to). They summarize a number of studies showing that social support may have indirect effects on health by reducing the impact of stress or by fostering a sense of meaning and purpose in life. While positive social relationships provide a central source of emotional support for most people, negative social relationships can be extremely stressful. (Marriage, for example, is a major source of both support and stress for many people, and poor marital quality can compromise both immune and endocrine functions as well as cause depression.) Relationship stress undermines health through behavioral, psychosocial, *and* physiological pathways.

Ostracism is a terrible experience. According McRaney[5] (p. 113), a person left on his or her own rarely, if ever, thrives—all too commonly, survivors are socially excluded and left on their own. When one feels ostracized and unwanted, that person naturally recoils, becomes much less cooperative, is unmotivated to work or produce, and is more likely to abuse drugs or alcohol, smoke cigarettes, or do other reality-escaping, self-destructive activities. Rejection typically erodes self-control, and lack of self-control leads to even greater rejection, which fosters a vicious cycle that without question is ego depleting.

Ego Depletion / Decision Fatigue

Think of ego as your mental battery and of ego depletion[13] as the drain of your charge, the burning up of your mental energy. The current

---

[13] According to David McRaney[5] (p. 116), *ego depletion* is a figure of speech for multiple elusive physiopsychological components that no one could fully

understanding is that all brain functions require energy and that many things besides rejection can significantly drain your charge—deplete your ego. McRaney[5] reports that common ego drains include the effort involved in making a choice or in focused concentration, fatigue, alcohol/drug use, overstimulation, lack of brain-healthy food, dehydration, and exercising executive function. (Executive function includes such skills as remembering instructions, multitasking, drawing logical comparisons, organizing and acting on information, making consequential decisions, etc.) Executive functions, McRaney explains, seem to require the most mental fuel, and the more significant any decision or choice involved is, the more fuel those functions will demand.

Given the need after a brain injury to deliberately make so many more choices about *everything*—from how and when to say what you want to say to how to walk and move the way you want to walk and move to how to respond in socially acceptable ways, all this while lacking the schema to place situations in their proper context and without a healthy self-esteem, without an internal locus of control to tell you when you are doing the right thing, without the capacity for self-regulation you formerly possessed, without awareness or self-knowledge, without your intuition, without knowing how you feel about your choices, without the support of family or friends, and *with each additional choice* made even more complicated by perplexity, distractibility, fatigue, short-term memory loss, and social isolation— the result is that those choices made easily, even "automatically," prior to brain-injury, can now feel nearly impossible. The effort involved in making choices, moreover, will accelerate your ego depletion. All this accounts for why executive functions commonly are the most difficult aspects of life for survivors.

The medical explanation of why, after brain injury, you have such difficulty with normal things is that pre-injury you had over 60 percent

---

explain. Further, when you need to be at your cognitive best and regulate your behaviors in alignment with your beliefs and desires, to avoid opting for the easy way out—self-destructive behaviors—it is important to be well rested and eat healthy foods.

of your brain's capacity available in reserve to handle higher than normal demands. (People normally use less than 40 percent of their brains for cognitive, emotional, and physical demands; they call on their reserve as needed and are able to function quite well under high-demand circumstances.) Post-brain-injury, you have to use as much as or more than 85 percent of your brain's capacity for normal cognitive, emotional, and physical demands. That leaves only 15 percent or less in reserve for higher demands. Lacking normal reserve brain capacity, a survivor can easily be overwhelmed by ordinary life—when a new task needs to be done or a question must be answered, he or she may simply shut down and be unable to perform. Lower brain reserves amount to lower stress capacity—so much so that even normal problems, normal background noise, normal daylight, normal activity, normal life can become absolutely overwhelming. More out-of-the-ordinary, stressful situations are simply impossible for many survivors to deal with. The result is that, just to survive, they avoid much of life, trying their best to avoid falling into a seemingly bottomless chasm of overstimulation and information overload (see chapter 14. *INTERNALIZING WHAT YOU SHOULD KNOW*).

In his book *The Ghost in My Brain: How a Concussion Stole My Life and How the New Science of Brain Plasticity Helped Me Get It Back*,[11] Dr. Clark Elliott explains very well the tendency of a broken brain to become overwhelmed and to shut down. Like McRaney, he encourages us to think of a survivor (a "concussive") as having batteries powering his or her brain. Developing the "fuel source" metaphor further, he suggests we conceive of three sets of batteries, each with a specific application. The first set is instantly available as the source of energy for the brain to draw on first to conduct its symphony of multiple operations and cognitions—this set is replenished quickly, in not more than a few hours. The second set is a reserve source, on the ready should the first set be depleted, but the second set takes longer to be replenished— sometimes more than three days. The last set is another reserve source, a safety net source, available should both the first and second sets be depleted, but this final set takes even longer to be replenished than the second set—up to fourteen days.

The first set, according to Elliot, does not replenish itself very well until the second set is replenished, and the second set does not replenish itself very well until the third set is replenished. Moreover, a concussed brain more quickly burns through the first source of energy in addressing normal demands and often has to rely on its reserves. So after the third reserve source of energy has been spent, it takes a very long time before a survivor's brain can function adequately in "conducting its symphony" moment by moment. Even normal life demands that a concussed brain be supported with regular break periods, where no demands are placed on it—no physical activity, no cognitive activity, and no sensory perceptions (no seeing, hearing, smelling, touching, or tasting).

About simply normal life, Elliott points out, "Some tasks require that our concussive stay focused for longer periods, or require more intense use of her brain than can be powered by the Set A batteries" (p. 58). Survivors may be able to follow a routine (to always clean up after themselves or their families after meals, for instance), but there are times when routines need to be set aside and a more pressing situation, or a relationship dynamic, attended to. However, this requires that a decision be made by the survivor, and decisions—executive functions that call on intuition and situational as well as emotional awareness—consumes an enormous amount of energy; the more consequential the decision, the more energy demanded. Hence, it can be very difficult for the pressed survivor to make good decisions concurrently while involved with more demanding situations. (With a brain injury so many situations are demanding.) Going shopping may no longer be a simple or enjoyable task on account of all the noise of public activity, all the multicolored product labels under bright lights, all the people with varied expressions that can no longer be understood, and all the extensive decision-making called for by every promotional offer displayed in every aisle and every new stranger caught sight of. Shopping, in other words, is now something so replete with audio, visual, relational, and cognitive overload that the survivor's brain capacity is quickly used up and all his or her "battery sets" drained.

To give a very different example, caring for children requires that a survivor be able to see the same situation from multiple perspectives and be able to respond appropriately even when his or her true emotions are the opposite of what will make for a desirable response. According to Elliott, during such times, the first set of batteries is quickly spent, and the concussive has to tap into the second set to keep thinking and operating. He or she can tap into the second set if there is adequate rest between such demands—several days—wherein he or she can rest and recharge. With adequate, compensatory rest, a survivor appears normal—other than requiring more rest than pre-injury. The problem is normal life is not typically "compensated" with rest breaks, etc., and when the reserve battery sources are used up, everything breaks down for the survivor. "But when the Set C batteries are used up, there is nothing else for our concussive to draw on. . . . Her life will not return to 'normal,'" Elliot stresses, "without a week or two of rejuvenating cognitive rest while the Set C batteries recharge" (p. 59).

In Greg Critser's 2014 article "Clocked![14]" UCLA researchers are redefining the science of concussion and David Hovda, PhD, builds on the "energy crisis" theme recalling, "When we looked at the film, we saw that the jolt to the head caused a massive flow of ions (needed for key brain functions). That in turn created a huge demand in the brain for glucose, for energy. And this massive burning of glucose was followed by a huge energy depression throughout the brain. There was no bleeding, swelling or wound. But these brains were in a *huge energy crisis.*" In addition to highlighting concussion's tremendous energy level deficits, the critical conclusion of Critser's publication—that every parent of an athlete should internalize—is that, initially, TBI did not cause noticeable problems but clearly interfered with youth "reaching their full cognitive potential."

---

[14] https://www.uclahealth.org/u-magazine/clocked

It is imperative that survivors respect their diminished brain energy capacity—their compromised battery sets—and schedule their lives with the regular rest periods necessary to keep themselves functioning safely and at a higher level. Among survivors I work with, no matter which of the "lifelong" consequences any one of them may suffer from, he or she always seems to overwork themselves and display an accompanying degree of anosognosia. What I have observed is more a mixture of denial and blind spots than an outright "not knowing that he or she does not know." Many of my high-achieving clients keep trying to be their old selves, their pre-injury selves, by taking on workloads that were routine for them before BI, only to get overstimulated after a number of days. Ultimately, they crash with all three sets of batteries drained and then find themselves unable to function either at work or at home for a significant period. I repeatedly advise them to reduce their workloads, their levels of responsibility, and the distractions they have to deal with around the jobsite while increasing their accommodations and rest periods until they find a balance point where they can consistently perform on the job to expected standards *and* have enough energy to live a satisfying social life at home.

When working "like they used to," survivors feel—*before* they crash—much like their old selves. They are performing well and getting good feedback from coworkers, family, and friends (all of which are what they want more than anything else). Consequently, they believe they can continue handling that level of responsibilities and workload while fostering satisfying relationships indefinitely—just as they used to. Predictably, when they exceed their new limits and consume all their energy reserves, they lose self-awareness as well as short-term memory capacity and become more distracted, fatigued, prone to error, perplexed, and irritable. The "appearance" of being their pre-BI selves was only a temporary illusion. It was an illusion that, unfortunately, survivors often cannot recognize as such. Consequently, they keep repeating the whole pattern as if unable to learn the lesson life is trying to teach them—success on the job for survivors is going to require changes, beginning with reduced hours and specific accommodations.

Without accommodations or rehabilitation, compromised brains simply do get overloaded. People with such brains do crash again and again and in the very same way. I call this tendency of survivors—our having to make the same mistake a "thousand times" before we learn our lesson—*Groundhog Day syndrome*. (The classic American comedy *Groundhog Day* tells the story of TV weatherman Phil Connors, played by Bill Murray, who is forced to live the same February 2 over and over again until he gains some karmic—and comic—insight into his life.) Survivors who repeatedly work beyond their current limits, get overstimulated, crash with fatigue, and have to sleep many days in a row, until they can function again, have Groundhog Day syndrome. It may take several years for a survivor to gain enough karmic insight about the reality of life with BI to learn to better accommodate his or her disability; work a consistent, albeit reduced, schedule with adequate rest periods; and also cultivate a healthy, even though limited, social life outside work.

The assertion made to me more than once that "everyone has the same problems" (that I, as a survivor, have) and that I "should just deal with them, like everyone else does," as well as the advice "You should not focus so much on your brain injury" are same things that millions of other survivors have also heard. In a sense, it is true that many mild/moderate survivors are only dealing with common, everyday life issues/problems, but it is *our capacity to handle those problems* that is drastically different. When a normal person is dealing with everyday life issues, it is as if he or she is "carrying his or her load" in two equally weighted suitcases—one in each hand. Granted, it is more difficult to walk carrying two suitcases than not, but a normal person can make great progress growing stronger and becoming more adept across his or her life span at having a suitcase in each hand—in fact, such progress and development in life is expected. A survivor, by comparison, is carrying his or her load all in one suitcase *with only one hand* the whole way. Being unbalanced, fatigued, and awkward, survivors find everyday life an enormous chore, *so much more difficult*, and the general public cannot understand *why*.

It can also be as if a survivor has to live with one hand tied behind his or her back. With hemiparesis, the affected hand is in effect "tied" behind the back. Moreover, even beyond physical hemiparesis, it may be social aptitude, cognitive skill, spiritual capacity, or vocational professionalism that is restricted or diminished and "tied behind the back" to the point of causing lifelong problems.

A common misconception on the part of both the general public and the medical/rehabilitation profession is that if the survivor can perform a vocational duty, learn a manufacturing procedure, or follow a social protocol a couple of times, he or she can always follow or perform the same in the same way—indefinitely—like everyone else. That may not be the case. After a brain injury, behavior and performance more often resemble a string of Christmas lights that work only occasionally. You have to shake the string to get all the lights to come on, but they do not all stay on all the time—so you have to shake them again. When the neurological connections in survivors' brains are "on," the survivors perform and relate normally—they seem just fine, like everyone else. Yet at other times, there are neurophysiological disconnections, and then—like a string of defective Christmas lights—they do not work or behave normally.

I myself, like many survivors, am able to perform high functions, demonstrate great comprehension, speak eloquently, solve difficult problems and follow work procedures satisfactorily for a long time; yet I have been known to, at random, completely forget a procedure and let down my boss and coworkers. Or I can learn my padlock's combination and remember it for a year and then inexplicably completely forget what it is. Or I can keep my balance standing in one place without thinking about it in a store's checkout line, in my church's choir loft, or by a coworker's desk; but all of a sudden, I may lose my balance and almost fall over. Or when fatigued, my speech pattern degrades, and connecting my thoughts becomes so difficult that it is hard for others to understand me. My brain's "Christmas lights" do not always have the connection needed to stay lit—to function normally.

How does a vocational rehabilitation specialist accommodate intermittent satisfactory job performance with unpredictable lapses in performance or behavior? There are no guidelines for such intervention. It is a shocking fact that I have never met a department of vocational rehabilitation counselor adequately trained to identify brain injury symptoms, work with brain injury survivors, and proactively accommodate the disabilities commonly associated with BI.

Loneliness

Psychosocial deprivation—which is a major BI consequence—involves loneliness and depression. Severe or moderate brain injury can be worse than being in the middle of an ocean all alone on a life raft. If you were in an ocean on a life raft, you would still be yourself, and you would simply wait for someone to come and save you, to bring you back to where you live. Rescue might not happen, *but it could*, and it seems reasonable to hope with all your heart that it will happen. After a severe closed head injury, however, you are not *yourself*, and you cannot go back to how you used to be; you cannot even hope for that. You are adrift on a virtual ocean with no land in sight. Your chagrin is palpable, and even the lines of Samuel Taylor Coleridge, the eighteenth-century English poet, in his best known poem, "The Rime of the Ancient Mariner," cannot adequately express your desperation: "Alone, alone, all, all alone, / Alone on a wide, wide sea."

Even in normal lives, there usually comes a time when people feel all alone, when they feel their worst. It might be during and after a divorce, a terminal diagnosis, or the loss of a loved one. But usually, when people go through such events, at least their mental and emotional faculties are intact to help them process whatever they face and to help them dialogue with friends and professionals who can, to some extent, understand what they are going through and be helpful. When people have a severe/moderate brain injury, however, most likely, their faculties are not intact. The professionals *do not* know how to completely rehabilitate a survivor, nor do they really understand him or her. How could they? How could your family or friends understand? Only those who have been brain damaged can understand brain damage. Then again, we survivors do not understand it either; we only know what it feels like (and that is *if* we are able to feel our feelings).

Brain injury *both* stresses relationships and isolates people from one another. In 2017, according to the former surgeon general Vivek H. Murthy, loneliness is now a public health crisis—an epidemic—a profound issue in the USA that affects people of all ages and socioeconomic backgrounds from coast to coast. Jena McGregor quoted Murthy in her *Washington Post* October 4, 2017, article[15] as saying, "When you look at the data, what's really interesting is loneliness has been found to be associated with a reduction of life span. The reduction in life span [for loneliness] is similar to that caused by smoking 15 cigarettes a day, and it's greater than the impact on life span of obesity. . . . Look even deeper, and you'll find loneliness is associated with a greater risk of heart disease, depression, anxiety and dementia." Nearly half of Americans report feeling alone.[16] Murthy went on to publish a book on April 21, 2020, *Together: The Healing Power of Human Connection in a Sometimes Lonely World*[14], that could prove valuable when working this aspect of brain injury.

The United Kingdom has recognized loneliness as one of the greatest public health challenges of our time. The prime minister Theresa May said she launched the first cross-government loneliness strategy to tackle it and confirmed "all GPs in England will be able to refer patients experiencing loneliness to community activities and voluntary services by 2023."[17]

---

[15] www.washingtonpost.com/news/this-former-surgeon-general-says-theres-a-loneliness-epidemic-and-work-is-partly-to-blame/.

[16] https://www.marketwatch.com/story/america-has-a-big-loneliness-problem-2018-05-02.

[17] www.gov.uk/government/news/pm-launches-governments-first-loneliness-strategy.

The prime minister admitted, "This strategy is only the beginning of delivering a long and far reaching social change in our country—but it is a vital first step in a national mission to end loneliness in our lifetimes."

The UK has further designated a minister for loneliness, Tracey Crouch, who said, "Nobody should feel alone or be left with no one to turn to. Loneliness is a serious issue that affects people of all ages and backgrounds and it is right that we tackle it head on."

As a young boy, I watched Jacques Cousteau on TV once when he was telling a story about the strange behavior of a dolphin sighted near Corsica in France. The dolphin was not swimming but just watching the boat. Cousteau's party decided the dolphin was sick, so they netted and examined it. The animal showed no sign of fear. There was no sign of a wound. They injected a stimulant, but that did not help, and an hour later, the dolphin was dead. The conclusion they reached was that the dolphin had perhaps been ostracized from the company of other dolphins. When excluded in this way, it is said dolphins become desperate—they attach themselves to anything and anyone, and sometimes they allow themselves to die. Are not people equally sensitive and vulnerable? Do we not need other people who care about us even more than animals need each other? Of course, we do. Dr. James Garbarino, codirector of the Family Life Development Center and professor of human development at Cornell University, writes in his book *Lost Boys*,[12] "Rejection is a psychological cancer" (p. 49).

With the social isolation, loneliness, reduced self-awareness, impaired situational comprehension, ego depletion, language difficulty, pain, fatigue, memory issues, involuntary emotions, distractibility, and perplexity associated with brain injury, an additional deficit is severe depression. Tyson Luke Fury is a British professional boxer who is a two-time heavyweight world champion having defeated some of the best fighters in the world. Out of all the challengers he has faced, Fury said his toughest opponent has been the clinical depression that he has struggled with his whole life. Depression may well be your greatest opponent as a survivor, for it magnifies all the negative consequences of a brain injury and quickly depletes energy reserves.

◆

Are you beginning to get the picture why a survivor is no longer him- or herself? Why he has reduced self-awareness, why she has an external locus of control, why he cannot pick up on the schema in conversations or express himself verbally, why she has social/vocational "blind spots," why he cannot foresee the consequences of his behavior, why she lacks self-regulation and is consequently rejected by different groups? Why do survivors' lives often fall apart no matter what? They are only operating with 15 percent reserve brain capacity, are commonly fatigued and depressed, are limited with partial situational awareness and only have intermittent connection to lifelong memories. They are no longer able to infer from past experience or make sense of what's currently happening; they flatly cannot remember the rules of social etiquette or the rhythm of life. Forced to function with depleted brain capacity and very little available energy, they simply cannot be their former normal selves. Survivors' brains are peppered with lacunae (gaps) and holes—black holes. Simply to cope on any given day, they have to use most of their brain's capacity because portions—even whole chapters—are missing from their brain's "book of life." Put a different way, survivors' "oceans" are replete with empty harbors and empty bays, and they often get lost in one of those. Once lost, self-preservation instincts kick in, and a survivor then uses even more brain energy *more rapidly* in an effort to find his or her way back to safety. Some survivors get lost in conversation every time they talk, others get lost whenever they walk alone around their neighborhood, and still others cannot find their way in social and vocational situations. Understandably, at times, a survivor may just fall apart, and then avoid contact with others altogether—with a BI you might react the same under such circumstances.

In addition, degrading negative mental health consequences, chronic pain, and low life satisfaction are common and troubling long-term effects of BI. Increased reports of psychiatric diagnosis, reduced subjective well-being measures, and poor quality-of-life outcomes can manifest decades post-injury (Corrigan et al., 2014; Hart et al., 2011; Hart et al., 2012).

Before ending this chapter, I want to say something about the suddenness with which people typically are thrown into the other world of brain injury. *It happens in a split second* without any warning or preparation. Boom! You fall, you crash, you stroke. If you live through it, you are a survivor. Then your whole world is turned on end.

The brutal abruptness of brain injury is something often overlooked by rehabilitation counselors, but it needs to be addressed. To some extent, everybody expects that mental decline may come with age. Over time, we can even, to some extent, prepare for that kind of decline; but in an "instant, an ordinary instant," brain injury unexpectedly changes everything in life. No matter what your age, you are never prepared for that. I borrowed the phrase "ordinary instant" from Joan Didion, who wrote in her book *The Year of Magical Thinking*[13] of her response to the sudden loss of her entire family within less than a year. She captured her experience with the words "Life changes in the instant. The ordinary instant." (At the time, Didion's husband unexpectedly died; their daughter, Quintana, was bedridden with critical pneumonia. Quintana recovered but only to suffer, one month after her father's funeral, a massive intracranial hematoma [a localized collection of blood inside the skull]. Her condition required six hours of brain surgery at UCLA Medical Center. Despite that surgery, Quintana also died—only eight months after her father). Didion's book (which was immediately acclaimed as a classic book about mourning) eloquently describes the change in her own life brought about by the loss in such rapid succession of both her husband and her daughter.

The changes that follow when death has taken loved ones away from us are quite different, however, from the changes met by those whose family member survived a brain injury. When I was injured, there was unfortunately no book to offer guidance. No one knew what to say to my family or the millions of other survivor families about what to expect and how best to structure life with a brain injury survivor.

Your experience of a brain injury, like your experience of most things, is to an extent predetermined by what your assumptions were before the event. When we are young or middle aged without any disabilities, we are likely to assume that our life, our spouse's life, or our child's life will be (with the possible exception of a few normal detours or setbacks) one of expanding possibilities—an almost never-ending upward spiral. We take it for granted that we/they will leave our/their unique mark on the world and enjoy our/their later years when we/they reach them. A downward spiral is nowhere in the picture. Then in an ordinary instant, all those normal assumptions become irrelevant because of the "most complicated disease"—a significant brain injury.

After a brain injury, as much as you may want to hold on to your normal assumptions, *nothing is normal.* In fact, you should no longer assume anything. You will simply have to begin groping your way through the worst quagmire ever, with the goal of reconstructing your own life or your spouse's or child's life as best you can but with scarcely a map to follow or a clue to help you find your way. A degree of anosognosia may well serve a survivor at the outset, but that survivor's family had best take a realistic approach and learn as much as they can as soon as they can to better navigate the BI journey that lies before them. Such an approach will enable them to set different yet hopeful and meaningful goals for both the survivor and the rest of the family.

4   P. S. Daniels, "Your Brain: A User's Guide, 100 Things You Never Knew" (Washington, DC: National Geographic Partners, LLC, 2018), https://www.amazon.com/National-Geographic-Your-Brain-Things/dp/B00AO70YGO

5   D. McRaney, *You Are Now Less Dumb: How to Conquer Mob Mentality, How to Buy Happiness, and All the Other Ways to Outsmart Yourself* (New York: Gotham Books, 2013.)

6   M. Mehl et al., "Eavesdropping on Happiness: Well-Being Is Related to Having Less Small Talk and More Substantive Conversations," *Psychological Science* 21, no. 4 (2010): 539–41,https://www.ncbi.nlm.nih.gov/pmc/articles/PMC2861779/?TB_iframe=true&width=921.6&height=921.6&mod=article_inline. For more information about this study, please contact Matthias R. Mehl at mehl@email.arizona.edu

7   N. Gibbs, "The EQ Factor," *Time* 146, no. 14 (June 24, 2001): 60–68, http://content.time.com/time/magazine/article/0,9171,133181,00.html.

8   A. Damasio, *The Feeling of What Happens* (New York, San Diego, London, 1999).

9   J. Twenge et al., "Social Exclusion Decreases Prosocial Behavior," *Journal of Personality and Social Psychology* 92, no. 1 (2007): 56–66.

10 D. Umberson and J. Karas Montez, "Social Relationships and Health: A Flashpoint for Health Policy," *Journal of Health and Social Behavior* 51 (Suppl., 2010): S54–S66, doi:10.1177/0022146510383501, https://www.ncbi.nlm.nih.gov/pmc/articles/PMC3150158/

11 C. Elliott, *The Ghost in My Brain: How a Concussion Stole My Life and How the New Science of Brain Plasticity Helped Me Get It Back* (New York: Penguin Publishing Group, 2015).

12 J. Garbarino, *Lost Boys: Why Our Sons Turn Violent and How We Can Save Them* (New York: Anchor Books, 1999).

13 Didion, *The Year of Magical Thinking* (First Vintage International Edition, 2007, 2006), www.vintagebooks.com.

14 V. Murthy, *Together: The Healing Power of Human Connection in a Sometimes Lonely World* (2020).

4

YOUR BRAIN INJURY RISK INCREASES

In view of the disability that can result from a brain injury, it is imperative to prevent that kind of injury as best we can. Prevention is the best medicine for brain injury as it is for most health issues, and it cannot be encouraged strongly enough. Those who have already been injured should not let down their guard in a false belief that "lighting never strikes twice in the same place." Statistics show that a survivor is more prone, in fact, to a second head trauma than the general population is to a first. That is because the consequences of a head injury may include diminished perception, compromised balance, slower reaction time, distractibility, neurological indebtedness, and more. (Neurological indebtedness is a metaphor for the lost neurons and missing neurological connections associated with brain damage.) Athletes who have had one concussion are four times more likely to have a second concussion, after which they are prone to permanent damage because of Second Impact Syndrome (SIS).

According to the American Academy of Neurology (AAN), a concussion is any "traumatically induced alteration in mental status that may or may not involve a loss of consciousness." A concussion is a mild traumatic brain injury (mTBI). The Center for Disease Control estimates that 1.6 to 3.8 million sports- and recreation-related concussions occur in the United States each year.[18] The CDC further reports that 90 percent of concussions do not involve a loss of consciousness. The number of unreported concussions occurring from

---

18   www.cdc.gov/media/pressrel/2007/r070607.htm.

falls, automobile/motorcycle/bicycle accidents, playground mishaps, and the like is projected to be over 2.2 million per year.

For neurological reasons, a second head trauma is not merely *additionally* worse than the first (5 + 5 = 10)—it is *exponentially* worse (5 × 5 = 25). If charted on a graph, the second impact does not increase the negative consequences in a straight line by addition; rather, it rapidly increases the negative consequences on an accelerated growth curve that increases by multiplication—which is to say "exponentially." For this reason, the second impact is called a "syndrome." Look at the picture on the inside flap of the back cover showing pieces of a puzzle out of place. After a mild head injury, the brain is working to pick up "500" missing pieces to put them back in their places, but because many of the "pieces" (brain cells) no longer work, the brain has to search for different brain cells to match or substitute for the ones that have been forever destroyed. Although the brain is very resourceful and does an amazing job of adjusting to damage, "substituting" for lost cells is very difficult. Depending on the injury, it may not even be possible. However, if a second injury occurs shortly after the first, the brain suffers much more than the loss of 500± additional pieces; it is up against the complications of SIS. The complications, or syndrome, of the second impact involve the fact that, in addition to the elimination of more brain cells, there is a loss of reference to the brain cells destroyed in both injuries. This loss of reference and neurological indebtedness can cause rapid brain swelling, massive damage, loss of cardiovascular regulation, make it absolutely impossible for recovery to occur, or result in sudden death, because the brain cannot match or substitute for cells it cannot identify. So again, SIS *exponentially* increases the severity of consequences caused by a combination of brain injuries. It is as if the person were not dealing with the loss of 1,000 brain cells (500 + 500) but the loss of 250,000 brain cells (500 × 500).

WARNING

—for a period of time following a concussion—

IT ONLY TAKES A LITTLE IMPACT TO THE
HEAD TO CAUSE A SECOND CONCUSSION

(see chapter 9, "Warriors on the Playing Field and Battlefield").

If everyone in the United States were aware of the initial brain injury threat and

- did not abuse alcohol or other psychoactive substances;
- drove their automobiles safely, sober, with seat belts on;
- wore a helmet when riding a bike, motorcycle, skateboard, or horse (or even for an elder when walking over uneven terrain);
- had worst-case scenario safety measures in place when taking risks;
- and if every athlete waited at least eight weeks after a concussion— or until their symptoms cleared—before returning to sports,

then each year our country would save more than half the $76.5 billion annual/lifetime cost of brain injury in our country.[19] Those who pay insurance premiums or the taxes that fund Supplemental Security Income (SSI), Medicaid, Social Security Disability Insurance (SSDI), and Medicare benefits—and who want to reduce those payments— need to know the enormous public cost of brain injury.

In addition, every politician and financial planner should accurately assess the huge financial burden BI lays on the American economy by relegating so many once abled wage earners/taxpayers to public

---

[19]   www.cdc.gov/traumaticbraininjury/severe.html

entitlements by effectively removing them from the workforce. (Two-thirds of people with disabilities never work again.) In a short time, our financial investment in decreasing the incidence of brain injury, and rehabilitating those so injured, will more than pay for itself. (*For every $1 spent on rehab care, $11 are saved on long-term disability costs.*)

Cost savings, however, are only one of the potential benefits of prevention. Prevention will also affect quality of life for the millions spared from this malady, including their extended families. In addition, by reducing the violence we are all subjected to, it will benefit the general public (see chapter 7, A Threat in More Ways Than Imagined").

5

THE EXTENDED IMPACT OF CLOSED HEAD INJURY

When survivors lose their internal locus of control and the essential ingredients of healthy self-esteem, it is the embrace of a loving family that has proved to be a central ingredient of the best adjustments. Yet the typical article on brain injury writes of the survivor alone, without mentioning his or her family, friends, and community. That is like trying to isolate a wave from its body of water, when actually it is the body of water and circumstances that "make" the wave. It was family/friends/community and circumstances that made up much of a person's life pre-injury, and it will be family/friends/community and associated circumstances that make up much of his or her life afterward. Research shows that, in the long run, the family ends up taking most of the responsibility for helping survivors, and family members suffer along with survivors, albeit in a different way. Consequently, it is fundamental to include a survivor's family in the rehabilitation process.

In March of 2000, Marisa Rodriguez[15] survived a solo accident caused by a Firestone tire failure with a severe brain injury as well as a broken neck. Marisa's four-year-old son, Joel Jr., would not afterward climb up to her bed or even go near her because he was scared of her. He told his father, "My mama is dead." Marisa could no longer hold Joel, talk to him, play with him, or understand him when he asked for something. The mom Joel Jr. had known was no longer present, so in his mind, she was dead. Family members commonly describe the state of their survivor in similar ways: "She is dead," "He is not himself," "She is not the normal Judy," "Kevin is gone."

The changes family members experience were first noted in the famous case of Phineas P. Gage. In the 1800s, Mr. Gage was an American railroad construction worker who is notably remembered for his improbable survival of an accident in which an explosion launched a large iron rod that was driven up from under his jaw all the way through the front top of his head. The rod destroyed much of his brain's left frontal lobe, resulting in such profound effects on his personality and behavior that his friends said he was "no longer Gage." Phineas's family and friends lost the relationship they had had with him before the brain injury. Phineas is now a part of medical folklore, and his story is taught to every neurological/neuropsychological student. Given the state of some survivors, death might—from at least one point of view—be easier on a family. Yet from another perspective, life—even disabled life—is precious and therefore worth protecting *with every effort.*

It is natural for everyone to feel terrible when they have to deal with the paradoxical joy/grief associated with BI. There is joy that a loved one has survived what was expected to be certain death, but at the same time, when the realization strikes home that the person who has survived is not the *same person*, there is grief. The grieving process is complex when it involves the ambiguous kind of loss that results from any form of BI (TBI, Parkinson's, Alzheimer's, stroke, anoxia, etc.). Compounding the post-brain-injury grieving process is the fact that, as a rule, a *survivor family's loss* is not acknowledged or even recognized by most people in their social circle.

Others have to be quite close to a family to understand just how much "family life loss" is associated with BI. According to the psychologist Herbert Gravitz, PhD,[16] "Mental illness can weave a web of doubt, confusion, and chaos around the family." And I have found this to be true for brain injury as well. Dr. Gravitz reports that five different factors bind families to the despair of a loved one's BI: stress, trauma, loss, grief, and exhaustion. The impact on families abruptly thrown into the other world of brain injury, which commonly isolates families from their communities, can certainly be overwhelming. The problems associated with brain injury are far too great, however, for anyone or any family to face alone. Fortunately, support groups can meet some of the emotional needs of survivor families. Support groups can offset a family's natural tendency to isolate once they discover that the larger community does not, and cannot, comprehend what they are dealing with.

Many professionals agree that adequate family intervention needs to include three components: *education* about the brain injury and its effects, *emotional support* for all involved, and—very important—*collaboration* among the family members with the medical, academic, and vocational professionals involved.

As mentioned earlier, Dr. Masel alerts us to the fact that medical schools are not teaching post-brain-injury treatments to health professionals and exhorts us, "Therefore, it is the educated patient and family who become the manager of the disease."[20] I cannot overstate the importance of *education*. The smartest thing anyone who is supporting a survivor can do is learn about the consequences of brain injury and what best supports the recovery process. Education can help people distinguish between behavior caused by brain damage and behavior that is truly personal choice. Making that kind of distinction requires both knowledge of the brain injury symptoms and extended experience with a survivor (ideally both pre- and post-injury).

The *emotional* component involves building for the family—by means of counseling and support groups—a foundation of community with others in a similar BI situation or with those empathetic about the matter. Emotional support for the survivor's family is essential because of the stress they undergo. For them, because—again—the defining characteristics of the survivor they knew are often no longer present, it can be as if the survivor were buried alive—alive but lost to the world and to those who love him or her. This horrible state is often more

---

[20] www.brainline.org/article/brain-injury-chronic-disease-interview-brent-masel-md.

torturous for those who are aware of it—family and friends—than for the survivor, who is unaware of the altered mental/physical state he or she is in. I strongly encourage family members to prioritize taking care of *themselves* emotionally and physically and to be involved in their local communities—if they are to support their survivor as best they can for as long as they can.

According to Gary Null, PhD, author of over seventy best-selling books on healthy living, caregivers have the highest mortality rate of any group of people in the world. For brain injury caregivers, the best supports available are well-connected extended families and friends, people who have been involved enough and who care enough to learn a bit about brain injury and who also, through experience, know best how to assist the survivor and his or her immediate family. For me, the "well-connected friends"—who were every bit as important to me as my amazing family and who were very important in protecting my family from burnout—were members of my wonderful church. After caring and involved family and friends, the best resource to help caregivers decompress, strategize, and stay healthy may well be a caregiver's support group.

Marci Drimmer, caregiver of an adult survivor, reported in her caregiver column article "Put on Your Own Oxygen Mask First," as found in the Brain Injury Alliance of Colorado (BIAC) quarterly newsletter *HeadSTRONG*,[21] that she loved and greatly needed every minute of a six-day vacation she took away from her survivor family member. If that sounds harsh or insensitive, she points out it is the healthiest thing a family caregiver can do for themselves—and for their survivor. BI caregivers are under the daily burden of "holding it all together" physically, emotionally, mentally, and many times financially as well. Dimmer wrote, "We become the rock for our families and forget that we have been injured as well. You may believe that it is absurd to stand next to the TBI survivor and claim you too

---

21   www.biacolorado.org/biac/wp-content/uploads/2017/06/HeadSTRONG-v1-i2-June-2017-FINAL.pdf.

have been injured." Yet that is exactly what happens—and as stated earlier, sometimes the family members suffer the greatest life-changing consequences.

Drimmer continued, "Our family life has been forever changed and we are working hard to adapt to all the changes." Many days, she was sad because of what her partner could no longer do. Other times, she was angry that they were even brain-injured in the first place because safety measure might have prevented the accident. Drimmer recognized the tremendous amount of energy it takes to manage one's fears and emotions while providing care for survivors. Caregivers may not give themselves room to express anger, frustration, or anxiety because they do not have a BI. Commonly, caregivers prioritize the survivor's needs, forgo their own, and give away their physical and emotional health, all for the injured loved one. Some feel obligated to give everything away for their survivor, not knowing that, in the end, doing so is the worst thing for the survivor, for themselves, and for the entire family.

Drimmer compared the gas and maintenance our cars need—that we recognize and provide—to caregiver's need to care for themselves in a similar fashion; however, we commonly fail to do that and expect ourselves to "drive on bald tires or run on empty." She gives us a clear picture with this next image: "When you board an airplane with children they always say, 'put on your own oxygen mask first.' We caregivers desperately need time to refuel and replenish ourselves *physically, emotionally and spiritually*." Drimmer expects some to be angry that she maintains caregivers should take time for themselves, and others to have no idea what *replenish* means. With time, experience, and success, she has grown in strength and conviction to preach that, for caregivers, "taking care of ourselves first is best for BI survivors in that it demonstrates to them that self-care needs to be a part of their life as well" (pp. 4–5). I applaud Marci Drimmer for helping her BI partner the best she can by first demonstrating self-care—making sure she herself is healthy and emotionally grounded, then faithfully applying herself for the betterment of her loved one.

"A-B-C's for Caregivers"[22]

A -   ACKNOWLEDGE and ADMIT things are different. ASK for help.

B -   BALANCE is essential to maintain strength and energy long-term.

C -   COMMUNICATE your needs. COPE through self-care.

D -   Don't get DETAINED in DENIAL or DEPRESSION. Don't DELAY getting help.

E -   EDUCATE yourself about available resources.

F -   FOLLOW coping strategies. Be FEARLESS about the future.

G -   GRIEVE appropriately for losses. GROW in new directions.

H -   HOPE, HUMOR, HONESTY

I -   INFORM your friends, extended family, and employer about your needs. INFORMATION is power.

J -   JOIN support groups.

K -   KNOW your limitations. KEEP your life simple.

L -   LISTEN to your body for its needs.

M -   MOVE beyond MEDICAL MODELS, if needed.

---

[22]   "A-B-C's for Caregivers," written by Debbie Leonhardt (2004), is reprinted here with her permission. Debbie Leonhardt is president/CEO of Alexandria Counseling and Consulting Services Inc. in Taylorsville, North Carolina. In 1992, she sustained a brain injury in a motor vehicle accident and has served multiple terms on the Brain Injury Association of North Carolina board of directors.

N - NEVER give up. Don't NEGLECT self-care.

O - OPEN yourself to new technologies to help your loved one. OBSERVE good health practices.

P - PRACTICE being PRO-ACTIVE to be heard by professionals.

Q - QUESTION things you don't understand.

R - RESTORE yourself through REST and RECREATION.

S - STAND FIRM on what you believe is best for your loved one. Reduce STRESS by following a SCHEDULE.

T - TAKE TIME for yourself.

U - USE every resource available.

V - VOCABULARY may be confusing. Learn medical terms as needed.

W - WILLINGLY accept assistance.

X - XEROX method—copy strategies and techniques that work for others.

Y - YELL for help when you need it. YOU are important too.

Z - ZEALOUSLY guard your private time.

The third component, *collaboration,* includes daily *documentation* (by the family and school) of a survivor's progress or lack of progress in resolving his or her symptoms and the *communication* of such observations to the medical staff. According to the REAP Project,[17] which promotes a "multidisciplinary team" approach as the foundation of good concussion management, better management of concussion is achieved through optimal collaboration among the four team members: family team, school physical team, school academic team, and medical team.

The best way to assess when a student/athlete is ready to start the step-wise process of "Returning-to-Play" is to ask these questions: 1) Does data from multiple perspectives and multiple sources suggest that all symptoms have resolved? 2) Do all symptoms stay "resolved" with exertion, when fatigue or under stress— even when medications are no longer being used? 3) Is the student/athlete functioning back to baseline academically (and/or on measures of cognitive abilities)? The answers to these questions can only be available on a daily basis to the student/athlete, the family and the school team(s). Even the most involved medical professional will likely not be able to see the student on a daily basis; therefore, periodic symptom assessment must be collected by the family and school team(s) and must be shared with the medical team. The key to success is **documentation and collaboration!** . . . . The best practice is clear . . . multiple points of data, from multiple sources MUST be considered to make the soundest decision. In other words, the initiation of the Return-to-Play decision must be made by consensus of the Multi-Disciplinary Concussion Management Team, in consultation with a medical professional. (p. 9)

15   R. Manor, "Firestone Settles Tire Suit in Texas: Paralyzed Woman Gets $7.5 Million," *Chicago Tribune*, August 25, 2001.

16   H. Gravitz, "The Binds That Tie—and Heal: How Families Cope with Mental Illness," *Psychology Today* 34, no. 2 (March/April 2001): 70–76.

17   REAP Project can be accessed by contacting Karen McAvoy, PsyD, coordinator of mental health services, coordinator of the Cherry Creek School District brain injury team, phone: 720-554-4252, fax: 720-554-4272, email: kmcavoy@ cherrycreekschools.org, www.concussiontreatment.com/images/REAP Program.pdf.

6

AWARENESS/ACCEPTANCE

Survivors and their families must be aware of the potential repercussions of brain injury if they are to set realistic goals and become capable of acceptance. The acceptance I am referring to is not of a kind that will make of disability something with which to barter for a "comfortable existence." ("Professional victims" are people who have become known for doing this, and they wear out friends faster than anyone else.) Nor is it the kind of attitude adjustment process that television talk shows sell as a form of entertainment. Acceptance of a disabled self is also not mere philosophical or mental acquiescence (the reluctant acceptance of something without protest) whereby a survivor embraces the role of victim and believes he or she is meant to suffer. Rather, an informed awareness of the consequences of brain injury—the kind of acceptance I urge, the kind that will benefit the survivor and his or her family—is one that (1) recognizes the disability caused by the brain injury, (2) separates that disability from the survivor's self, (3) affirms the survivor's self, and then (4) works to develop lifelong compensatory strategies to minimize the consequences of the brain injury and maximize the remaining or newfound strengths and abilities.

An integral part of acceptance is grieving/mourning what has been lost. Usually, a survivor's perception is distorted in such a way that, for a time, he or she does not realize the full extent of his or her loss and naturally feels no need to grieve it. That is probably a good thing initially. *Temporary* survivor denial protects a survivor from being overwhelmed and altogether giving up. Denial on the part of the family, however—family denial—is never a good thing. Denial has been described as a wonderfully effective coping tool for people in the middle of turmoil or disorder—as long as those around them are not in denial.

Nonetheless, there should come a time later in a survivor's recovery when he or she honestly faces all that has been lost and grieves it. That probably will not happen without the help of well-informed, caring people who can provide a safety net of sorts within which the survivor can grieve. (Well-informed people do better in so many ways.) Mental-health-care professionals around the world recognize how necessary grieving/mourning a significant loss is for a healthy adjustment. Survivors and family members have to grieve their loss to move toward acceptance. Just how soon a survivor or his or her family members will be able to grieve the loss is difficult to say. (In my case, it took ten years.)

What complicates mourning a loss suffered from BI is, again, its ambiguous, paradoxical nature. Survivors typically show no visible signs of injury, yet they have suffered one of the most complicated and pervasive injuries. They have not died, but they are not fully present; they have lost a significant degree of their defining, personal characteristics, and the reality is friends and family *have* lost the person they knew. The important things to remember are (1) each person has to be aware of the loss before he or she can grieve it, (2) grieving/mourning the loss is necessary before it can be truly accepted, *and* (3) acceptance on everyone's part is essential to fostering the positive relationships that are associated with the best brain injury rehabilitation outcomes.

If someone is to be transformed by grief and accept it rather than be crushed by it, he or she has to share it with another. The great Russian short story writer and playwright Anton Chekhov unforgettably portrays this truth in his classic short story "The Lament." When Iona Potapov's son has died and no one will listen to her grief, she finally, in desperation, tries to get relief by telling the story of her grief to her horse. Grief cannot be allowed to "fester." If it is to be healed, it must be brought out into the open and shared with someone who cares and will listen. Shakespeare[23] said it well: "Give sorrow words; the grief that does not speak / Whispers the o'er-fraught heart and bids it break." There is consolation and strength in finding someone to talk to who will not avoid discussing the cause of your grief. When brain injury losses are being mourned, it is better if a listener does not give advice (listeners, please do not feel you have to give advice); rather, it is better to listen reflectively[24] and ask questions that help survivors work through their grief—they are the ones who need to "give sorrow words." The best thing you can do, as a listener, is help a survivor by writing down his or her story, adding to it over time, capturing all the important happenings with their consequences, noting the different people who have come and gone, editing the narrative, until the survivor feels it captures and tells his or her story. That way, the survivor will have the full typed account on file and can share the whole ordeal with anyone *who sincerely wants to know.* Then a survivor becomes able to engage in normal, everyday conversation and does not overwhelm others by repeatedly reciting at length all his or her brain injury woes. Many survivors feel they have to tell their BI tale again and again, but doing that pushes people away and can, in fact, keep survivors *stuck* in their own story. With his or her account heard and put in print, however, the survivor can move on to talk about *what he or she is doing about it today* in response to the all-important life question "Now what?"—or simply talk about the

---

23   Shakespeare tragedies—*Macbeth* Act IV, Scene III.

24   Reflective listening is a strong communication style involving two key steps: working to hear and understand a speaker's idea or proposition and then reflecting/restating what has been said back to the speaker to confirm that you understand him or her correctly. A more specific strategy than active listening, reflective listening uses the speaker's own words (rather than merely paraphrasing them) to summarize the essential concept of what has been said. Reflective listening genuinely embraces the speaker's perspective without necessarily agreeing with it. Begin with stating, "What I hear you saying is . . ." "Sounds like what you are saying is . . ." "So what happened to you was . . ." Then mirroring the mood of the speaker, reflecting his or her emotional state, and using the very words with the nonverbal communications he or she has used, restate what you have heard. This technique shows great respect and perfectively eliminates misunderstandings and miscommunications.

weather, the news, sports, and common interests—the way everyone else connects through daily conversations.

I believe acceptance is the most important variable affecting a survivor's and a family's adjustment to brain injury. In true acceptance, survivors admit that they will never be the "same" as they were before being injured, they undertake to relearn how to operate within the norms of the community, and they allow themselves to be guided by others as may be necessary in relearning how to walk the "walk of life." When survivors and families accept life with a brain injury and all its consequences, they throw away old measuring sticks that measure people by what they are able to do, how well they are able to think, or what they look like. They find new measuring sticks, new approaches, that esteem people for who they are in light of what they have been through, regardless of abilities or appearance. Families that are accepting (1) embrace and sustain struggling survivors, (2) attempt to understand brain injury, and (3) encourage survivors to set realistic, meaningful goals. With true acceptance, people enlarge the scope of their values, downplay physical and intellectual prowess, contain/accommodate a disability's effects, and do not allow those limitations to dominate their lives. They integrate brain injury rehabilitation into their lives without focusing on it exclusively.

Dennis Prager, the nationally syndicated radio talk show host, developed the "missing tile" analogy that I will use here to illustrate what a hindrance it is when survivors and their families make the mistake of continuing to center their lives *exclusively* on the brain injury or on rehabilitation *after* the first few years. (During the early years, it is critical to primarily focus on such.) According to Mr. Prager, when all the tiles on your ceiling are in place except for one, you naturally focus on the one missing tile. That's all right in the case of a ceiling because you will be motivated to replace the tile (to fix the problem), but it is no way to live life. We all have missing tiles of different sizes and shapes in our lives. Some people have physical disabilities, some cannot bear children, and others have failed in business. If we focus only on the missing tile, whatever it may be, we will never be happy, and an unhappy life is a hard life to live—or live with. The lesson of this tile analogy is that if you cannot replace a missing tile in your life, you cannot afford to *exclusively* focus on it.

With a similar insight C.S. Lewis wrote, "Getting over a painful experience is much like crossing the monkey bars. You have to let go at some point in order to move forward." Lewis' monkey bars analogy clearly communicates that there will come a time when you will have to let go of a painful memory in order to grow from, and progress beyond it. While I am not advising one to become cavalier and pretend his or her brain injury did not happen, every survivor, along with members of his or her family, should (1) work to accept that a brain injury is a lifelong condition that will never be "completely fixed," (2) seek out remarkable rehabilitation therapies/therapists that have been found to be unmatched in improving physical, cognitive and emotional health, (3) accommodate the resulting disabilities as best he or she can without focusing on them exclusively, and then (4) proceed to find the strength and courage to become a better person, not a broken one—a better family, not a broken one.

7

MY PROGRESSING BRAIN-INJURED LIFE

Although for more than ten years things were only becoming more and more discouraging, I still hoped to regain a normal life. Then in an unexpected development ten years after the accident, a friend (with no medical training whatsoever) heard a cassette tape recording about the successful brain injury therapy offered by Dr. Bernard S. Brucker (see "Remarkable Professionals and Their Therapies," chapter 10) in Miami, Florida, and this friend gave me the tape to listen to:

> Dr. Brucker, it turned out, had developed a method to facilitate re-education of the muscle coordination and movement patterns necessary for activities of daily living after a brain injury. The Brucker Method/Brucker biofeedback center grew out of the *Miami Project to Cure Paralysis* (www.themiamiproject.org—1-800-STAND UP), that was founded in 1985 with the help of Barth A. Green, M.D. and NFL Hall of Fame linebacker Nick Buoniconti—after Nick's son Marc sustained a spinal cord injury during a college football game. The Miami Project to Cure Paralysis is housed in the Lois Pope LIFE Center, a Center of Excellence at the University of Miami Miller School of Medicine that is the world's most comprehensive spinal cord injury research center. The Brucker Method went on to develop and use the Neuroeducator II Electromyography Biofeedback System to measure the motor unit action potentials that are generated by a patient's active muscles. These signals

are detected, then amplified and converted into audio and visual signals that serve to reinforce the patient's voluntary muscle control.

The Brucker biofeedback center has reported great success with both adults and children who are facing permanent paralysis from damage to the brain, brain stem, or spinal cord resulting from brain injuries, strokes, cerebral palsy, brain tumors, brain stem injuries, spinal cord injuries, multiple sclerosis, certain neurological diseases, or other types of central nervous system damage. When I listened to the tape my friend had heard, I did not understand Dr. Brucker's method and didn't think it would help me, so I dismissed it. However, when my parents listened to the same recording of Dr. Brucker speaking to a medical school, they called his office and got me on the waiting list for an initial assessment. (The wait time then was a year and a half.)

Gerald McIntosh, MD, a neurology specialist who served as the chief of staff at Poudre Valley Hospital in Fort Collins, Colorado, was the treating doctor who prescribed Brucker biofeedback therapy for me ten years post-TBI, along with many of the other therapies that I have participated in since 1991. Dr. McIntosh, an amazing man with more than forty years of medical experience, has taken the time to understand me—and my BI. In my experience and in that of others, his professionalism is unmatched. (He has received the coveted Patients' Choice Award; see the website Vitals.com, which *Forbes* magazine has called one of the "five health shopping websites worth watching.") Without Dr. McIntosh's help, I would not have been able to identify which therapies would be (and are) truly beneficial for me or to have prescriptions written for them. If only there were more BI professionals like Dr. Gerald McIntosh. If only every survivor could be as privileged as I have been to receive the quality of care he offers, the "brain injury world" will be a better place. I cannot predict what his care can do for anyone else, of course, but his medical approach has certainly helped me.

After completing my first visit to Dr. Brucker's biofeedback center, I could walk much better—not altogether normally but *much better*—and my hope was rekindled. One of my first thoughts was *Why didn't any of the health-care professionals I had worked with for the preceding ten years, know of and tell me about the Brucker biofeedback method?* I made more progress in one week at Dr. Brucker's center than I had made in ten years with all other therapies. I am not exaggerating; my family and friends agree with this assessment.

I have continued with annual and then semiannual therapy in Dr. Brucker's center at the Miami Jewish Home and Hospital in Florida, and my gradual improvement continues with each visit (i.e., I am able to increase my neuromotor action signal potentials each time, and I am better able to coordinate the left side of my body). Dr. Brucker's biofeedback therapy did not replace all my other therapies, but it made them all more effective.

Through this therapeutic process, my physical abilities improved so much that I was able to get a full-time job in a grocery store as a sacker. In the course of that job, which I held for five years, I learned some invaluable things—modesty, teamwork, the importance of being on time, and the benefits of a daily routine, among others. During the same period, I joined a functioning BI support group. The supervising psychologist, Doug Strachan, observed my group interactions for a year; and when my involvement proved to be of significant benefit to fellow members, he encouraged me to pursue the counseling field professionally. On the basis of that positive feedback—not only from Mr. Strachan but also from many in the support group and my family—I reapplied to the University of Northern Colorado's Graduate School and was again accepted into their rehabilitation counseling master's degree program.

Within the same eventful time frame, I became as if a son to an older woman named Elsha who was motivated to help me pursue this graduate degree. How that came about is a whole new story in itself. When I met Elsha, I was constantly moving from one housing situation to another because of either relational difficulties or financial hardship. (I would either take a room in a friend's house for a while until the friendship wore thin or have my own apartment until I could no longer afford it.) When Elsha learned I had been accepted into the master's degree program and that the college housing arrangements I made had fallen through, she opened her home to me and gave me a bedroom to live in.

After I moved in, one of the first things she did was to read books on brain injury to help her better understand and relate to me (the smartest thing anyone could do). Even with the advantage of the valuable perspective she gained in this way, we still had some really frustrating exchanges. We were able, fortunately, to work through them because of our common goal—getting me through graduate school. Elsha helped me with personal focus, housing arrangements, food preparation, laundry and transportation. She even typed my graduate school projects—all so that I could pursue a professional career in counseling. She used tough love, had a realistic approach, and helped me through that stage of my healing journey more than anyone else.

Around that same time, in addition to the tremendous involvement of Elsha in my life, many other factors supporting a turnaround also began to align themselves in my favor both internally and externally. You will find that story in chapter 11, "My Catharsis to a New Normal."

8

A THREAT IN MORE WAYS THAN IMAGINED

Another consequence of brain injury (which can befall you no matter how safely you play sports or drive automobiles) is VIOLENCE. The national and personal cost of continuing to ignore the association between brain injury and violent behavior is beyond measure. If you are concerned for your own safety and that of children, you need to be aware of how brain injury/brain impairment can contribute to the violence that threatens everyone. Centers for Disease Control and Prevention reports that "according to jail and prison studies, 25–87% of inmates report having experienced a head injury or TBI as compared to 8.5% in the general population reporting a history of TBI." You probably will not hear anyone explore this subject at a brain injury conference or see anyone weave together the factors that contribute to violence, but allow me to do so here. For I am ethically bound to illustrate critically negative behaviors that contribute to violence and that survivors should avoid if they are to achieve optimum rehabilitation outcomes.

Dr. James Garbarino writes about the spread of youth violence across America in his book *Lost Boys*.[12] He reports researchers have found that a boy's chances of committing murder are *twice as high* if, among other factors, he has a *history of being abused*. The odds *triple* if he also has additional "risk factors," one of which is a neurological problem that impairs thinking and feeling. Medical records show that many children today are living with neurological difficulties that can impair thinking and feeling. That single factor, however, according to Dr. Garbarino, "rarely if ever tells the whole story or determines a person's future" (p. 10). All murders and violent people do not have brain injury, and not nearly every survivor is violent. He maintains that it is the "buildup of negative influences and negative experiences that accounts for the variation in how individual youths turn out. . . . It is important to recognize the central importance of risk accumulation" (p. 10). Yet unlike other negative influences, he says, violence endured or experienced at home early in life is a critical component in the psychological makeup of the violent youth throughout our society.

A 1977 study (*predating* Dr. Garbarino's *Lost Boys*) of juvenile offenders incarcerated at a reform school in Connecticut documented the same connection between brain impairment and violence. The Connecticut study found that 81 percent of the more violent offenders had either minor or major neurological problems, compared with 41 percent of the less violent offenders. The one social factor that differentiated more violent from less violent juveniles was a *history of extreme physical or emotional abuse by parents or surrogate parents*. The authors of this study felt it was apparent that enduring or experiencing violence (e.g., being shaken as a baby, violently threatened or beaten as a child), rather than viewing it on television, predisposes a person to violent behavior. (This finding in no way absolves violent, explicit, or offensive media that minimize the value of people by depicting them as if they were bugs on a wall to be killed or maimed. In fact, Michael Lavery has documented in his book *Whole Brain Power* how viewing such media does, indeed, damage a person's brain. More on Lavery's work later in this chapter.) The Connecticut reform school study concluded that, without a doubt, extreme physical or emotional abuse by parents or parent substitutes damages the "neuropsychological/perceptual filter" in a child that can distinguish violent entertainment from appropriate real-life behavior. Damage to the brain's perceptual filter can generate a juvenile with an arsenal of parent-taught, media-modeled, violent behaviors, from which that juvenile will indiscriminately draw his or her own behaviors.

Exposure to lead may also be implicated. The *negative influence* of lead has long been recognized as a cause of brain damage in children across America. The AMA, in 2001, released research by Colorado State University sociologists Paul Stretesky and Michael Lynch[18] showing a connection between lead exposure and violent behavior/homicides. This study by Stretesky and Lynch found that in US counties with the highest lead levels in the atmosphere, the murder rates were correspondingly high. The study carefully factored out race, levels of poverty and education, and other air pollutants, leaving the connection between lead-caused BI and violent behavior hard to deny.

According to Michael J. Lavery, author of the exceptional book *Whole Brain Power*,[19] additional significant negative influences are *violent video games, television shows, and movies,* as well as visuals that are "hyper-edited with frenetic camera work and intense sound tracks" (p. 168). Lavery found that such entertainment can have serious consequences for your brain and your body's health—that the impact on the brain of prolonged viewing of violent or hyper-edited video games, television, and movies is strongly correlated to the impact of post-traumatic stress disorder (PTSD) on the brain of a soldier returning from war. Showing further that the hippocampus of a soldier's brain will have shrunk from the "uncontrollable passive stress" he or she has experienced on the battlefield, Lavery maintains that a consumer of violent, hyper-edited audiovisual entertainment may also have a shrunken hippocampus. Such a consumer comes to have, in essence, a mild case of PTSD not unlike that of a soldier because anyone viewing intense entertainment will have beta-endorphins pumped into his or her brain by the brain itself as it attempts to deal with this kind of "passive virtual stress." According to Lavery, "Such viewing has been measured to be 18% to 48% more powerful a narcotic than morphine" (p. 169).

He believes that five to ten minutes a day of this kind of "endogenously produced high is probably harmless" but notes, "Gamers are glued to their screens two to six hours a day, movies last two hours, and Nielsen research indicates that Americans average 4.5 hours of television per day" (p. 169). Lavery is certain a brain cannot be in this white-knuckle, edge-of-seat state of high tension for so long, especially daily, without serious negative consequences.

Lavery does not, it should be noted, condemn all television, film, or computer-based entertainment. Quality storytelling that does not pander to an appetite for gratuitous violence and that incorporates slower-paced editing and camerawork and thought-provoking content, he believes, can even have a positive impact on the brain. Nevertheless, Lavery reports, according to a compilation of research studies documented by Aric Sigman in his book *Remotely Controlled: How Television is Damaging our Lives*,[20] "Television is a major factor in the decline of our brain health and strongly correlated to a decline in the health of our bodies" (p. 172). Sigman's research supports Lavery's theory that television

- may retard brain cell development and damage function in the dentate gyrus, hippocampus, temporal and frontal lobes and cerebral cortex;
- is positively linked to Alzheimer's disease in people ages 20–60;
- is linked to ADHD in pre-adolescent and adolescent children;
- is a major independent cause of clinical depression
- is positively linked to significant negative physical consequences. (p. 173)

Lavery wrote that Sigman's findings are "based on clinical evidence that has been buried in academic journals, and has not been splashed on the front pages of *USA Today* or the *New York Times*" (p. 173).

Sigman and Lavery independently arrived at the same conclusion about what they both believe is *the greatest health scandal of our time— television*. Their reports state that viewing television (in even moderate amounts) can produce a broad spectrum of the diseases prevalent in American society and that these diseases have been on the increase ever since the mass production of televisions. Thanks to Lavery and Sigman, I now understand the significant negative consequences of television and violent video games, and I'm glad to hear other "experts" also proclaim in many venues that *watching six hours of TV per day is as bad for a person as smoking cigarettes*. I only hope they may be able to "splash" that news on the front pages of newspapers until it becomes more widely known by my fellow Americans.

Wade Mackey and Nancy Coney wrote in their article "The Enigma of Father Presence in Relationship to Son's Violence,[21] published in the *Journal of Men's Studies*, spring 2000, that the rate of violent crime could be predicted by the percentage of out-of-wedlock infants. These researchers found that, in the United States, the relationship between murder rates and illegitimacy rates was significant. As illegitimacy percentages increased, so did murder rates. Mackey and Coney reported that nearly two-thirds of the variance in murder rates could be accounted for by corresponding changes in illegitimacy rates. They postulated that people have often and correctly drawn a correlation between fatherlessness and violence. I cannot help thinking that this correlation exists because the absence of a father from a boy's life (and, to a degree, a girl's life) somehow impedes his or her psychosocial development and may compromise the function of the brain's temporal and frontal lobes. Mackey and Coney concluded that

> to the extent that a son's early experiences do affect his later behavior, a boy who is socialized with his co-resident father, even for just his first few years, is relatively inoculated against engaging in violent behavior. Such a boy has an added layer of "self-inhibition." His conscience is more potent.

◆

This next point does not deal with violence directly, but it does call attention to a possible *significant negative influence* on your brain's health, especially during recovery—namely, high-volume sound. Dr. Ron Minson told me about Dr. Alfred Tomatis (1920–2001), who grew up in France and worked with opera singers helping them regain their voices. The singers he worked with were no longer able to sing on key because they had lost a degree of their hearing from repeated exposure to high volumes (primarily their own singing voice). Dr. Tomatis was able to successfully restore the voices of many great singers through a process he developed called the "Listening System." The Listening System restores the ear's ability to hear frequencies missing in the voice. Not only did the opera singers recover their voices but their marriages, relationships, and overall life functioning significantly improved as well. Again and again after treatment, the singers found that—in addition to regaining their voices—their mood, energy, communication and relationships also improved.

Dr. Tomatis took his Listening System out into the world and used it successfully to help children and adults with learning disabilities, mood disorders, and speech/language problems. The ear has been called the window to the brain, influencing many aspects of learning/cognition and mental health: It plays a critical role all through life but especially during early brain development in childhood. *The ear is also a critical component of rehabilitation after a brain injury*: It should be treated as such. Dr. Tomatis's work has also taught us that loud music, industrial noise, or any other source of high volume is a negative influence from which you should protect both yourself and your children.

Dr. Ron Minson of Denver, Colorado, who was professionally trained in France by Dr. Tomatis, introduced me to the Listening System, and later to the Integrated Listening System (iLs),[25] a portable, effective, and affordable evolution of the Listening System. iLs incorporates a simultaneous, multi-sensory approach that combines movement, visual, and vestibular input, along with listening therapy. iLs trains for brain/body integration through a staged approach, starting with the fundamentals of sensory integration and then extending through more complex cognitive functions, including language, self-expression, and social skills. Today in America, iLs is being used in hospitals, schools, clinics, and homes to help both children and adults recover from loud-noise-induced hearing loss as well as autism. Yet millions of parents and

---

[25]   https://integratedlistening.com.

their children still remain unaware of the Integrated Listening System, and unfortunately, they will suffer the consequences of hearing loss or poor auditory processing for the rest of their lives. Even for those who have benefited from iLs therapy, it would definitely be preferable if they had never needed such therapy in the first place. Please protect your hearing and your children's hearing from loud-noise auditory degradation.

In 2010, the ABC News medical unit published a report by Kim Carollo, "Loud Music Causing More Teens to Lose Hearing, Experts Say,"[26] showing that in the United States, children between the ages of twelve and nineteen have a 30 percent increase in hearing loss compared with children in the same age group fourteen years ago. Carollo quoted Dr. John W. House, president of the House Ear Institute in Los Angeles, who observed that "[t]eenagers are experiencing high-frequency hearing loss which is most consistent with noise exposure." In Dr. House's opinion, "We're seeing that trend now because of iPods and other personal listening devices that teenagers listen to at high volumes for long periods of time." Carollo also quoted Tommie L. Robinson, president of the American Speech-Language Hearing Association, who said:

> We've got to get people to do three things: turn down the volume, take listening breaks, and use ear protection when they're in an environment with loud noises for extended periods of time, such as concerts or doing yard work. . . . Once you lose your hearing, you cannot get it back. It's gone for good.

Unfortunately, today's children who have lost 30 percent or more of their hearing are on the fast track to brain atrophy and dementia and will likely have a significant degree of difficulty with learning, behavior regulation, and communication for the rest of their lives. I

---

[26]   https://abcnews.go.com/Health/Wellness/hearing-loss-teens-prevalent/story?id=11419424.

learned from Dr. Barbara Jenkins that hearing loss very likely causes the brain to shrink—lose volume. Dr. Jenkins was the state of Colorado's first board-certified doctor of audiology. She has more than twenty-five years of hospital and clinical experience treating both hearing loss and tinnitus. She was named National Audiologist of the Year in 2010 for her clinical expertise and humanitarian efforts, and in 2015, her practice—Advanced Audiology Inc.—was rated as the most ethical small business in the Denver-Boulder area by the Better Business Bureau (BBB). Advanced Audiology was also given the 2015 Humanitarian Audiology Practice of the Year designation by the Signia Aspire Award. Dr. Jenkins referred me to an online study and article that unmistakably connect hearing loss and brain atrophy. The online study "Hearing Loss Linked to Accelerated Brain Tissue Loss,"[27] authored by Frank Lin, MD, PhD, and his colleagues, was conducted at the Johns Hopkins Hospital. After analyzing the MRIs of participants in a Baltimore Longitudinal Study of Aging, Lin and colleagues reported, .

> Although the brain becomes smaller with age, the shrinkage seems to be fast-tracked in older adults with hearing loss, according to the results of a study by researchers from Johns Hopkins and the National Institute on Aging. The findings add to a growing list of health consequences associated with hearing loss, including increased risk of dementia, falls, hospitalizations, and diminished physical and mental health overall. (p. 1)

Further, Dr. Lin found that participants who had hearing impairment before entering the study lost more brain volume faster than those with normal hearing. "Those with impaired hearing lost more than an additional cubic centimeter of brain tissue each year compared with those with normal hearing." This Johns Hopkins study makes a convincing case for the urgency of treating hearing loss as soon as possible. "If you want to

---

[27]   http://www.hopkinsmedicine.org/news/media/releases/hearing_loss_linked_
to_accelerated_brain_tissue_loss .

address hearing loss well," Dr. Lin said, "you want to do it sooner rather than later. If hearing loss is potentially contributing to these differences we're seeing on MRI, you want to treat it before these brain structural changes take place."

The article in the *Hearing Journal* "Preventing Cognitive Decline: Hearing Interventions Promising"[22] is authored by Barbara E. Weinstein, PhD. Weinstein reports that both decreased brain volume and accelerated whole brain atrophy have a direct correlation with hearing impairment. People with advancing degrees of hearing impairment have a proportionally increased risk of "incident all-cause dementia" compared with those without hearing loss. Weinstein asserts that, worldwide, age-related hearing loss and senile dementia go hand in hand and have numerous features in common, although regrettably this correlation slips the attention of most health-care professionals. She believes there is a way to treat and prevent such cognitive impairment with hearing aids or cochlear implants combined with auditory-based cognitive rehabilitation. "Audiologists," Dr. Weinstein urges, "must assume responsibility for sharing clinical evidence that restoration of communication contributes to successful aging." The World Health Organization[28] reports around 466 million people worldwide are suffering from disabling hearing loss and that unaddressed hearing loss poses an annual global cost of US $750 billion. Further, that disabling hearing loss is expected to affect 900 million people in the world by 2050, socially isolating most of them and, without exception, challenging all their relationships, plus collectively costing as much as $1.5 trillion.

Nathan D. Zasler, Douglas I. Katz, and Ross D. Zafonte reported in their excellent 2013 book, *Brain Injury Medicine: Principles and Practice*, second edition,[23] "Common Risk Factors of TBI:

28　　www.who.int/news-room/fact-sheets/detail/deafness-and-hearing-loss.

Young or advanced age (< 25 or > 70 years)
Male gender
Abuse of alcohol or other psychoactive substances
Risk-taking personality
Certain sports (e.g., professional boxing, alpine skiing,
snowboarding, roller skating, ice hockey, American
football, many motor sports)
Speeding or other negligence in traffic
Cycling without a helmet
Car driving without a seatbelt
Low social class
Psychiatric disorders
Proneness to violence
Low intelligence
Previous brain injuries" (p. 43)

A combination of risk factors—a buildup of negative influences—contributes to producing the more violent offenders in our society. I want to hypothesize that—without excluding lead-caused BI or hearing loss—it is repeated concussions/brain injuries; violence endured or experienced at home; alcohol or psychoactive substances abuse; driving under the influence or over the speed limit; moderate/prolonged viewing of violent video games, television, or movies; contact sports; playing soccer or volleyball or cycling without a helmet; and fatherlessness can be significant contributing negative cofactors in the violence equation. My hope is that someone will pick up on this hypothesis and develop it further to help clarify what sort of multifaceted intervention program is needed. It is an undisputed fact that abuse and violence today are rampant, many boys are fatherless, brain injuries are epidemic, and the content of teenage entertainment is primarily violence accompanied with loud music. It seems to me that society will be well served by a holistic approach to counter all these negative influences. Addressing only one of the risk factors will be, in my opinion, a flawed approach.

The BrainWise Method founded by Patricia Gorman Barry, PhD, which is based on the latest understanding of how the brain works, appears to be on the right track. This method teaches children and adults to use their "wizard brains" (cerebral cortex) rather than their "lizard brains" (the limbic system). The limbic system is where animalistic responses like fight or flight and lust are generated, whereas the cerebral cortex, referred to as the human brain, brings into consciousness diplomatic responses, love, the capacity for comparative analysis, and other such higher mental functions. The integrity of the cerebral cortex is at risk from the negative influences examined in this chapter. Repeated exposure to such influences causes people to rely more and more on their lizard brains. Consequently, just like the majority of our prison convicts, people who have suffered multiple negative influences choose more often to respond with "animalistic instinct" and less often with human compassion or understanding. Learning how to (1) control impulsive behavior, (2) accurately identify choices, (3) assess the consequences of intended actions before taking them, and then (4) make responsible decisions is what Gorman Barry's program is all about. The BrainWise Method is reported to be appropriate for almost every child; it may also be appropriate for some adult survivors. (Learn more by visiting Dr. Gorman Barry's website.[29])

Everyone should be taken aback to learn how far-reaching the effects of every insult to your brain and your neighbor's brain are on the quality/safety of your life and on the well-being of society in general. Equally striking is the multitude of things that can compromise a brain's recovery from injury. According to a 2014 report published by the National Research Council, "The Growth of Incarceration in the United States: Exploring Causes and Consequences,"[30] "After decades of stability from the 1920s to the early 1970s, the rate of imprisonment in the United States more than quadrupled during the last four decades. The US penal population of 2.2 million adults is by far the largest

---

[29]   www.brainwise-plc.org.

[30]   https://www.nap.edu/catalog/18613/the-growth-of-incarceration-in-the-united-states-exploring-causes

in the world. Just under one-quarter of the world's prisoners are held in American prisons." Marlena M. Wald, MPH, MLS, Sharyl R. Helgeson, RN, BAN, PHN, and Jean A. Langlois, ScD, MPH, report in their article "Traumatic Brain Injury Among Prisoners"[24, 31] that the prevalence of a TBI history among inmates may be ten times higher than in the general population. Nearly a thousand male prisoners were surveyed, and 83 percent reported having had one or more head injuries. Since approximately 95 percent of people incarcerated in prison or jail will be released into the general public at some point, BI among this population represents a serious public health threat.

Related problems that complicate the management and treatment of BI prisoners while they are incarcerated include (1) a wide range of problems in thinking, sensation, learning, language, behavior, or emotions; (2) mental health problems such as severe depression, anxiety, and anger control issues; (3) alcohol or substance abuse; and (4) a range of difficulties in performing activities of daily living. To these should be added the increased risk for Alzheimer's and Parkinson's diseases and other age-related brain disorders. All these problems pose challenges to people in the general public when these former inmates return to the community. As reported in the article "Traumatic Brain Injury in Prisons and Jails: An Unrecognized Problem,[32] "The Centers for Disease Control and Prevention (CDC) recognizes TBI in prisons and jails as an important public health problem" (p. 1). They support new research to develop better methods for identifying inmates with a history of TBI and related problems and for determining how many of them are living with such injuries. "A recent report from the Commission on Safety and Abuse in America's Prisons recommends increased health screenings, evaluations, and treatment for inmates" (p. 2).

◆

---

[31] www.brainline.org/article/traumatic-brain-injury-among-prisoners.

[32] www.cdc.gov/traumaticbraininjury/pdf/Prisoner_TBI_Prof-a.pdf.

Most everyone is well aware of the negative effects of alcohol on the general public. Those effects obviously have even greater negative carryover consequences for survivors. Angela Chen's April 27, 2015, *Wall Street Journal* article, "Adolescents' Drinking Takes Lasting Toll on Memory: Even Moderate Drinking by Adolescents on a Regular Basis can Cause Potentially Lasting Changes to the Brain,"[25] reported that a Duke University study on the long-term outcomes of "intermittent" drinking on cognitive functioning and the circuitry of the adolescent brain found those exposed to alcohol had worse cognitive functioning in the hippocampus, a brain region responsible for learning. According to Dr. Scott Swartzwelder at Duke University, the lead scientist in the study, "Adolescence does not end on our 18th birthday. Rather, the adolescent brain continues to develop until the age of 25, with several key areas of the brain still being 'built' or undergoing processes of maturation."

During this stage of development, our brains are more vulnerable to the toxic effects of both drugs and alcohol, as well as to concussion. Without question, every brain injury survivor, *especially those under twenty-five years of age*, should avoid drinking alcohol altogether during the critical first three years of their rehabilitation journey and should drink only in moderation—if at all—after that.

◆

With regard to brain injury rehabilitation, the point to take away from this chapter is *subjecting yourself as a survivor to an identified negative influence or risk factor or to any combination thereof can further damage your brain and obstruct your rehabilitation progress.* Any such exposure is counterproductive to brain health, and it will hinder neurological recovery. Again, watching violent television, playing violent video games, being abused or exposed to abuse, listening to loud music, drinking alcohol, using psychoactive drugs, and so on can retard your brain's recovery from injury and likely exacerbate your brain's disabilities. If you are unable to find positive, cognition-enhancing television, then do not watch television. Do not remain in environments with loud noise or music for more than a few minutes. Turn down the volume, take listening breaks, and make it a habit to wear ear protection.

Or better yet, stay away from such negative influences altogether. *Avoid all such negative influences like the plague.* To reach the highest levels of success in rehabilitation, each survivor as well as his or her family must understand how crucial this matter is and take the necessary steps to replace all detrimental influences in his or her life with positive ones.

18   M. Lynch and P. Stretesky, *Exploring Green Criminology* (Farnham, England; Burlington, VT: Ashgate Publishing, 2014), https://core.ac.uk/download/pdf/41071488.pdf.

19   M. J. Lavery, *Whole Brain Power: The Fountain of Youth for the Mind and Body* (Blaine, WA: LULU.com), www.wholebrainpowercoaching.com.

20   A. Sigman, *Remotely Controlled: How Television Is Damaging Our Lives*, new ed. (Vermilion, 2007), https://www.amazon.com/Remotely-Controlled-Television-Damaging-Lives/dp/0091906903.

21   W. Mackey and N. Coney, "The Enigma of Father Presence in Relationship to Son's Violence." *Journal of Men's Studies* 8, no. 3 (Spring 2000): 349–73, www.journals.sagepub.com/doi/abs/10.3149/jms.0803.349https://www.questia.com/library/journal/1P3-650097751/the-presence-of-the-social-father-in-inhibiting-young.

22   B. Weinstein, PhD, "Preventing Cognitive Decline: Hearing Interventions Promising," *Hearing Journal* 68, no. 9 (September 2015): 22–24, 26, https://journals.lww.com/thehearingjournal/Fulltext/2015/09000/Article.4.aspx.

23   N. Zasler, D. Katz, and R. Zafonte, *Brain Injury Medicine: Principles and Practice*, 2nd ed. (Demos Medical Publishing, 2013), www.demosmedpub.com.

24   M. M. Wald, S. R. Helgeson, and J. A. Langlois, "Traumatic Brain Injury Among Prisoners," *Brain Injury Professional | NABIS*, 22–25, 216.97.226.57/node/66, https://www.brainline.org/article/traumatic-brain-injury-among-prisoners.

25   A. Chen, "Adolescents' Drinking Takes Lasting Toll on Memory: Even Moderate Drinking by Adolescents on a Regular Basis Can Cause Potentially Lasting Changes to the Brain," *Wall Street Journal* (April 27, 2015), https://www.wsj.com/articles/adolescents-drinking-takes-lasting-toll-on-memory-1430173521.

9

WARRIORS ON THE PLAYING FIELD AND BATTLEFIELD

Staff writer Tommy Tomlinson asked the question in his Reader's Digest article "The Greatest Sports Moment I Ever Saw"[26] why do most people share such a great love for sports? Why do we get fixated on the competition of athletic games? Why is it important for us to know the outcome? He postulated that in contact sports, someone is going to get floored, knocked down, after which everyone will be looking to see who gets back up and keeps competing or fighting and who doesn't—who the winner and loser will be. What Mr. Tomlinson failed to recognize is that in sports, it is usually a headshot that "knocks down" an athlete, and no matter how good the athlete is at getting up, he or she does not get up as the same person. Athletes who endure repetitive headshots all lose a significant part of themselves, regardless of whether they do or do not get back up to keep playing or fighting.

William Nack reported in his *Sports Illustrated* article "The Wrecking Yard"[27] that Harry Carson, former linebacker of the New York Giants who had suffered a number of concussions, said he had great difficulty with communication (finding and pronouncing words) and completing his thoughts. Simple things would confuse Carson; he would forget why and what he was doing and worry that he was losing his mind. He believes that post-concussion syndrome (PCS) is far more common among ex-football-players than anyone wants to admit.

According to Carson, when he played, football-concussed players were not educated on the complications stemming from brain injury and were completely in the dark about the symptoms that can manifest.

In 2010, twelve-time Pro Bowl player Junior Seau retired from pro football after playing for twenty years. A standout on the San Diego Chargers' only Super Bowl team, he was named to the NFL's 1990s All-Decade Team and later inducted into the Chargers' Hall of Fame. Junior Seau was better than most at getting up after being knocked down, and he did that over and over again; then he committed suicide in 2012 at the age of forty-three. Later studies by the National Institutes of Health (NIH) concluded that he had suffered from chronic traumatic encephalopathy (CTE), a type of brain damage that has also been found in other deceased NFL players and boxers.

Dr. Bennet Omalu, a Nigerian immigrant, was the first to publish research on degenerative brain disease in contact sports (Omalu et al., 2005). Dr. Omalu, a forensic pathologist, noticed something strange in 2002 when performing an autopsy on Mike Webster, "Iron Mike," the famous former Pittsburgh Steelers football player. Dr. Omalu discovered that concussive blows to the head cause the formation of chemically modified tau protein deposits. Further, that exposure to repetitive concussions peppers the brain with these deposits—choking the brain until they eventually kill the person. Dr. Omalu named the disease "chronic traumatic encephalopathy or CTE," which can be diagnosed only with an autopsy after death.

According to Boston University's CTE Center, the symptoms of CTE include memory loss, confusion, impaired judgment, impulse-control problems, aggression, depression, anxiety, suicidality, parkinsonism, and eventually progressive dementia. These symptoms often do not manifest until years or even decades after the last brain trauma or active athletic involvement. It is important to keep in mind that identified symptoms are only the tip of the iceberg. Ninety percent of this brain disease and its life-robbing complications progress unseen beneath the surface.

Mark Fainaru-Wada and his brother, Steve Fainaru, write in their groundbreaking book *League of Denial*[28] that, in 2005, Terry Long—who played eight seasons in the NFL for the Pittsburgh Steelers—killed himself by drinking antifreeze; Andre Waters, a former Philadelphia

Eagles safety, committed suicide in 2006 by shooting himself in the head; and Merril Hoge, who played for the Chicago Bears, retired at twenty-nine after a concussion left him unable to recall his daughter's name and caused him to go blind briefly. The wife of legendary Colts tight end John Mackey, Sylvia Mackey, wrote a letter to the then NFL commissioner Paul Tagliabue describing her husband's condition as "a slow, deteriorating, ugly, caregiver-killing, degenerative, brain-destroying tragic horror" (p. 215). Steve Fainaru said the fate of those men was all too familiar. A hard-hitting football player, successful businessman after retirement, and once thoughtful, friendly, fully functioning, good-humored husband, father, and neighbor eventually becomes a withdrawn, forgetful, angry, unpredictable, bankrupt, and tortured shell of his former self.

The Fainaru brothers further report that, out of concern for his clients, superagent Leigh Steinberg—who at one time represented practically every starting quarterback in the NFL—gathered research material describing concussions as "a health epidemic, the consequences of which are a ticking time bomb that may not be seen in their totality for 10, 15 or 20 years" (p. 232). Dr. Robert Cantu, who has been looking into the relationship between sports and head injuries for as long as anyone alive (several researchers call him "the King of Concussion"), is cited throughout *League of Denial*. He greatly helped the Fainaru brothers "connect the dots" in exposing the long-term consequences of accumulated concussions and subconcussive blows to the head. According to the Fainarus, neuropathologist Ann McKee says she has "never seen this disease in the general population, only in contact-sport athletes. It's a crisis" and admonishes that "[a]nyone who doesn't recognize the severity of the problem is in tremendous denial" (p. 265).

In 2015, the NFL was startled to hear that San Francisco 49ers linebacker Chris Borland was retiring because of concerns about the long-term effects of repetitive head trauma. ESPN's 2015 *Outside the*

Lines article "SF's Borland Quits over Safety Issues"[33] reported, "He [Borland] made his decision after consulting with family members, concussion researchers, friends, and current and former teammates, as well as after studying what is known about the relationship between football and neurodegenerative disease." Borland said that with the long-term health of his brain and body in mind, his best choice was to not continue playing football—for him, the risk was too great. According to *Outside the Lines*, "Borland becomes the most prominent NFL player to retire from the game because of brain injury concerns." ESPN recognized that many retired football players have been diagnosed with CTE after their deaths and that multiple studies have shown a direct correlation between football's inherent concussions and subconcussive blows to the head, with significantly negative consequences that diminish the quality of life and all too often shorten life itself. Borland said, "I'm concerned that if you wait 'til you have symptoms, it's too late. . . . I just want to live a long, healthy life, and I don't want to have any neurological diseases or die younger than I would otherwise."

Andrew Luck made a similar decision, retiring just before the 2019 season began. To the chagrin of Indianapolis Colt fans who were looking forward to a promising season (and career for their franchise quarterback), Luck walked away from the game because, he said, he could no longer live with the constant pain from the many injuries he had endured. Luck had excelled at playing football all his life. To put in perspective the enormity of what he walked away from, Luck would have earned as much as $500 million over his career. He was certain, however, that being able to live a life free of pain and with full cognitive abilities—being able to fully be with and love his family—was worth more than half a billion dollars.

On November 25, 2015, the Associated Press ran a story on the family of Pro Football Hall of Fame hero Frank Gifford titled "Frank Gifford's family says CTE found in his brain." According to Gifford's

---

[33]   https://www.espn.com/espn/otl/story/_/id/12496480/san-francisco-49ers-linebacker-chris-borland-retires-head-injury-concerns.

family, signs of the degenerative disease CTE were found in the player's brain after his death. The AP account said the family "made the difficult decision to have his brain studied in hopes of contributing to the advancement of medical research on the link between football and traumatic brain injury."[34] The resilient family who survived Gifford was encouraged that going public with his condition would help break the silence surrounding the epidemic of concussions associated with football at all levels. They looked forward to the sorely needed, open, and unequivocal dialogue that may serve as the foundation of a viable solution for this urgent problem. Further, they found solace in realizing Frank Gifford might be an inspiration for others experiencing early signs of degenerative CTE and for those interested in taking the steps necessary to prevent the disease.

Chris Casey's article "Back to Class for Former Denver Broncos Star," published by University Communications[35] on September 1, 2017, tells the story of professional football player David Bruton Jr., a member of the 2015 Denver Broncos Super Bowl 50 team. After Bruton suffered his sixth concussion in 2016, he decided to walk away from the game he had loved his whole life, despite having cleared the doctor's protocol and having been given the green light to keep playing. Within a week of announcing his retirement, the headline in *Sporting News* read that "CTE was found in 99 percent of deceased NFL players' brains that were donated to scientific research." Pursuing his great interest in health—both his own and others'—Burton went on to study medicine at CU Denver. Being able to serve others as a professional health-care provider will be a lifelong pursuit for him, one that makes up for having set aside his love for the game of football and the camaraderie of the Bronco team.

Coaches and professionals owe it to our youth to educate them about traumatic brain injury, second impact syndrome (SIS), and

---

[34]   https://apnews.com/b4905a1293e440f693514a7f770b60c4/frank-giffords-family-says-cte-found-his-brain.

[35]   https://www.cudenvertoday.org/.

chronic traumatic encephalopathy (CTE); to teach them to play by the rules, to change the rules when necessary; and, in case of injury, to see to it that they follow a multifaceted intervention similar to the CHAMP BRANDISE protocol (see "Remarkable Professionals and Their Therapies," chapter 10). Increasing knowledge about the far-reaching negative consequences of head injuries in sports should do away with our "love" for headshots in sports and change our eager appetite for seeing athletes "get up *or not*" after being knocked down into revulsion. *Take head injuries out of sports wherever possible—beginning with practice. Let's be amazed and entertained by the skills and strength of our amazing athletes—not their head-bashing gladiator spectacles. And let's help athletes keep their cognitive abilities, their personalities, and their quality of life for many years after retirement.*

In view of the mounting evidence associated with the deaths of contact sport athletes, I pray and believe Comm. Roger Goodell with the NFL conglomerate—out of basic human compassion—will become the biggest proponents of brain injury prevention/rehabilitation—when they see that there *is* a way to accomplish this while maintaining the popularity and profitability of the game of football. I think the NFL will not delay in making the necessary, positive and practical changes once they better understand them. I was delighted to learn that, for the 2014/15 season, Mr. Goodell had instituted the most robust to date "post-concussion protocol before resuming play/practice" for NFL players.

The NFL's evolving post-concussion protocol will also become the prototype, I hope, for college and high school football policy, making the sport a safer game for every athlete who plays on the gridiron. The NFL's concussion assessment tool[36] is a two-page, nine-section document that combines a visual diagnostic test and several cognitive tests to measure a player's responsiveness, with timed gaps between the first test and the delayed-recall test. It takes "at least" fifteen to twenty minutes to administer. If the NFL is serious about player safety, which

---

36   www.static.nfl.com/static/content/public/photo/2014/02/20/0ap2000000327062.pdf.

they claim to value over all else, it will take action against any team that violates the league-mandated concussion assessment protocol. We will see the NFL impose huge fines on teams that return players to the playing field without truly assessing if those athletes have suffered a brain injury—*without*, that is, taking the full twenty minutes required to go through the concussion assessment tool, which is still today's best medical practice.

Having the best post-concussion protocol is one thing, and implementing it is another. It is disappointing that, so far, the NFL has not been able to bring their excellent policy, their "best practice protocol," and actual implementation of it into congruency. Sports columnist Sally Jenkins's 2015 *Washington Post* article titled "NFL's Concussion Priorities: Dodging Blame, Making Players Responsible"[37] reported dizzy players were told not to "hide their symptoms" —as if that would make the game safer. The problem is professional football's brain damage problems grow out of its monetary recompensation arrangement, which in effect *forces* players to play when hurt—that is, to hide their symptoms or lose their job. The NFL Players Association (NFLPA) has worked diligently to do away with the onus placed on the players to "self-report." They have also insisted that independent neurological evaluators be a part of the game. Their demands have been recognized and even included in the agreement, yet those safeguards have not been enforced by the league. According to Jenkins, the NFL has a detached attitude when it comes to player protection from head injury and seems to think telling players to self-report covers all NFL liability. Even when a player has obviously been head-injured (as was the case, for example, once when—after a helmet-to-helmet hit— quarterback Case Keenum grabbed his head and lurched sideways), the medical and coaching staffs brazenly ignored basic precautions and kept him in the game.

---

[37] www.washingtonpost.com/sports/redskins/nfls-concussion-priorities-dodging-blame-making-players-responsible/2015/12/03/1b8752f8-99d2-11e5-94f0-9eeaff906ef3_story.html.

Jenkins suggests there is a foundational corruption in football that has been camouflaged in many ways yet absolutely must be exposed if it is to be remedied. "NFL management invariably ducks its failures on health and safety by framing injuries as something for which players signed up," she says. However, washing their hands by maintaining that it is the players' fault for (1) playing the game in the first place, (2) using their helmets headfirst when they block or make tackles, and (3) not self-reporting when concussed—does not absolve the NFL of their culpability for CTE nor of their responsibility to make the game safer. The all-time great Pittsburgh Steelers quarterback Ben Roethlisberger did self-report and took himself out of a game when he had concussion symptoms. He admonishes his fellow quarterbacks that a concussion is not an injury anyone should overlook or continue playing with. Roethlisberger is of the opinion that the game of football "is not worth" having to live with the terrible consequences of brain injury when he retires.

Jenkins commends Cincinnati Bengals tackle Eric Winston, the NFLPA president, for exposing the fact that the NFL accepts and surreptitiously promotes a disregard for "professionalism when it comes to medical misconduct." She quotes Winston as saying the NFL allows deviation from medical/pharmaceutical laws, sending players back to play after having a joint tapped and pain relievers injected (doing so only to doom them to future debilitating injuries) or looking away from players like the quarterback Case Keenum (even after they saw him take a serious headshot and wobble around dazed) because with him in the game, "they could win." She ends her excellent article by saying that the NFL's insistence on calling their concussion policy a "protocol" is a joke that could be laughed at if the consequences are not enough to make a person cry. Protocols should be enforced; else, they are a mockery. Jenkins spells it out plainly: "Until a team doctor and coach are suspended for leaving a wobbly player in a game, then all the spotters and independent neurologists in the world are just window-dressing. And it will remain clear what NFL management's interest really is: liability, not player longevity."

In April 2016, a paper titled, "Study: More Than 40 Percent of Retired NFL Players Had Brain Injury" [38] was delivered at the Sixty-Eighth Annual American Academy of Neurology (AAN) Meeting in Vancouver, Canada. The author of the study in question, Francis X. Conidi, MD, DO, of the Florida Center for Headache and Sports Neurology and the Florida State University College of Medicine in Tallahassee, Florida, said, "This is one of the largest studies to date in living retired NFL players and one of the first to demonstrate significant objective evidence for traumatic brain injury in these former players." An AAN press release further explained that MRI diffusion tensor imaging scans

> measure . . . damage to the brain's white matter [which connects different brain regions] . . . with a less than one percent error rate. Seventeen players, or 43 percent, had evidence of traumatic brain injury. On tests of thinking skills, about 50 percent had significant problems on executive function, 45 percent on learning or memory, 42 percent on attention and concentration, and 24 percent on spatial and perceptual function.

According to a parallel April 2016 article in the *Washington Post*, as we become more and more aware of CTE and the long-term consequences of concussions and subconcussive blows to the head, "tackle football—as America knows it—is doomed in the long run."[39] Unfortunately, despite our "increased awareness," an NFL 2015 official document showed that "reported concussions" increased by "32 percent from 2014 to 2015." The *Washington Post* article claims that when Jeff Miller, NFL vice president for health and safety, told Rep. Janice Schakowsky (D-Ill) publicly that there is a definite link between brain injury and football, it was the first known time an NFL official made such a proclamation. Unfortunately yet almost predictably, other high-

---

[38] www.aan.com/PressRoom/Home/PressRelease/1453.

[39] https://www.washingtonpost.com/news/morning-mix/wp/2016/04/12/40-percent-of-former-nfl-players-suffer-from-brain-damage-new-study-shows/.

ranking NFL officials watered down Miller's acknowledgment and "were far less definitive on the subject." Comm. Roger Goodell evaded directly answering the question about the glaring brain damage/football link. "At least two influential team owners said they were not certain about the relationship between football and brain diseases such as CTE." The *Post* article refers to legal experts who maintain that if the NFL admits there is a definite link between brain injury and football, it will sabotage its position in court and potentially create an open-ended liability with current and future players.

I believe that for the NFL to save their game from being doomed, they will first have to flatly admit there is a problem with the high rate of brain injuries and long-term brain diseases—then work with Dr. Omalu, Dr. Cantu, and others to fix that problem, make the game safer on player's brains, and by so doing resurrect our wonderful American football tradition, bigger and better than before.

Shortly after the *Washington Post* article was published in 2016, the NFL concussion litigation was settled and an agreement reached. The settlement, worth over a billion dollars, was "not perfect, but it was fair," according to federal district court judge Anita Brody, who approved it. The historic agreement will provide payments of up to $5 million to players who have one of a handful of neurological disorders, medical monitoring for all players (to determine if they qualify for payment), and money for education about concussions. Retired players who could potentially be awarded the most money include those who have been diagnosed with ALS (Lou Gehrig's disease), Parkinson's disease, or Alzheimer's disease. All retired NFL players may be eligible for compensation. Family members of deceased former players may also be eligible to file a claim and receive compensation on behalf of their loved one. This court-upheld concussion agreement sets the stage for the NFL to become known in the future as one of the biggest proponents of brain health, player longevity, and TBI prevention/rehabilitation—but only *if,* as a result of the legal agreement, the NFL actually eliminates headfirst tackling/blocking techniques, starts suspending team doctors and coaches for leaving a concussed player in a game, and makes available the most effective rehabilitation protocol plus facilities to its players and to the communities where they live.

◆

Dave Mirra was a BMX legend. For two decades, he was—to the mainstream—his sport's "steely-eyed, strong-jawed representative." He posed for covers, hosted a show on MTV, and fronted his own video game series. As action sports took off, there was Tony Hawk, and there was Dave Mirra, who was the first rider to land a double backflip as well as the first to win three gold medals at a single X Game. After his death from a self-inflicted gunshot wound on February 4, 2016, he became the first action sports athlete to be diagnosed with CTE. Mirra, who was forty-one, had suffered a fractured skull when a car hit him at age nineteen. He went on to endure countless concussions during his BMX career and had dabbled in boxing as well after his retirement from BMX.

In an exclusive article, "A Hero's Death and CTE's Arrival,"[40] *ESPN Magazine* talked to Dave's wife, Lauren Mirra, about changes in his behaviors. According to her, Dave had always been a nice guy who got along with everyone. Then his mood started to change for no reason. He became inappropriate in various social situations, his intensity increased as well as his fatigue both physically and emotionally, and no one knew what the reason(s) for all these changes could be. The last sixty to ninety days before Dave took his life were the worst for him and the family—involving, on Dave's part, forgetfulness, mood swings, frustration, bewilderment, and crying. No one had ever seen Dave cry for so long at any earlier time in his life. Like most Americans, the Mirras had had no idea what CTE was, but then a friend asked them to watch the *Concussion* movie. Dave could only watch part of the movie before he left the room. Lauren, however, intently watched the whole

---

[40] https://abcnews.go.com/Sports/dave-mirra-heros-death-ctes-arrival/story?id=39331389.

movie, for she saw and recognized Dave's symptoms playing out in the film, and she very much wanted to understand CTE—to understand Dave—and to help him, if she could.

Like others suffering with CTE, Dave was desperate for help but didn't know what was wrong or who could help. At times aware something was awful, he just couldn't figure it out. His train of thought would randomly switch tracks, or his mood would change, and before he could make any sense out of the changes he was experiencing, he would forget what he was even pondering—all of which caused him even greater confusion. Even those around him who had full cognition and were in control of their thought process could not understand his symptoms—*until* they learned about brain damage and CTE.

As things progressed, Dave became a mere shadow of his former self. It was as if Lauren could see straight through him—he was empty. Anyone with the same concussion history would be equally empty. Dave was lost to himself and to those closest to him, his communication skills were gone, and he was no longer present in the moment. All his relationships suffered greatly. Everyone was challenged with the Silent Epidemic. Lauren said she would ask Dave, "Where are you? Where are you? What is wrong? Are you OK?" She felt the most difficult thing to experience in life is looking at someone you love, someone who loves you, and not being able to talk to that person, not being able to communicate because he or she cannot understand you, cannot even understand himself or herself yet cannot explain why. He or she just fades away before being gone forever.

Lauren wanted other action sports athletes and their families to understand that CTE is a real disease and to teach younger athletes about it and then work to prevent CTE from happening. She wanted to turn Dave's life with CTE into something good for others. "'Stay strong,'" Lauren said. "Dave autographed that on everything. When I sat down and talked to our girls, I said, 'You know how Daddy always said to stay strong? Well, it's our turn to be brave now.' So that's our motto. 'Be brave. Stay strong.'"

Some doctors quibble about CTE and SIS and cite information that calls into question the prevalence and consequence of both. Robert Cantu,[9a] MA, MD, FACS, FACSM, codirector of the Center for the Study of Traumatic Encephalopathy, clinical professor of neurosurgery at Boston University School of Medicine, international speaker, and author of more than 415 medical journal articles and 30 books, told me that anyone who wants to look at research data "in a certain way" can find support for their predetermined proposition and miss the bigger picture. It doesn't matter, he says, if you do not want to call it CTE, SIS, or something else. Call it what you will—just do not deny that with second impact syndrome, there is "loss of auto-regulation in the brain arterials that causes them to dilate when they should constrict, which leads to rapid brain swelling, massive brain damage, and death (50% of the time)." Even before the "first documented impact," Dr. Cantu explains, "an accumulation of sub-concussive blows to the head may have predisposed an athlete to SIS—especially a young athlete, who is more susceptible to brain injuries and SIS than adult athletes."

Again, for a period of time following a concussion

IT ONLY TAKES A LITTLE IMPACT TO THE HEAD TO CAUSE A SECOND CONCUSSION.

What this means is *an athlete may get up after taking a headshot, say he/she is fine and even seem fine, but if he or she continues to play in the same game or next week's or next month's game, even one additional minor impact to the head can kill or permanently disable that athlete.*

For this reason, it should be obvious why sports head injuries are so dangerous if injured athletes (1) reenter the same game, (2) resume

practice/competition sooner than the eight weeks or longer of "rest/
rehabilitation" after a concussion as recommended by Dr. Cantu, or
(3) in some cases if they play or practice contact sports ever again.
Resuming practice or competition before being cleared to do so by a
neurologist can cost athletes their lives or tragically impair their quality
of life *and their family's quality of life*, until the day he or she dies from
complications.

◆

Up to this point in this chapter, my focus has been on adult
professional athletes. Concussions are more of a danger, however,
for children and teenagers, whose injured brains require additional
accommodations in their rehabilitation programs. Schools will do well
to have a verified concussion treatment and management protocol that
is followed with each athlete before they return to play—if they return
to play.

REAP[17] stands for the four essential elements of concussion
treatment and management:

R - Reduce physical, cognitive, and mental demands

E - Educate the student athletes, families, educators, coaches,
and medical professionals on all the possible symptoms

A - Accommodate the student athletes academically

P - Pace the student athletes back to activity, play, and
learning

REAP helps families, schools, and medical professionals develop a
multidisciplinary team approach around a student athlete to help ensure

his or her best recovery from concussion. Every athlete must avoid any activity—without exception—that potentially could cause another head injury until the current concussion is resolved. REAP recommends three weeks minimum of such inactivity.

Managed rest after a brain injury is essential, especially so in the case of young athletes. According to a medical note written by Sue Kirelik, MD (director of pediatric emergency medicine at Sky Ridge Medical Center in Lone Tree, Colorado, and REAP Project medical adviser), "Newer recommendations are that children and teens should be treated much more conservatively than adults when it comes to a head injury. The developing brain is very different from the adult brain; when injured it is much more likely to manifest symptoms later and have long-term problems, especially if the child is not allowed to rest and recover"[41] (p.1). Part of the difference between adult and youth brains is that the young brain's neurons are not fully myelinated. (Myelin is an electrical insulating material that forms a layer, the myelin sheath, usually around only the axon of a neuron. It is essential for the proper functioning of the nervous system.) For this reason, it is easier for the fiber tracks and neurons in a young brain to be torn apart. Also, because youths have disproportionately larger heads and weaker necks, they are more prone to brain damage in the first place.

According to Kirelik, if you want to maximize your child's recovery from a concussion, "[i]mmediately double up on your R's: REDUCE and REST! Insist that your child rest, especially for the first few days post-concussion and throughout the three-week recovery period. . . . Plenty of sleep and quiet, restful activities after a concussion maximize your child's chances for a great recovery" (p.1). When managed well from the onset and during the first three to eight weeks, more than 80 percent of concussions resolve without complications. Kirelik points out that "[a]pproximately 10% to 20% of concussions do not resolve in one to three weeks. When, and if, symptoms (*physical, cognitive, emotional or maintenance*) do not resolve as expected, it is suggested

---

[41]   www.concussiontreatment.com/images/REAP_Program.pdf.

that the student/athlete work with their medical professional to pursue a more specialized outpatient evaluation (*medical, neuropsychological or psychosocial*)" (p. 11).

At the annual conference of the Brain Injury Alliance of Colorado in 1998, James P. Kelly, MD, MA, FAAN, FANA—clinical professor of neurosurgery and director of the University of Colorado School of Medicine, associate professor of rehabilitation medicine and neurology at Northwestern University Medical School, and director of the Brain Injury Program at the Rehabilitation Institute of Chicago—reported that "on American football fields the average is seven deaths each year from head injuries—primarily second head injuries." I met Dr. Kelly at that particular conference and learned he was referring to a fourteen-year study by Joseph S. Torg, MD; Joseph J. Vegso, MS, ATC; Brian Sennett; et al.[29] in the *Journal of the American Medical Association* (*JAMA*)[42] that reported the high for one year was twelve craniocerebral (skull/brain) deaths and thirty-four permanent quadriplegias; the low for one year was four craniocerebral deaths and five permanent quadriplegias. Over 80 percent of all incidents occurred at the high school level, and nearly every injury could have been prevented if coaches and players had only *followed* either the rule book of the high school athletic association or the football rule book of the NCAA. Both sports authorities have created rules intended to control the headfirst techniques that cause untimely deaths and terrible injuries. Dr. Kelly concluded his presentation by admonishing athletes and coaches to *wait eight weeks* after a first head injury before resuming competition to avoid the terrible consequences of SIS.

Thanks to Dr. Kelly's work, the REAP Project, and the efforts of other health-care workers, "Go home and rest" is now the advice commonly given to mild TBI patients. However, according to Dr.

---

[42]   *JAMA: Journal of the American Medical Association*, "To promote the science and art of medicine and the betterment of the public health." PO Box 10946, Chicago, IL 60654. Phone: 1-800-262-2350/1-312-670-7827, www.jama.ama-assn.org.

Jeffrey J. Bazarian—an emergency physician with an active concussion clinic and research program—"'Go home and rest' alone is no longer acceptable. The disability associated with mild TBI has sparked an intense effort to develop treatments for this injury *in addition to resting*." Dietary/supplemental nutrition, for example, can be very important early in the brain injury recovery process; medical teams working with military survivors have found that nutritional supplementation can have a positive effect on outcomes. In the interest of achieving optimum recoveries for survivors, I intend to bring to the table what I know has helped me personally and to work with other professionals in developing evidence-based post-brain-injury standards of care that will combine best treatment programs to achieve optimum recoveries.

Parents who want to protect their children from suffering for the rest of their lives with the effects of brain damage should work to limit full-contact practice and entirely eliminate headfirst techniques. They should also employ commonsense safety measures to prevent brain damage outside of sports. Whenever a child takes a blow to the head, even if there is no immediate indication of injury (concussion symptoms are often delayed), responsible adults should use Dr. Cantu's twenty-six-symptom checklist at the end of chapter 9, noting any evident cognitive, behavioral, or physical changes. If changes worsen, the parent or guardian should immediately take the affected athlete to a doctor specializing in brain injury. (Keep in mind that symptoms may not manifest for months—continue keeping accurate records for at least six months.)

As for the three to eight weeks' recommended interval of rest before returning to play, Dr. Cantu implores parents and coaches, "The longer you wait the better!" He takes this position because scientific technology has shown that for two to four months or more after a person is asymptomatic (no longer showing signs of concussion), the brain still shows specific indicators of injury and remains prone to SIS. That fact, combined with the fact "no two brain injuries are alike," has led him to recommend that an athlete should return to learn (i.e., to school) before he or she returns to play. If the neurological demands of schoolwork provoke symptoms, then the athlete is not ready for sports or practice. Dr. Cantu wants everyone involved to avoid all stress to a damaged brain either physically or cognitively during its critical recovery stage. Again and again, he repeats, "The longer you rest after a concussion—the longer you wait to resume normal activity—the better."

If ever the fable of *The Hare and the Tortoise* applies, it does after a brain injury. While there are conflicting interpretations of this universal story, the similar theme among them is the wisdom of making slow but steady progress as opposed to hurrying to reach a goal with no regard of pace. Although the overconfident hare takes off at a high speed and races far ahead, he has to then stop and rest from exhaustion before finishing; the tortoise, meanwhile, keeping up a slow but consistent pace, passes by the napping hare, gets to the finish line first, and is proclaimed the winner because he never had to quit. Put another way, the moral of the story if applied to brain injury recovery is "The greater the haste, the farther one falls behind, and the worse the outcome."

I use the tortoise fable to remind myself and other survivors that when it comes to life with a brain injury, the deliberate CHAMP BRANDISE regimen or one like it, combined with gradually expanding, measured activity over the first two plus years will win the race for a survivor. Be perfectly clear—it is not the one who gets back to work the fastest, or the one who picks up where he or she left off in academic or relational endeavors the fastest who wins. Rather, the winner is the survivor who understands and respects the limits of a damaged brain's ability to recover—the survivor who reduces the demands placed on an injured brain during the first two years, the survivor who slowly reactivates the cognitive connections in a damaged brain and the neuromuscular connections in the body, and the survivor who shows resilience by doggedly building on those rehabilitated connections to eventually get as close to 90-95 percent of his or her original ability as possible. Epictetus, The Greek Stoic philosopher who was born a slave, learned that, "No great thing is created suddenly, any more than a bunch of grapes or a fig. If you tell me that you desire a fig, I answer that there must be time. Let it first blossom, then bear fruit, then ripen." If the insight of Epictetus and the biblical observation "The race is not to the swift" in Ecclesiastes 9:11 can encourage you as it has encouraged me—to slowly but steadily keep moving forward, making incremental improvements—then use it to your advantage as I have used it to mine.

The sports media need to understand their responsibility for the promotion of violence. Instead of presenting sports as "do or die" struggles, the media, coaches, and athletes will do well to build awareness of participation in sports as a life-enriching/team-building/competitive edge experience—one that can and should be kept free of brain injuries. In football, the smartest thing the media could do would be to build a consensus in support of the admonition of Notre Dame's retired football coach Lou Holtz that the helmet/head should never be used for making a block, getting a tackle, running up the middle, or playing football in any fashion. To think our thoughts and feel our feelings—as well as solve our problems (personal as well as local and national)—we human beings, athletes and non-athletes alike, need *all* of our brain's abilities.

◆

Do you think because you would never play such an aggressive sport as American football you are safe? Dr. Frank Abreau[30] reported in his 1990 dissertation, "Neuropsychological Assessment of Attention and Concentration in Soccer Players," that there is a measurable loss in intellectual ability with each soccer game played. Soccer players in the study showed a "significant negative correlation" between the number of soccer balls headed and performance on the Paced Auditory Serial Addition Test. "Significant negative correlation" means that the more soccer balls players headed, the worse their test performance. Since Dr. Abreau's study, which was published in *Neuropsychology*, others have confirmed that brain injury is a consequence of heading a soccer ball. John T. Matser, A. G. H. Kessels, B. D. Jordan, M. D. Lezak, and J. Troost reported in their 1998 *Neurology* article, "Chronic traumatic brain injury in professional soccer players,"[31] that soccer players exhibited impaired performance in memory, planning, and visuoperceptual processing compared with other athletes. A soccer player's poor performance was directly related to the number of concussions incurred in a game and to the frequency with which that player headed the ball. It is obvious, Matser notes, that brain damage results from heading the ball in soccer games. This fact should be thoroughly investigated and exposed. Others have said that the danger involved from heading soccer balls is an area that is still "disgracefully avoided by purveyors of the sport."

Dr. Travis Ring's September 11, 2018, article, "Chiropractic and spinal care protects soccer players from long-term health hazards associated with sports injury and neck degeneration,"[43] said, "Research showed the amount of force generated while completing a header averages as much as 450 lbs. on the head, neck, and spine. The study revealed that the cervical spine absorbs a significant amount of force when a player uses their head to strike the ball. Degeneration of the cervical spine (neck vertebrae) for some soccer players occurs as much as 10–20 years earlier than that of the normal population. The advanced health deterioration originates from the high impact trauma to the neck vertebrae caused by heading the ball." Ring's finding that heading a soccer ball can subject a player's head to 450 lbs. of force must be brought to everyone's attention— youth soccer coaches, players, parents and especially the purveyors of the soccer.

Michael L. Lipton, MD, PhD, FACR, reports that repeated, deliberate subconcussive hits from heading soccer balls damage the brains of soccer players and lead to cognitive and memory problems. (Dr. Lipton, a neuroradiologist and neuroscientist, is associate director of the Gruss Magnetic Resonance Research Center at Einstein College of Medicine and medical director of MRI Services for Montefiore Health,

---

[43]   http://www.easternoklahomachiropractic.com/chiropractic-and-spinal-care-protects-soccer-players-from-long-term-health-hazards-associated-with-neck-degeneration/.

both in New York.) Dr. Lipton divides his professional time among the clinical practice of neuroradiology, teaching, and research. His research broadly addresses the use of advanced noninvasive imaging technology to reveal heretofore inaccessible substrates of brain dysfunction, particularly in the realms of behavior and cognition. More specifically, his research has focused for nearly a decade on detecting and characterizing the effects of mild brain injury/concussion. Both the Dana Foundation and the National Institutes of Health have funded his work on the impact of subconcussive heading on brain structure and function in amateur soccer players, and it has been reported extensively in the press worldwide.

With lower levels of heading, Dr. Lipton explains, the adult brain *may* be able to repair itself most of the time. However, there appears to be a tipping point in adult brains—approximately 1,000 to 1,500 headers per year—where trauma results in long-term problems, such as memory loss. Depending on the direction of the header and on the soccer player, some headers are many times worse than others and should not be "counted" the same. Moreover, damage to a young brain from heading a soccer ball is magnified and has more far-reaching complications because of the greater susceptibility of young brains. (Please see Dr. Lipton's "Einstein Soccer Study,"[9b] which, while preserving the game's beauty, has the goal of eliminating major injuries.) Every young soccer player who has aspirations to continue playing recreational or college soccer and then maybe professional league soccer and who wants to be cognitively intact—without memory and relationship problems as an adult—should avoid heading soccer balls *altogether* until he or she is over twenty-two years old.

Dr. R. Dawn Comstock's 2015 study "An Evidence-Based Discussion of Heading the Ball and Concussions in High School Soccer" documents, "Although heading is the most common activity associated with concussions, the most frequent mechanism was athlete-athlete contact. Such information is needed to drive evidence-based, targeted prevention efforts to effectively reduce soccer-related concussions. Although banning heading from youth soccer would likely prevent some concussions, reducing athlete-athlete contact across all phases of play would likely be a more effective way to prevent concussions as well as other injuries."[44]

Every soccer mom who has not, up to now, been told this critical information may want to address her child's coach and soccer association regarding their dereliction of duty. Statistics show that 6.2 percent of all girls playing soccer suffer a mild traumatic brain injury during a game or practice and that 5.7 percent of boy soccer players do also. The higher percentage among girls is not because they head more soccer balls than boys (in fact, they head fewer); it is because the basic morphological structure of the female skull is different from that of the male skull and because female necks are weaker, a combination that makes girls more vulnerable to brain injuries than boys whether they are participating in soccer, boxing, or other sports. (Girls are especially vulnerable to rotational injuries, which are worse than direct frontal injuries because rotation stretches neurons.)

According to Gretchen Voss's article "Women and Concussions," in *Dr. Oz the Good Life*,[32] researcher Tracey Covassin, PhD—an associate professor of kinesiology at my alma mater Michigan State University—reports, "The general public is not aware of the average person's risk, let alone the average woman's risk (*of a TBI*). But we're starting to discover that females not only have greater chance of sustaining a concussion, they also tend to have more symptoms—and more severe symptoms" (p. 46). High school football players have the highest rates of concussion in youth athletics, but in sports played by both genders (basketball, soccer, and softball), girls suffer more concussions and take longer to recover. For more information, look into Tracey Covassin, C. Buz Swanik, and Michael L. Sachs's 2003 *NATA Journals* article "Sex Differences and the Incidence of Concussions Among Collegiate Athletes."[45]

---

[44] https://www.google.com/search?client=safari&rls=en&q=www.srf.ch+%E2%80%BA+file+%_E2%80%BA+Comstock%2B2015_JAMA%2BHeading%2BHigh%2BSchool&ie=UTF-8&oe=UTF-8.

[45] https://www.ncbi.nlm.nih.gov/pmc/articles/PMC233178/

Sports-related brain injuries are more common than I realized. In 2020, Jamie Butler brought to my attention how she was brain-injured as a spectator at her daughter's volleyball game. Further, many of the young female volleyball players in the league have been concussed, and some have had to stop playing volleyball altogether. Lee Feinswog's 2018 article "Volleyball Concussions: 'It's scary. It's a hard injury to deal with'" recognizes that "[v]olleyball has a concussion problem. It's not new, but it's there, and, from all accounts, it's worse than ever. When we asked longtime Arizona women's coach Dave Rubio if he'd ever dealt with concussions, he said simply, 'We all have.'" Feinswog was compelled to ask other coaches, "You think it's because it's becoming an epidemic or the game is becoming more dangerous?" No one knew the answer.[46] GameBreaker.com's article "Common Injuries in Volleyball" found concussions in volleyball are very serious with more permanent, lifelong consequences compared with extremity injuries (hands, feet, ankles, ACL, etc.). Even with the physical demands of jumping, spiking, serving, and blocking, "more trauma can occur both from taking a volleyball to the face or head area, as well as the occasional fall on your back on the hard floor hitting your head. This is why many teams are requiring, and individual players are now wearing protective headgear."[47]

Clearly, not only soccer and volleyball parents but also *every* survivor, athlete, coach, assistant coach, and parent must know about traumatic brain injuries and second impact syndrome and then be equipped with reasonable precautionary guidelines before—and effective interventions after a concussion. Even if it is determined that a player who has just been concussed seems able to play again, he or she should, nonetheless, wait *at least eight weeks* before playing again. It is paramount to repeat and keep repeating this until everyone concerned about the health of athletes gets it. *For a period of time following a concussion, it only takes a little impact to the head to cause a second concussion, and its consequences*

---

[46]   https://volleyballmag.com/concussions-081318/

[47]   https://gamebreaker.com/common-injuries-in-volleyball/

can be a thousand times worse than that of the first. During that period after a concussion, it is as if a sword of Damocles is hanging over the head of a survivor in that he or she is in a situation of constant and imminent peril. All coaches and assistant coaches should learn by heart Dr. Cantu's twenty-six-TBI-symptom checklist (see end of this chapter) and insist that athletes who have been concussed sit out for 56 days or more to ensure they have the best chance for returning to sports and for a lifetime free of significant brain injury consequences.

Athletic fields are not the only setting where concussions and brain injuries are all too frequent. Tragically, the incidence of such injuries is far higher on contemporary battlefields. In 2015, Caroline Alexander authored "Behind the Mask: Revealing the Trauma of War," [48]–[49] a *National Geographic* cover story. She reported that hundreds of thousands of US active soldiers and both army and air force veterans are suffering with the invisible disabilities that go hand in hand with the "signature injury of the Afghanistan and Iraq war"— brain injuries from explosions. Back in 1951, the US Atomic Energy Commission studied the effects of very large explosions on animals. Lt. Col. Kevin "Kit" Parker, the Tarr family professor of bioengineering and applied physics at Harvard, told Alexander that brain damage from large explosions was "completely overlooked." He admitted that, in war, it was natural to bypass the soldier in an army combat support hospital who was confused or having memory issues when the soldier next to him or her was bleeding profusely or missing an arm. In retrospect, Lieutenant Colonel Parker admitted the soldier more likely to have lifelong debilitating consequences is going to be the man or woman with brain injury rather than the amputee.

According to Alexander, Lee E. Goldstein, Andrew M. Fisher, and Ann C. McKee's May 2012 article, "Chronic Traumatic Encephalopathy

---

[48]   www.nationalgeographic.com/healing-soldiers/

[49]   www.nationalgeographic.com/healing-soldiers/blast-force.html

in Blast-Exposed Military Veterans and a Blast Neurotrauma Mouse Model,"[50] results of studies showed a possible association between blast-induced neurotrauma and CTE. With high-speed cameras, Goldstein's team recorded what happens to a mouse brain exposed to a moderate-sized explosion. In less than a second, "the oscillating wind from a blast caused a 'rapid bobblehead effect.'" In a fraction of a second, one moderate-sized explosion inflicts multiple "hits" on a brain, after which that brain manifests the tau protein tangles associated with CTE—the same CTE that comes from years of contact sport concussions and subconcussive blows to the head. The May 2012 report documented that when multiple hits are inflicted on a brain in a split second, "SIS consequences are multiplied exponentially."

In the field of war, when soldiers are exposed to the shock waves coming off an explosion, they immediately check themselves for blood and ability to hear, see, feel with their hands, move all their limbs, and so on. If there is no sign of blood and "everything" is working, soldiers think they are good to go. After questioning and checking them, their partners and the medic concur with the assessment—"good to go!"— and the soldiers are sent back into the field. It is all too common, however, that seven weeks or seven months after exposure to a blast event, concussion symptoms start to manifest: headaches, migraines, anger control issues, seizures, memory loss, fatigue, and clinical depression. According to Alexander, the Defense Department reported that between 2001 and 2014, as many as or more than "230,000 soldiers and veterans who served in Iraq and Afghanistan were identified as suffering from so-called mild traumatic brain injury."

Having no previous exposure to anyone with a brain injury and not provided with adequate, relevant post-injury education, the military men and women afflicted with this invisible disability would rather have suffered physical deformation or loss of a body part. At least people would then be able to see their injury and understand why they are having problems. Instead, when people cannot see an injury, they think

---

50   https://www.ncbi.nlm.nih.gov/pmc/articles/PMC3739428/

there should be no problem; they ask these soldiers, "What's wrong with you?" Brain-injured soldiers feel they do not have a good answer because they themselves do not understand why they are having problems. The stress of this conundrum increases their depression and often causes veterans to withdraw or, worse, commit suicide.

Alexander concludes her excellent article by telling of her family's own experience with blast exposure. Her brother, Ron Haskins, had endured two brain injuries from IED attacks in Iraq, where he served in the Army Special Forces. As a veteran, Haskins suffered from headaches, ringing in his ears, and sleeplessness. For a time after leaving the military, he stayed on in Iraq, where he was employed by a private security force. When he came back home, he started his own security company and contracted with the Department of Homeland Security supervising "breacher training courses." But "one night in the summer of 2011," Alexander says, "for some reason no one could fathom, he picked up a gun and ended his life."

In contrast, Travis J. Tritten reported in his article "Veteran suicides called 'Horrible Human Costs' of VA dysfunction," published in *Stars and Stripes*,[51] that Iraq War veteran Daniel Somers tried desperately to get VA mental health care for years before committing suicide in the summer of 2013. "Despite his diagnosed post-traumatic stress and brain injury, Howard and Jean Somers told House lawmakers Thursday, again and again their son was met with 'uncaring, insensitive and adversarial' staff in the Department of Veterans Affairs, which is mired in a nationwide scandal over deep dysfunction and records manipulation in its health care system."

Kyle Buckley reported in the June 18, 2013, National Center for Policy Analysis (NCPA, a nonprofit American think tank) article titled "Veterans Affairs Fails to Curb Suicide Epidemic,"[52] there were over

---

[51]   www.stripes.com/news/veteran-suicides-called-horrible-human-costs-of-va-dysfunction-1.292743

[52]   http://www.ncpathinktank.org/pub/ib122

125,000 reported suicide attempts in a five-year time span, 55,000+ of which were "successful" suicides. Buckley points out that the VA relies on two different noncomprehensive measures to track veteran suicides, leaving the actual number of veterans at risk for, or who commit suicide each year, uncertain.

Margaret Esiri, DM, FRCPath, Oxford University's emeritus professor of neuropathology, and Daniel Perl, professor of pathology at the Uniformed Services University of the Health Sciences in Bethesda, Maryland, coauthored the third edition of *Oppenheimer's Diagnostic Neuropathology*[33] (a modern classic in its field, covering the practical aspects of the work of the neuropathologist). Sharon Baughman Shively, MD, and colleagues reported in a *Lancet Neurology*[34] 2016 article, "Characterization of interface astroglial scarring in the human brain after blast exposure: a post-mortem case series."[53] They worked to discover if blast exposure produces unique brain damage compared with impact induced, non-blast traumatic brain injuries and found that chronic blast exposure showed a distinct and "previously undescribed pattern of interface astroglial scarring" and had an "antemortem diagnosis of post traumatic stress disorder." The prominent brain-scarring pattern from blast exposure was consistent with known principles of blast biophysics and "could account for aspects of the neuropsychiatric clinical sequelae[54] reported." However, "[t]he generalisability of these findings needs to be explored in future studies." With that in mind, they implore we need *now* to design such a study, with a view to identify the best ways to rehabilitate the survivors of such injuries and begin treating our enlisted military and veterans with the "respect and dignity they deserve."

Former US secretary of defense, retired Marine Corps general James Mattis has said, "The most important six inches on the battlefield are between your ears." General Mattis brought great leadership to the effort to put therapeutic systems in place for our servicemen and women both pre- and post-active-duty. If in fact the brain, the "six inches between

---

[53]   www.thelancet.com/journals/laneur/article/PIIS1474-4422(16)30057-6/fulltext

[54]   Sequelae: conditions that are the consequence of a previous disease or injury

your ears," is recognized as the most important aspect of success on the battlefield, as well as in life after service, the US Department of Defense will invest in *and* support the brain health of our active-duty military men and women proportionally more than it does that of other parts of their bodies and will also invest in brain health for all discharged, honorable military veterans.

ROBERT C. CANTU, MA, MD, FACS,FAANS, FICS, FACSM
TODAY'S CONCUSSION SIGNS/SYMPTOMS CHECKLIST

Patient Name:_____Date:_____

Today's Date Date of Concussion	None	Mild	Moderate	Severe				Today's Date Date of Concussion	None	Mild	Moderate	Severe			
	0	1	2	3	4	5	6		0	1	2	3	4	5	6
Balance Issues								Nausea/Vomiting							
Confusion								Neck Pain							
Difficulty Concentrating								Nervous/Anxious							
Difficulty Remembering								Numbness/ Tingling							
Dizziness								Ringing in the Ears							
Don't Feel Right/Dinged/ Bell Rung								Sadness							
Drowsy								Sensitivity to Light							
Fatigue/Low Energy								Sensitivity to Noise							
Feeling In A Fog								Sleeping Less than Usual							
Feeling More Emotional								Sleeping More than Usual							
Feeling Slowed Down								Trouble Falling Asleep							
Headache/Head Pressure								Visual Problems/Blurred Vision							
Irritability															
Loss of Consciousness	No Loc	<15 sec	15-30 sec	30-45 sec	45-60 sec	>60 sec									

The athlete should score themselves on the above symptoms based on how they feel today.
(i.e. 0 = not present, 1-2 = mild, 3-4 = moderate, 5-6 = severe).

©Copyright – No reproductions without permission   *For Dr. Cantu's Use Only:*

Symptom Load _____/26   Symptom Score_____ /156

Concussion Grade_____

9a. I had the great pleasure of meeting Dr. Cantu at one of the Brain Injury Alliance of Colorado's annual conferences. When I told him I was writing a book about my brain injury experience as well as the national brain injury epidemic and that, in one chapter, I had quoted him several times, Dr. Cantu asked me to send him a copy of it when I could. When I did that in 2017, Dr. Cantu called me and said, "I was so pleased to read your book. I was impressed by the amount of work that went into it. Your references are excellent." Working with me afterward, Dr. Cantu helped me complete this book. He wrote me, "It was my pleasure to meet you at the Brain Injury Alliance of Colorado's Annual Convention in downtown Denver, and to be able to read a copy of your book before it is published. Your book is incredible! I agree everyone should read it! I would like you to add my 26 Symptom Concussion Check List to your book and invite readers interested in working with it, to contact me for reproduction privileges, *and* to understand how to use the checklist for triaging medical care, identifying rehabilitation protocols, and/or litigating compensation settlements." Dr. Cantu ended his letter with these words: "Thank you Mark for what you have accomplished with your book and the sacrifices you have made along the way—if there is anything I can do to help you with your mission of reducing the incidence of brain injury and helping survivors reach the highest level of rehabilitation possible, do not hesitate to let me know. Please be sure to put Massachusetts on your book launch/speaking tour—I look forward to hearing you in person." Contact Dr. Cantu directly at the Cantu Concussion Center, 310 Baker Avenue, Concord, MA 01742; call 978-287-8250 or email info@concussionfoundation.org.

9b. The Einstein Soccer Study examines the impact of soccer heading on the brain over the short and long term. Integrating neuroimaging, cognitive testing, and genomics, the Einstein Soccer Study aims to determine the relationship among subconcussive head injury in adult amateur soccer players, their brain structure, and its relationship to functioning. Are you an active adult soccer player interested in participating in this study? For questions about this study, please visit https://www.cnn.com/2015/07/14/health/youth-soccer-safety/ and then call 718-430-8712 or go to: https://www.einstein.yu.edu/centers/gruss-magnetic-resonance-research/einstein-soccer-study/.

26 T. Tomlinson, "The Greatest Sports Moment I Ever Saw," *Reader's Digest* 100 (September 2012).

27 W. Nack, "The Wrecking Yard," *Sports Illustrated* 94, no. 19 (May 7, 2001): 60–75, https://vault.si.com/vault/2001/05/07/the-wrecking-yard-as-they-limp-into-the-sunset-retired-nfl-players-struggle-with-the-games-grim-legacy-a-lifetime-of-disability-and-pain.

28 M. Fainaru-Wada and S. Fainaru, *League of Denial* (New York: Crown Archetype, a division of Random House LLC, 2013), https://www.penguinrandomhouse.com/books/221286/league-of-denial-by-mark-fainaru-wada-and-steve-fainaru/.

29 J. Torg et al., "The National Football Head and Neck Injury Registry14-Year Report on Cervical Quadriplegia, 1971 Through 1984," *Journal of the American Medical Association* 254, no. 24 (December 27, 1985): 3439–43, doi:10.1001/jama.1985.03360240051033, https://jamanetwork.com/journals/jama/article-abstract/402289.

30 F. Abreau, "Neuropsychological Assessment of Attention and Concentration in Soccer Players" (PhD dissertation, California School of Professional Psychology, 1989; reproduction: photocopy, Ann Arbor, Michigan: University Microfilms International, 2000), viii, https://psycnet.apa.org/buy/1991-26117-001.

31 J. Matser, A. Kessels, and J. Troost, "Chronic Traumatic Brain Injury in Professional Soccer Players," *Neurology* 51, no. 3 (September 1, 1998): 791, https://n.neurology.org/content/51/3/791.abstract.

32 G. Voss, "Women and Concussions," *Dr. Oz the Good Life* 2, no. 5 (June 2015): 44–49.

33 M. Esiri and D. Perl, *Oppenheimer's Diagnostic Neuropathology: A Practical Manual* (London: Hodder Arnold, Hodder Headline Group, 2006), http://www.hoddereducation.com.

34 S. Baughman Shively et al., "Characterization of Interface Astroglial Scarring in the Human Brain after Blast Exposure: A Post-Mortem Case Series," *Lancet Neurology* 15, no. 9 (August 1, 2016): P944–53, https://www.ncbi.nlm.nih.gov/pubmed/27291520.

10

REMARKABLE PROFESSIONALS AND THEIR THERAPIES

For three days in October 2005, over sixty top neuroscientists and physicians from across the United States and twelve nations met to review the progress, or lack of progress, in brain injury research and recovery since the congressionally mandated National Institute of Health consensus conference held in 1998. Their review resulted in a document titled "Report to Congress: Toward Successful Recovery from Traumatic Brain Injury, March 2006."[55] The report's executive summary wastes not a word with its verdict. "What emerged was a very bleak conclusion. Little has been accomplished to substantially improve recovery from brain injury. While the numbers of survivors have increased significantly, and the cost of care continues to rise." For everyone's sake, we have to do better.

I cannot speak of the remarkable professionals and of their valid, promising concussion therapies that have lifted me to greater levels of functional ability and cognitive skill than most mainstream health-care workers believe is possible without remarking on how these people with their breakthrough therapies have come into my life over the years and decades after my brain injury.

---

55   www.brainline.org/article/report-congress-toward-successful-recovery-traumatic-brain-injury

Brucker Biofeedback Therapy, Hoshino Therapy, Holistic Care, and Acupuncture

When I began working with Dr. Brucker[10a] and his biofeedback method in 1991 (again—on the recommendation of a friend with no medical training—see full story in chapter 7), I was simultaneously introduced to Bodhi F. Kocica and a specific modality of massage therapy called Hoshino therapy.[56] Each time I participated in Brucker biofeedback therapy in Miami, I was able also to receive Hoshino therapy delivered through the hands of Bodhi Kocica. This therapy's creator, Prof. Tomezo Hoshino, was born and raised in Japan. He was on the last boat leaving Japan before World War I broke out in that country. Settling in Argentina, he lived between there and Miami, Florida, for the remainder of his life. Professor Hoshino taught that "[n]othing surpasses the hands" in the evaluation and solution of "arthrosis," which encompasses the many types of pain and disability associated with aging. Professor Hoshino developed unique manual techniques for palpating 270 selected "acu-points" that relate to the biomechanical functioning of the body. Remaining vigorous and healthy into his nineties, he was a prime example of his own therapy's powerful benefits. I believe that Hoshino therapy helped me achieve the great results I did through the Brucker biofeedback method.

Bodhi Kocica—personally trained by Professor Hoshino—became owner and operator of the Hoshino Therapy Clinic, d.b.a. Center for BioTherapeutics, in Florida and the national director of the Hoshino training program. With over fifty years of Hoshino therapy experience, Kocica carried on the legacy and was the leading practitioner of Hoshino's work in North America. Currently at the Center for BioTherapeutic in Coral Gables, Hoshino therapists Susana Vazques and Jennifer Roch provide this effective therapy for the solution of a myriad of disorders, including bursitis, tendinitis, sciatica, TMJ, joint pain, tennis elbow, sports injuries, osteoarthritis, headaches, and more.

---

[56]   www.facebook.com/Hoshino.Therapy/

When I was in Miami for my 2005 Brucker biofeedback therapy series, I met as well the gifted Dr. Emilia Cabrera.[10b] She has helped me with her healing technique ever since. Dr. Cabrera has developed a unique protocol that utilizes a complex psychological method to unblock the trapped emotional energy that often disturbs normal functioning of the body's bio-mechanisms, while simultaneously strengthening the immune function of the cells to operate at optimal capacity. Each time I was in town for the Brucker biofeedback method, I underwent Dr. Cabrera's therapy,[57] and it did, in fact, help me as well.

Denver in 2008, I met Dr. Lixin Zhang[10c] at a Brain Injury Alliance of Colorado conference, and I have benefited from his treatments for many years. Through weekly acupuncture treatments at Lixin Acupuncture,[58] Dr. Zhang has significantly improved my health and well-being. He has been able to restore my ability to flare out my left little toe—something I had not been able to do for twenty-seven since my accident. In 2008, after many years of overusing my right hand and arm (compensating my left hemiparesis), I developed severe tendonitis in my right elbow to the extent that I could no longer exercise or work with my right arm. With both arms disabled, I was scared and desperate. Dr. Zhang used his family's unique "fire needle" technique on the tendonitis and completely restored the health and function of my right elbow and right arm—in one treatment.

Far Infrared Light Therapy

My first experience with far-infrared (FIR) light therapy[10d] was more than twenty-five years after my brain injury. At the time, I was experiencing secondary TBI consequences, including overuse syndrome on my right side (my "good side") and multiple joint discomfort in my left foot from an abnormal gait pattern. My condition had deteriorated to such an extent that I could no longer participate in weight training

---

[57] www.holisticcaresolutions.com.

[58] www.lixinacupuncture.com.

or walk free of pain. I began receiving FIR light therapy on a Vigen 9500 bed for forty minutes a day, five days a week, at Vigen USA's clinic in Denver. Soon thereafter, people noticed (and told me) that my balance and gait pattern had improved. After four months of regular treatments, I was back to my regular workouts with no pain and no loss of strength. I have since used the Vigen 9500 bed daily and sleep on the Vigen Hygiea pillow every night, which has helped my straightened neck regain its natural curve.

MojoFeet Custom Orthotics and the Pettibon System for Spine

Then one day the best massage therapist in Colorado for me—Roann Riedel—referred me to Bradley Bosick, DC,[10e] for his chiropractic technique and custom orthotics. Wonderfully, Dr. Bosick's technique proved better able to help me than any of the other twelve chiropractors I had seen since my brain injury.

Years of walking with a broken gait had suddenly caused my left foot to stop working altogether without excruciating pain. When I met Dr. Bosick, I could not walk any distance, even five yards, without screaming pain in the instep of my left foot. Some standard orthotics had been prescribed by an MD, but they were not the solution and failed to relieve the pain. Dr. Bosick's custom MojoFeet orthotics,[59] however, were able immediately and completely to correct the pain in my left foot. MojoFeet orthotics have continued to enable me to walk pain-free and more correctly ever since I began wearing them.

I also learned of the Pettibon system,[60] which is a comprehensive rehabilitation program for the spine's hard and soft tissues. It uses seated X-rays for diagnosis, assessing progress, and proof of treatment effectiveness. Developed in the 1980s by Dr. Burl Pettibon, his

---

[59]   www.mojofeet.com.

[60]   www.pettibonsystem.com.

system enables the human spine to maintain its optimal structure for normal function. The Pettibon system is based on specially developed weights and exercises that directly affect lasting spinal correction by strengthening targeted muscles. Dr. Pettibon continues to train doctors and therapists with cutting-edge developments in the field.

Whole Brain Power Training, Communication Game, and Mnemonics for Cognitive Skills

William White, MD, [10f] a fellow member of my church, is someone else who has led me to invaluable therapies. (One of the humblest, highly intelligent doctors I have ever met, Dr. White has helped me in countless ways. He does more good for more people than anyone else I personally know.) He gave me a copy of *Whole Brain* Power,[18] authored by his family friend Michael J. Lavery. [10g] The Whole Brain Power left-handed exercises developed by Lavery are ingenious. They recruit many areas of the brain, including the basal ganglia (or basal nuclei). This group of nuclei are essential elements in Whole Brain Power training because they directly control such output activities as spoken language, gesture preparation, and mastery of *Perfect Penmanship*.[61]

"Penmanship practice," Lavery declares, "is for the health of your brain, to help attain the fine-motor-control exercise it needs for impulse control, neurogenesis, and even steroidogenesis." He quotes a 2007 article in *Newsweek* by Raina Kelley, titled "The Writing on the Wall,"[35] that posits penmanship is more than penmanship. "Evidence is growing, that handwriting fluency is a fundamental building block of learning. Emily Knapton, director of program development at Handwriting Without Tears, believes that 'when kids struggle with handwriting, it filters into all their academics'" (p. 90). Lavery adds "Dr. David Snowdon found another fascinating reason to practice cursive penmanship daily. His exhaustive study as reported in his book, *Aging with Grace*,[36] analyzed

---

[61] www.perfectpenmanship.com.

the brains of more than 400 Catholic nuns. The results found that nuns who *exhibited superlative language acuity* (that is, who were articulate, who were storytellers, and who had facile memories) *and who also expressed that language acuity through penmanship skill, maintained a healthy brain into old age*" (p. 91). Lavery sums it up:

> When you write cursive penmanship you're lighting up your brain, forcing it to maintain a high degree of focus, fine motor skill, and a host of other active responses. You're unleashing long-term potentiation in the hippocampus, firing neurons across the pre-frontal cortex. If you're writing mirror-image with your left hand then you're opening up your center of imagination and creative thought in your right hemisphere. Remember it was Da Vinci who was famous for writing left-handed mirror image in his journals, and he was arguably the most creative mind in the history of humanity. (p. 92)

Lavery's inspired exercises engage the brain and rehabilitate it in a way that other physical therapies and cognitive therapies simply cannot, and I feel they should be a part of every survivor's repertoire.

When Lavery read a draft of my book in 2018, he told Dr. White that he was "fascinated by it," and he reached out to me personally. In a conversation we had over the phone, he awakened me to the concept of how significant our speech behavior is—in addition to left-handed exercises. Coach Lavery challenged me to play his *Communication Game* and quickly identified some of my "lazy-brain speech production." He told me, "Allow yourself to slow down and develop your thoughts before you speak. Breathe in deeply through your nose, filling your lungs full of air, oxygenating your brain, and swallow your saliva. Tell your brain, 'I control you.' Stay cool, calm, and contemplative as you speak relevant words to the benefit of your listeners and the edification of yourself. Be observant of people's speech pattern as well as your own."

When Lavery recognized that "non-descriptive language dulls the brain," he began working on his Communication Game to supplement the Whole Brain program. Lavery's Communication Game is simply brilliant—literally, both simple and brilliant, in that on the surface it is merely speaking grammatically -correct English (or Spanish, French, etc.) with a subject and verb in each sentence. In practice, however, it demands memory, forethought, and preparation, making it difficult to do *correctly*. It is one of the most ingenious cognitive therapies available today. He would have each of us stop using one-word responses and provided the acronym LORY (like, OK, right, yeah) to remember "the most abused words in our language" that he said dominate our speaking patterns. Rather than these one-word knee-jerk communications, he would have us say, "That is as if . . ." or "That is comparable with . . ." or "I agree [wholeheartedly, somewhat, in principle, at this point] with . . ." and then reflectively rephrase what we just heard said. Additionally, we should not use the all-too-common "ah" between sentences or repeat ourselves when speaking.

He told me that highly descriptive language sharpens the brain. "When your speech is sloppy, you are not using your whole brain; rather, you are going on 'automatic pilot.'" According to Lavery, "The more you are engaged in storytelling and the more descriptive your storytelling is, the more plasticity spreads throughout your brain. Correcting your speech is the fastest way to get the brain to change its plasticity for the better."

Lavery challenged me, "Why aren't you constantly sharpening your ax [your brain via your communication patterns]?" He encouraged me to "fill up [my] quiver with more arrows—more words that are expressive and filled with meaning—[to] become familiar with four-, five-, and six-syllable words; to overcome word poverty and avoid redundancy; and to remember always to speak in complete sentences."

When I thought about it, I realized speech production is our most sacred skill—language is one of our most godlike attributes, for God *spoke* the universe and all of creation into existence. It has been said that three things cannot be taken back and can never come again: (1) a spent arrow, (2) a spoken word, and (3) a lost opportunity. Being awakened to the importance of my spoken words, I have accepted Coach Lavery's challenge to make my most sacred skill—my language and my ability to communicate intelligently—a priority. He encouraged me also to listen more intently to the speech patterns of others and to think more deeply before I speak. I am making the behavior changes necessary to accomplish this. I am choosing my words more wisely, with conscious intent, and trying to express myself with regard to how I would like to be remembered.

BI survivors comfortable with expressing themselves with broken sentences and one-word responses are missing a valuable opportunity to improve their brains' plasticity and are limiting the substance of their conversations, thus limiting their "happiness and well-being" as documented by Matthias Mehl (cited earlier). "Are you agreeing to be civilized with your speech production or do you not really care? Think of it," Lavery implores. "You are probably very conscious of dinner table etiquette and keep working at it throughout your life. Your speech behavior is more important than table manners and is something you should also work on throughout your life."

An important addendum: No matter how descriptive and complete our language is, no matter how much we avoid using the LORY words, if we think that what we are about to say will benefit the person we are talking to but then after reflecting on our word choice, we discern those words will only hurt him or her, it is better to remain silent. Everyone on the earth would be better off if they took the time to say and do all things with discernment. Our best thoughts must accompany our attention and our attention must precede our speech: Then we have the greatest likelihood of saying and doing the right thing. To habitually employ our discernment requires vigilance, and vigilance requires energy. A brain injury is, without question, an especially challenging drain on energy— and almost always distorts a survivor's discernment—making it all the more difficult to speak edifying, relationship-building complete sentences. No matter the challenge, the effort to eloquently speak meaningful and kind words to one another will nurture and build our brain's resilience while enhancing relationships—today and throughout our lives.

"The heart of the wise teaches his mouth, and adds persuasiveness to his lips" (Proverbs 16:23). According to Daniels,[4] "Language, including speech and reading, is so important to human survival that it accounts for a massive amount of cranial space" (p. 42). "Although some scientists believe the mind can exist without language, others argue that language produces mind. 'Without language, I wouldn't say that it is impossible to have mental experiences, but I'd say the mental experiences would not be very coherent,' said Derek Bickerton, an expert on Creole languages" (p. 45). If each one of us were to practice a higher level of communication, choose our words more wisely, be contemplative as we speak, eliminate lazy-brain speech production, and forgo the unnecessary, redundant, sarcastic, and divisive speech that alienates us from our neighbor, plasticity would improve throughout our brains, our "cognitive ax" sharper, and our understanding more complete. How much better our relationships would then be!

The benefits of substantial conversations using language-specific (English, French, Spanish, etc.), grammatically correct dialogue are quadrupled when occurring in face-to-face encounters. It is widely recognized that face-to-face communication (involving eye gaze with retinal eye lock) and physical touch are two central components magnifying the neurophysiological effect of human-to-human relations. According to the 2019 *JBI Database of Systematic Reviews and Implementation Reports* study titled "Neurophysiology of human touch and eye gaze in therapeutic relationships and healing: a scoping review"[62] by Fiona Kerr, Rick Wiechula, and Alison Kitson, "One of the most powerful human interactions is face-to-face contact involving eye gaze. The interaction between trusted individuals creates a *neural*

---

[62] https://www.ncbi.nlm.nih.gov/pmc/articles/PMC6382052/.

duet between brains due to the reciprocal firing of the brain's social networking areas, with a powerful effect on the level of trust and empathy as well as a positive attitudinal shift." Kerr et al. gathered that a healthy brain releases a number of chemicals when we interact with trusted friends and colleagues, two of which are oxytocin and vasopressin, that help reduce the physiological stress response while supporting health and healing. Proactive face-to-face communication with eye gazing and physical touch becomes a self-reinforcing positive feedback loop whereby more oxytocin encourages even more eye gazing. Kerr emphasized this dynamic naturally increases the trust and empathy between participants, which in turn stimulates the release of several chemicals that facilitate neuroplasticity and neurogenesis.

Oxytocin is often referred to as the "cuddle hormone" or the "love hormone" because, in addition to and especially when combined with eye gazing, oxytocin is released when people physically snuggle or bond socially. It makes social information more notable and important to each of us so that after being "tagged" and stored in areas of the brain that are closely related to the perception of emotion and empathy, this information is available for immediate recall. Larry Young, a behavioral neuroscientist at Emory University in Atlanta, Georgia, said, "[Oxytocin] connects brain areas involved in processing social information—whether it's sights, faces, sounds or smells—and helps link those areas to the brain's reward system."[63] Vasopressin, also called an antidiuretic hormone (ADH), may be released directly into the brain from the hypothalamus and likely plays an important role in *social behavior, sexual motivation, pair bonding,* and maternal responses to stress.[64]

Without human interactions and significant conversations involving eye gazing and physical touch (i.e., secretion of oxytocin and complimentary chemicals), it may be near impossible for a survivor to achieve the neuroplasticity and neurogenesis that is a key factor in

---

63   https://www.livescience.com/42198-what-is-oxytocin.html.

64   https://en.wikipedia.org/wiki/Vasopressin.

brain injury rehabilitation. Many survivors who are socially isolated and deprived of significant, stimulating communication seldom gaze into the eyes of a friend, rarely experience a *neural duet* between his or her brain and another's, or find a reassuring hand on their shoulder. Such isolation makes it ever so difficult to establish a sufficient level of trust and empathy among family and friends, or profit from a positive attitudinal shift. Consequently, those survivors—significantly deprived of oxytocin and vasopressin—may not be able to feel love either from or for another. Damage to specific brain structures hinders or prevents the secretion or transmission of oxytocin and vasopressin and may render a survivor socially numb, depressed, unable to bond with his or her significant other, incapable of experiencing sexual intimacy, and oblivious to foreplay—all through no fault of his or her own.

Katherine Harmon's May 2010 article, "How Important Is Physical Contact with Your Infant?,"[65] reported today it is universally recognized that children who have not had sufficient physical touch and emotional attention are at higher risk for behavioral, emotional, and social problems as they grow up. Further, such children have *significantly different hormone levels* —even into adulthood—from their parent-raised peers. According to Harmon, research has documented that children who experienced early deprivation also have lower levels of oxytocin and vasopressin. Further, that generous skin-to-skin contact between baby and parents can be a great benefit to all. Regular emotional engagement can speed a baby's self-recognition and facilitate their brain development.

Harry Harlow[66] is an American psychologist best known for his maternal separation, dependency needs, and social isolation experiments on rhesus monkeys. His empirical work with primates is now considered a "classic" in behavioral science—it revolutionized our understanding of the importance social relationships have in our lives. Harlow and other social cognitive psychologists discovered—and then championed—

---

[65]   https://www.scientificamerican.com/article/infant-touch/.

[66]   https://www.psychologicalscience.org/publications/observer/obsonline/harlows-classic-studies-revealed-the-importance-of-maternal-contact.html.

the importance of comfort, companionship, and love in promoting healthy development. In the studies, monkeys subjected to social isolation showed "disturbed behavior, staring blankly, circling their cages, and engaging in self-mutilation." Infant monkeys confined to isolation chambers for up to twenty-four months emerged "intensely disturbed." Harlow's research "produced groundbreaking empirical evidence for the primacy of the parent-child attachment relationship and the importance of maternal touch in infant development." More than seventy years later, Harlow's discoveries made him the twenty-sixth most cited psychologist of the twentieth century[67] and continue to "inform the scientific understanding of the fundamental building blocks of human behavior."

I maintain that a fundamental building block in every brain injury rehabilitation protocol has to be communication and social skill building. Grammatically correct language that is well thought out, well enunciated, and spoken clearly in face-to-face encounters with a good amount of eye contact is a wellspring of neuroplasticity and neurogenesis that gives rise to the spread of oxytocin and vasopressin throughout a brain's social networking areas. Further, such personal relationships generate the positive attitudinal shift so necessary with many survivors to help him or her continue "picking up the pieces" after the injury and remain disciplined in following a daily rehabilitation program. The importance of companionship, regular emotional engagement, and love in promoting healthy development post-BI cannot be understated. I certainly would not have made it as far as I have—and I will not be able to make the future progress that I have in mind—without the same. Are there other ways to enhance the social skills of survivors?

I had the opportunity to meet Dr. Parente at a Brain Injury Alliance of Colorado Conference in 2017. Rick (Frederick) Parente, PhD; Janet Anderson Parente, PhD; and Mary Stapleton, MA, have recognized a need to enhance the social skills of survivors. For many years, they have taught such skills, along with memory techniques, with good results.

---

[67]   https://en.wikipedia.org/wiki/Harry_Harlow.

They explain in their article "The Use of Rhymes and Mnemonics for Teaching Cognitive Skills to Persons with Acquired Brain Injury" that the two "biggest impediments to employment" have always been poor social skills and the inability to solve problems or make decisions. Social skills have such a far-reaching impact on our health, quality of life, earning potential, and vocational success that they must be emphasized in every rehabilitation program—with language and communication being the very foundation of social skill building.

After investigating several approaches to teaching social skills, attention, and problem solving, Parente et al. found that if they presented essential lessons as rhymes in good mnemonic form, survivors learned them faster and retained them longer. Throughout history, language in poetic form has been used to help people understand the nature of a psychiatric disorder, accept a disability, and understand a mental illness. Poetic verse is memorable and easy to learn and can express feelings in ways that simple written text cannot. Parente et al. maintain that these characteristics of poetry are useful for teaching social and cognitive skills to persons with BI. They have composed some excellent rhymes to address common BI problems and teach social skills that help survivors adapt in different social settings. The following rhymes are reprinted with Parente's permission and are offered as examples of ones that could be useful not only for survivors but also for people with learning disabilities and young children.

LISTENING SKILLS

Poor listening skills are a common problem reported by persons with BI. Survivors often have difficulty remembering what others say because they inevitably respond before they hear another person's entire statement. Survivors' responses commonly are premature and tangential, further detracting from their ability to remember or even grasp the gist of the original exchange. The following mnemonic teaches the skill of listening rather than speaking and of studying facial expressions while in conversation:

> Listening is the social grace
> Of hearing the words and watching the face;
> Good listeners speak less than half the time
> They evaluate the reason and the rhyme.
> So open your eyes and close your mouth,
> Study the face east, west, north, and south;
> Listening is both a skill and a choice,
> So choose not to hear the sound of your own voice.

EYE CONTACT

As stated, significant eye contact while in conversation generates neuroplasticity, aids in bonding and gives rise to the spread of oxytocin that facilitates the processing of social information while encouraging a positive attitudinal shift. Poor eye contact is prevalent among survivors. They often find it difficult to look into a person's face while carrying on a conversation, or else, they may stare uncomfortably. Without appropriate eye contact, it is not possible to notice the subtle facial expressions that add shades of meaning to a conversation. Even worse, poor eye contact can convey lack of confidence or suggest to others that a survivor is not interested or not entirely truthful. The following rhyme emphasizes the skill of maintaining eye contact:

> Maintain eye contact when you speak;
> Eye contact tells others that you are not meek.
> Notice changes in posture along with changes in the face;
> These signal disgust, awkwardness, or even disgrace.
> So study the details of the body and face;
> Remember, eye contact is a big part of our social grace.

CONTROLLING ANGER

Low frustration tolerance is another major problem after BI. This problem includes a number of different behaviors such as quickness to anger, giving up easily, and poor impulse control. Anger control issues—angry communication—commonly is a significant problem for survivors because it often results in being fired from a job or being avoided by family and friends and labeled as someone too uncomfortable to associate with.

Parente et al. address this problem with two rhymes; both combine a rhyming verse with a word mnemonic to help survivors control their anger. The ANGER verse emphasizes anticipation of the type of situation that provokes the survivor, combined with preventative action to avoid uncontrolled anger or to better deal with it when it arises. If anger does gain control, however, then a survivor can go through the second mnemonic—the CALM sequence.

ANGER

Anticipate those situations that trigger your rage.
Never act in anger—act your age.
Go through the CALM sequence below, then peacefully return assuaged.
Evaluate the situation in retrospect.
Review how you coped—review and reflect.

A survivor begins the CALM sequence by venting emotions in the presence of, or on the phone with, a sympathetic friend. He or she also learns to *leave* an anger-provoking situation and *move about*—because physical motion helps dissipate anxiety. Once calm, the survivor then returns to the *E* portion of the ANGER mnemonic to "Evaluate" the situation in retrospect. They "Review and Reflect" on what exactly it was they allowed to ignite their anger and also on the results of their response. In this way, each new anger-provoking situation that is met with a diplomatic, calming response that keeps the peace and can serve as a learning experience.

CALM

Call on someone you know.
Allow your emotions to confidentially flow.
Leave the situation—avoid the fray.
Move about—get out of anger's way.

(The person now returns to the *E* letter of the ANGER mnemonic above.)

In support of Dr. Parente's work to help survivors regulate their emotions, I want to include reference to James Gross—the pioneer of emotional regulation and director of the Stanford psychophysiology laboratory. The concept of emotional intelligence has four cornerstones: (1) recognizing the emotions of others, (2) understanding one's own emotions, (3) allowing emotions to influence reasoning and decision-making, and (4) regulating emotions in a way that is "situationally appropriate." Gross explains that different types of regulation strategies can benefit different goals and situations. Being self-aware of situations that evoke unwanted emotional reactions is a great advantage. *Reappraisal* is an effective strategy that examines the initial emotion and quickly reframes it to minimize its negative impact. For example, we can reappraise a terse, hurtful comment from a lady in the checkout line using compassion. ("Perhaps she has just lost her job and was let go abruptly with disrespect.") People who habitually reappraise do not take things personally, experience lower stress, have better social relationships and more positive emotions compared with those who do not use reappraisal.

Non-alkalized Cocoa

Dr. William White's own work over the last twenty years has focused specifically on vascular health and cardiology. Decades of research and investigation of natural food-based products that have a significant medical benefit to patients have led him to endorse non-processed/non-alkalized cocoa as a new ingredient base for healthy energy drinks. "The health benefits of using non-processed/non-alkalized cocoa," he reports, "are documented by clinical trials and research at leading universities including Harvard and Johns Hopkins.[10f1] The arterial dilation within the human body after consuming cocoa-rich flavanols is extremely impressive, serving as a natural stimulant that also promotes brain health." He adds:

> Non-processed/non-alkalyzed cocoa improves vascular function, including the heart and brain, and significantly supports overall health in general. An estimated six hundred nutrients can be found in unprocessed, no-sugar-added cocoa, including many anti-oxidants such as catechins, epicatechins, resveratrol, and the "feel good" nutrient anandamide, which is abundant in unprocessed cocoa.

Dr. White discovered adding sugar to cocoa diminishes or completely eradicates the benefits of natural, unprocessed cocoa, and alkalizing strips the cacao bean of many of its nutritional benefits. He therefore recommends *only* non-processed/non-alkalized cocoa and healthy herbal sweeteners such as stevia to assuage the strong taste of traditionally produced cocoa and maintain its subsequent health benefits. Standing on his research and credentials as a physician, he enjoins a daily intake of flavanol-containing cocoa for improving vascular function and brain health. Dr. White and I both use Hershey's Cocoa (100% natural, unsweetened cacao) and Pyure organic stevia.

Ketogenic Diet

Keto stands for "ketosis," a metabolic process that occurs when the body does *not* have enough glucose for energy. The ketogenic diet,[10h] or keto diet, is a very low-carb, high-fat diet that actually burns fat from our bodies at an accelerated pace. It replaces excessive carbohydrates with 80–90 percent fat, adequate protein, and limited carbohydrates (Gasior et al.)[10h1] Following the keto diet plan puts your body into a metabolic state similar to starvation—which is being in *ketosis*—and that is what generates the neurological benefits of the ketogenic diet. When ketosis is brought on by a keto diet, according to Erdman et al.,[10h2] glucose (our body's and brain's preferred energy source) is not available, which forces the liver to convert fats into three ketone bodies that are readily used as fuel by brain cells. The three newly converted ketone bodies can cross the blood-brain barrier and enter the brain to serve as a viable energy source.

Ketogenic diets were first developed in 1921 to treat epileptic children and have since been most studied in this context (Kossoff et al.[10h3]). However, additional neuroprotective benefits have been documented in animal models of several central nervous system disorders (Prins[10h4]). While admittedly the mechanisms by which a keto diet confers neuroprotection benefits are beyond our comprehension at this time, its good clinical track record and safety encourages its implementation. Mayumi Prins summarizes her study as follows:

> Cerebral metabolism of glucose has been shown to be altered after head injury, and increasing cerebral metabolism of alternative substrates (ketones) has been shown to be neuroprotective in several models of traumatic brain injury. This altered dietary approach may have tremendous therapeutic potential for both the pediatric and adult head-injured populations.

BI survivors may want to explore with their health-care providers the wisdom of making the ketogenic diet a part of their recovery regimen.

Probiotics

Dr. Mark Hyman, in his Broken Brain[68] series (Broken Brain, 55 Pittsfield Road, Suite 9 Lenox Commons, Lenox, MA 01240), said that the "gut-brain connection" is one of the most important pieces in the brain injury/restoration puzzle. According to Dr. Hyman, the healthy bacteria in our gut is going to benefit our brain and entire body. Our gut bacteria communicate with our brain's neurons. By sending and receiving signals, they influence one another. Further, the majority of dopamine, GABA, norepinephrine, neurotransmitters, and serotonin are made in our alimentary tract (digestive tract)—our guts. The new book *Psychobiotic Revolution: Mood, Food, and the New Science of the Gut-Brain Connection* by Scott C. Anderson[37] adds scientific evidence to the groundbreaking medical narrative that depression, anxiety, and obesity—even autism, Alzheimer's, and Parkinson's disease—may be treated by improving digestive bacteria.

I had never heard that a gut-brain connection even existed or that it was important for my brain's rehabilitation program. However, I had experienced constipation ever since my brain was injured. I was unable to find a solution until I came across the probiotic in Colorado called inner-ēco. Inner-ēco[69] is made from the living water of fresh young green coconuts and is completely dairy/gluten-free. It is a fermented, 100% natural, effervescent beverage full of billions of *live cultures*. Cultured foods were the first probiotics—long before capsules were invented or sold. Food-based probiotics are significantly more bioavailable than capsulated formulas. Furthermore, experts say we all need more fermented/cultured food in our diet. Inner-ēco is absorbed immediately and begins its work in your mouth, delivering prebiotics,

---

[68] https://brokenbrain.com.

[69] www.inner-eco.com.

probiotics, enzymes, and electrolytes throughout your entire system. The effectiveness of inner-ēco for promoting regularity is unmistakable and has made it the fastest-growing probiotic on the market since 2008.

I haven't stopped using inner-ēco since I started, and only now, thanks to Dr. Hyman, have I realized that it has probably been a significant part of my accelerated brain trauma recovery—a recovery that is still ongoing after more than forty years Inner-ēco was invented by my daughter Lia Salomē's godmother Niki Price and by Barb Vogel, who together came up with their own version of a health-restoring ancient probiotic beverage. They started the business in a garage, and today inner-ēco is available nationally at Whole Foods, other natural food stores, and many conventional retailers. Please see if making it a part of your health routine (to cultivate optimal gut bacteria, promote neuron activity in your brain, and nourish all the organs in your body) can be as effective for you as it is for me.

The Concussion Healing Solution

Garrett Bussiere[10i] wrote the book *The Concussion Healing Solution: Clarity Amid the Confusion*.[38] The book explains what he did to regain a normal life after his brain injury and develop what he calls the "HYH Concussion Healing Solution."[70] Honoring my request, Bussiere has shared much of his wisdom—to be included in my book—for the benefit my readers. He told me that the immense progress made in the medical research domains such as nutritional neuroscience, exercise physiology, and cognitive science has profound implications for the advancement of the human condition and even more so for those suffering from a brain injury. Therefore, the importance of proper nutrition, carefully executed exercise, and specific techniques for stress management and psychological resiliency—after a brain injury—cannot be overstated. As the research continues to pile up, it is clear—beyond any doubt— that what we put in our body, how and how often we move our body,

---

[70]   http://www.healingyourhead.com.

and whether we take or relinquish control of our mind determine the quality of our existence. Fortunately, these decisions are all up to us, all within our control, and how consistently we can stay the course of healthfulness determines our future brain health and overall quality of life.

Bussiere continued explaining to me that three consistent conditions of mild traumatic brain injury—inflammation, oxidation, and toxicity—are inevitable responses that torment a brain after injury. According to Drs. Christopher C. Giza, and David A. Hovda's, article, "The Neurometabolic Cascade of Concussion,"[10i1] oxidative stress and chronic inflammation are two immediate and consistent characteristics of mild traumatic brain injuries. They are immediate and complex reactions within a brain that lead to a myriad of acute and chronic symptoms such as foggy cognition and memory, sluggishness, irritability, aggression, apathy, and even depression, which oftentimes can last for years. The human brain after trauma is also extremely dehydrated and in need of proper hydration to heal and restore homeostasis. Giza and Hovda reported, "Important components of post-traumatic cerebral pathophysiology (repercussions of TBI) include, but are not limited to, free radical production (oxidative stress), inflammatory response (inflammation) and altered neurotransmission." The good news is that we all have anti-inflammation, antioxidant, and detoxification allies both within our brains and in a natural, nutritious, and organic diet that, when combined, work amazingly well to combat these conditions.

Regarding a nutritious and organic diet, Bussiere emphasized to me there is convincing scientific research that suggests that certain natural foods, herbs, and spices contain "neuroprotective properties" that have the ability to regenerate brain cells as well as protect and restore a brain after head trauma.[10i2] There are studies that conclude foods and other nutraceuticals containing healthy compounds assist in breaking up the accumulation of plaques in a brain and body to accelerate the process of restoring cognitive abilities.[10i3] By ingesting all eight essential amino acids in optimal proportions, you can restore neurotransmitter function.

By following the Concussion Healing Solution, you can enhance learning and memory, increase concentration, reverse apathy, and defeat post-concussion depression. Further, by eating and supplementing the proper balance of fatty acids, you can rebuild and create new cell membranes, reduce inflammation, decrease oxidative stress, enhance detoxification, and balance blood sugar to restore your brain to its ideal equilibrium—homeostasis.[104]

Wrapping things up, Bussiere pointed out that the encouraging news is that the power of nature provides us with the essential remedies to promote proper hydration, anti-inflammation, antioxidation, and detoxification. Our brains rely on the right balance of all eight essential amino fatty acids, complex carbohydrates, neuroprotective compounds, and natural detoxifiers to effectively maintain homeostasis and function at peak performance. Synergistically combining certain superfoods beautifully compliments a brain's homeostasis and enhances our peak performance. You can proactively choose to combat the aforementioned conditions with the formula presented in the Concussion Healing Solution, or you can choose to encourage these detrimental conditions by eating processed, high-fat, high-sugar foods and beverages that further complicate and prolong concussion recovery.

◆

Before introducing the next few remarkable professionals and breakthrough therapies I have had the good fortune to encounter, I must bring up a certain well-known phenomenon in the long-term experience of many brain injury survivors. There comes a time, some twenty-plus years post-brain-injury, when survivors are apt to undergo a decline in their functional abilities, both physical and mental. In my case, it took longer. Thirty-three years after my brain injury, decreased microcirculation in the shoulder on my left side resulted in a labrum tear that brought about a large paravertebral cyst and other complications in that shoulder. On account of atrophy/denervation caused by the cyst, I had lost all function in my left arm and shoulder—I could not raise my left arm to wash my hair, brush my teeth, or dress myself. In 2014, Dr. Armando Vidal (a Colorado "top doctor" according to *5280 magazine[71]*) performed orthoscopic shoulder surgery on me at Colorado University's Sports Medicine Hospital (one of the top five orthoscopic surgery hospitals in the nation; Dr. Vidal has since taken his practice to the renowned Steadman Clinic in Colorado).

After the successful surgery, I had to be in rehabilitation for a year and a half, working to regain function. According to Dr. Vidal, increasing the microcirculation in my left shoulder and throughout my body was medically necessary to heal the labrum repair operation, prevent additional injuries, and thwart the decline in function that most survivors experience two decades post-injury. I looked at the need to increase microcirculation as an opportunity to find a method, a therapy, a way to restore my abilities and continue independently caring for myself—and as an opportunity to play catch again with my daughter, who loves playing softball. I knew that if such a method to increase microcirculation is available, it will help other survivors' brains and bodies as well as mine.

Muscle Activation Technique (MAT)

Greg Roskopf[10j] came into my life in 2014 when Atty. Steve Shapiro of the law firm Fleishman & Shapiro PC, a former president of the Brain Injury Alliance of Colorado's board of directors—with whom, over the years, I have had many positive exchanges—introduced me to Roskopf and recommended Muscle Activation Technique (MAT)[72] to restore my shoulder as it recovered from surgery on the torn labrum. The skilled hands of an MAT Rx specialist, proved to be just what was needed for the restoration of my shoulder. It has also enabled me to continue making significant progress throughout my entire body more than thirty-three years post-injury. MAT sessions have tremendously

---

[71] https://directory.5280.com/doctor-category/orthopedic-sports-medicine/

[72] https://muscleactivation.com.

helped me rehabilitate not only my torn labrum *but also* much of my whole body's left hemiparesis. It takes Hoshino therapy to another level altogether and has made Brucker biofeedback therapy many times more effective for me.

Muscle Activation Technique is a system designed to evaluate and correct the muscle imbalances that contribute to chronic pain, injury, and altered performance/functional abilities. This technique takes basic components of physiology and biomechanics and transfers them into a systematic approach for evaluating and treating the multiple factors relating to diminished ability/disability. The evaluation and treatment protocols developed by Roskopf are biomechanically based procedures substantiated and validated by many factors of muscle physiology. The program is based on monitoring and restoring the capability of muscles to contract (i.e., restoring the neuromuscular connection—the brain/muscle contract/relax function). MAT corrects neuromuscular alignment to prepare the body for what it is being asked to do.

No matter the type of physical demand—golf, tennis, or just walking upstairs—the MAT procedure addresses the weak links. It thereby allows the body to function most efficiently, creating an environment in which the body can receive the positive side effects that result from optimal muscle contractile ability. The systematic MAT evaluation procedure, which correlates limitations in range of motion to muscle weakness, addresses the weak or atrophied muscles to correct diminished ability/disability. *5280* magazine reported in an April 2015 article, entitled "Muscling Through,"[73] "When the body senses instability, as with an imbalance or injury, Roskopf says, the brain sends a message to tighten the muscles in that area. Over time, this constant contracting can lead to inflammation and biochemical changes that can alter communication between the brain and muscles. Roskopf likens it to a loose car-battery cable. Your brain sends a message to the muscles to contract, but they don't always receive it. So other parts of your body compensate, and the cycle of imbalance continues. MAT

---

[73]   https://muscleactivation.com/latest-news/muscling-through/

seeks to end the broken cycle by stimulating those non-firing muscle fibers." Addressing contractile weakness with MAT sessions typically results in an increase in the range of motion of a joint or joints. The result is not only increased joint range of motion but also the stability of joints throughout their range of motion (i.e., mobility and stability).

Genius Brain Habits

I am always interested in learning of proven therapies like MAT and other effective programs with which to enhance my own recovery program or that of my clients. A *Reader's Digest* article, "Eight Genius Habits Your Eighty-Year-Old Brain Will Thank You for Doing Today: Senior moments? Not Anymore"[74] by Kimberly Hiss, reported on a useful resource, a 2017 book by Kenneth Kosik, MD, titled *Outsmarting Alzheimer's: What You Can Do to Reduce Your Risk*,[39] which offers *tips for a healthy brain*. Of Dr. Kosik's top eight medically recommended genius brain habits, four involve increased blood circulation:

1. *Meditation*: The daily habit of a twelve-minute centering, a meditation session can improve blood flow throughout the brain.
2. *Heart-Healthy Factors* (i.e., not smoking, being physically active, healthy blood pressure, balanced diet, etc.): The more "heart-healthy habits people have," the longer they maintain cognitive skills and independence. A healthy heart has a strong cardiovascular system with all its arteries, veins, and capillaries cooperating in the optimal delivery of nutrients to the brain.
3. *Strength Training*: Senior women who strength-trained two times every seven days showed "significantly less progression of white matter brain lesions."
4. *Moderate-Intensity Exercise*: Exercising thirty minutes (plus or minus) a day has documented brain health benefits by improving circulation via vascular health and anti-inflammatory effects.

---

[74] www.rd.com/health/wellness/brain-health-habits/

Increasing Microcirculation

In 2018, when I learned of the modulation of inflammatory effects and the *tremendous increased microcirculation* benefits associated with use of a pulsed electromagnetic field (PEMF)[10k] device manufactured in Europe, I felt certain that it would significantly benefit my brain injury and left hemiparesis. Blood circulation supplies the brain, tissues, and organs with oxygen, nutrients, chemical messengers (e.g. hormones), immune cells, and the like while removing and disposing of the resulting metabolic waste products. Of this process, 75 percent takes place in the smallest blood vessels, the smallest capillaries—the microcapillaries—the only place where such exchanges can occur. The capillary network is more than seventy-four thousand miles long. The heart cannot circulate this network alone; it gets help from the smaller blood vessels themselves, which propel blood cells along the way with their own self-pumping movements, called vasomotions, thereby completing the circulatory cycle. The vasomotions of the capillaries—their self-pumping movements—also regulate blood flow in such a way that areas with higher supply needs at a given moment are better supplied with blood than areas that happen to have a lower need at the same moment. For example, the brain's need for blood supplies is high during learning activities, while the muscles are less in need. In physical activities, exactly the opposite is the case. With healthy neurological function, the pumping movements of the smaller blood vessels help the blood cells do their work precisely where they are most needed.

The results of optimal circulation are evident: ideal cardiac function, increased mental and physical performance, improved nutrient supply and waste disposal, strengthened disease-fighting and immune capabilities, and greater oxygen utilization/optimal circulation. Only when all our brain and body cells are adequately nourished and all metabolic waste products removed can our brains and bodies function properly. The optimal regulation of circulation is a prerequisite for the best recovery from brain injury or stroke and for ensuring a lifetime of overall vitality and well-being. Deficient supply of nutrients to, or removal of waste products from, the brain, tissues, and organs over the long term leads to a decline in mental and physical abilities, increased disorders, more pain, inflammation, and disease.

Thankfully, I was able to participate in the continued use of the PEMF device before returning to Florida for a scheduled round of Brucker biofeedback therapy sessions on May 31, 2018. In their evaluation of me upon my arrival at that time, the Miami doctors noted, "Patient emerge into the EMG Biofeedback program with the greatest retention and carryover of neuromuscular differentiation from one session series to the next with a serious commitment towards functional restoration." According to those doctors—who have been involved in my rehabilitation therapy since 1991—I was entering therapy there walking better, demonstrating better fine finger dexterity, and with better balance than I ever had. Later that year when I returned for my second series of therapies, I had increased my function even further and demonstrated normal neuromuscular recruitment in a couple of areas. I have to attribute my historic progress to the combination of daily microcirculation enhancement, weekly MAT sessions, and biannual Brucker biofeedback therapy sessions.

Again, when I added the microcirculation enhancement to my rehabilitation protocol, I made the greatest scientifically measured improvement in neuromuscular recruitment and control since my accident in 1981. How is it that combining Brucker biofeedback therapy with MAT sessions and enhanced microcirculation via the PEMF device had such an exponential, synergistic effect? Ohm's law, I believe, explains well just how it happens that when these three therapies are combined, their positive effects multiply one another instead of just adding to one another. Ohm's law, a principle in electricity, states that the amount of electricity flowing through a wire depends first on the strength of the source of power and second on the resistance coming from the wire. If the source of power is increased, the flow of current is increased. If the resistance of the wire is increased, the flow of current is decreased. However, if resistance of the wire is decreased, the flow of current is increased.

When a muscle is nonresponsive/inactive/atrophied—resistant—after a brain injury, there is a limit to how much it can be rehabilitated. MAT sessions, however, can activate a dysfunctional muscle—turn it on—and significantly decrease the resistance to the electrical signal being sent from the brain. *An active, healthy muscle naturally responds to a neuromuscular electrical signal many times better than it does when in an atrophied or resistant state.* Brucker biofeedback therapy, for its part, educates the brain-body connection—the neuromuscular connection—efficiently increasing the electrical signal recruiting the targeted muscle while relaxing the opposing muscle and, by so doing, substantially increasing coordination. And finally, optimizing microcirculation throughout the body and brain delivers more nutrition and removes more waste products from each and every cell—significantly improving the neural signal strength, reducing the muscular resistance and better preparing the body for physical performance.

Combining the three treatments has effectively enabled me to reach my greatest rehabilitation results ever—thirty-nine years after severe brain injury. MAT has activated my dysfunctional muscles, Brucker biofeedback therapy has educated them, and the PEMF device has greatly enhanced the microcirculation throughout my damaged brain and my dysfunctional muscles, enabling me to retain the neuromuscular differentiation leaned in Brucker biofeedback therapy longer than I ever have since beginning treatment twenty-seven years prior. *The synergistic effect of combining Brucker biofeedback therapy with MAT sessions and enhanced microcirculation is, in my opinion, something of a trifecta marvel that should be replicated for every brain injury survivor with compromised motor functions.*

◆

While I have no personal experience with the medical professionals and therapies in the following section, my communication with colleagues and research disposes me to include them in my protocol and for your consideration.

Brain Retraining and Custom Optometry
Combining Neuroscience with Eye Care

In 2015, my brother Jeff gave me Dr. Clark Elliott's[101] newly released book for my birthday, and I read for the first time of a groundbreaking cognitive therapy that helped restore Elliott's mind after a car accident/ TBI. In the book *The Ghost in My Brain: How a Concussion Stole My Life and How the New Science of Brain Plasticity Helped Me Get It Back*,[11] Elliott told of how he went from one doctor or medical professional to the next for eight years after his car accident but found all of them, put together, had little to offer. "Once they got a look at me, no one has ever called me back." Disappointment after disappointment was pushing him toward a very bleak conclusion—"I was once again just going to have to face the fact that my life as I had known it, now almost a decade ago, was well and truly over." Then he was introduced to Donalee Markus, PhD,[10m] and Deborah Zelinsky, OD, FNORA, FCOVD.[10n]

Dr. Markus, according to Elliott, is an amazing person full of compassion and goodwill. Markus (a.k.a. Dr. Dots) received her PhD from Northwestern University in Evanston, Illinois, in 1983. She did postdoctoral work under Reuven Feuerstein at the Hadassah- WIZO Research Institute, Jerusalem, Israel. A master educator, she has effectively worked in the brain-training field for over thirty years and is the author of *Retrain your Business Brain: Outsmart the Corporate Competition*, as well as the originator of the Designs for Strong Minds program.[75] Having recognized an association between brain injury and vision issues, Markus herself acknowledges the work in optometry of Deborah Zelinsky. "In my 33 years of experience with Traumatic Brain Injuries, I have never seen a patient whose visual systems were not affected by the injury. Therapeutic lenses by Dr. Zelinsky accelerate my work, and I refer my patients to her."

---

[75]   www.designsforstrongminds.com.

Optometrist Zelinsky founded the Mind-Eye Institute[76] based on research that led to the discovery of how eyeglasses could alter listening ability. One of her books, *An Insight to Vision*, describes how optometry bridges the gap between neuroscience and eye care and explains how customized eyeglasses can calm the nervous system for faster recovery after injury. Zelinsky, according to Elliott, is primarily focused on how the various visual systems interact with brain function and how the various visual/spatial functions and auditory/temporal functions in the brain are integrated with the higher-order brain processing that makes us human.

Elliot reports in *The Ghost in My Brain* that within a week of getting his first pair of "brain glasses" from Zelinsky, his cognitive functioning improved so remarkably well that he felt normal for the first time since his brain injury eight years earlier. "The effect of the new glasses," he says, "along with the work I had started pursuing with Donalee, was stunning. Importantly, although it was tiring and challenging for me to make the transition, it also felt *right*. . . . For the price of an office visit and a pair of glasses and within the course of ten short days what some of the leading neurologists in Chicago, a famous rehabilitation center, and many others, had claimed would never happen, happened: I started to get better" (pp. 215–16).

It is astounding to me that I had not heard of Dr. Dot's cognitive therapy nor Zelinsky's Mind-Eye prescription glasses and "neuro-optometric rehabilitation" until 2015. I had been in the brain injury rehabilitation field for twenty years, attended many conferences, and consulted with many doctors but unfortunately had never heard of these two remarkable practitioners or their programs despite the fact that they may very well help me reach another level higher in rehabilitation. After reading Elliott's book, I felt it was imperative to include reference to it as well as to Markus's and Zelinsky's programs. Still other effective brain injury diagnosis/rehabilitation programs, such as CereScan, are also just now breaking to the surface of public awareness.

---

[76]   www.mindeye.com.

FocusBand

FocusBand uses EEG technology (electroencephalography) via an electrophysiological frequency-monitoring device to record electrical activity of the brain ranging from one to forty-four hertz. The brain produces electrical waves from the lowest range—delta (one to four hertz), theta (four to eight hertz), alpha (eight to twelve hertz), beta (twelve to twenty-four hertz)—up to the highest range—gamma (twenty-four to more than one hundred hertz). The brain is constantly generating different analog brain wave frequency patterns: delta during deep sleep and restful slumber, theta when approaching sleep or in deeper meditation, alpha in deep relaxation, beta during awake conscious and reasoning activities, and while currently little is known about the gamma waves, initial research shows they are associated with bursts of insight and high-level information processing.

FocusBand detects different frequencies emanating from a brain's frontal cortex through three sensors/contact points on the forehead and then generates an accurate reading of the brain waves and transmits this biofeedback information, via Bluetooth, to a digital mobile device. On the mobile device, FocusBand presents the user with an easily understood avatar for visual feedback, plus clear audio feedback to maximize effectiveness. This technology is remarkably effective for moving people away from their normal anxiety-prone thought patterns and behaviors into the flow state of mind where alpha waves predominate. When the FocusBand avatar shows the right hemisphere of the brain lighting up with a green display, the user has entered the *mushin* state (Japanese word meaning "no mind")—a clear mind without worries and preoccupations, on which he or she can establish a calm mind and enter the quiet-eye state of mind with positive, honest, upbuilding thoughts.

FocusBand does not produce this healthy state of mind; it detects it, and at that moment with the avatar displaying green, nothing is bothering the person or preventing them from staying cool, calm, and contemplative. The user generates healthy brain waves with their preferred technique (i.e., deep breathing, Whole Brain Power, visualizing peaceful-joyful times, Tapping Solution, etc.). FocusBand displays all brain wave frequencies so the user can learn how to reach the ideal state of mind whenever he or she chooses.

FocusBand was originally developed for professional golfers by Graham Boulton[10o] and has since spread its influence into the neuro-self-care field with several specific FocusBand apps now available on Amazon or in IT stores. Graham Boulton is currently working with large mental health companies around the world that want to use FocusBand for measurement of effectiveness with different mental health and well-being strategies. To learn more, visit https://focusband.com.

Brain Analytics and CereScan

CereScan[10p] (the world's leader in brain analytics) should be the first step in every brain injury rehabilitation program, for it provides the most precise brain diagnostics and makes available critical anatomical information to help doctors and brain injury survivors better structure rehabilitation programs and track progress. My opinion is based on that of top neuroscientists and physicians from across the United States and around the world (as reported in *Oppenheimer's Diagnostic Neuropathology: A Practical Manual*[32]), who all agree that improving brain injury survivor outcomes begins with improving brain injury diagnosis. For how can anyone know what's really wrong with a damaged brain without a look inside it?

At the time of my accident and for twenty-eight years afterward, it was impossible to "look inside" a living brain. In 2009, however, CereScan began incorporating advanced software, functional brain imaging—such as qSPECT, qEEG, and PET—and an extensive library of clinical data to help physicians analyze up to 120 regions of the brain. As the nation's current leader in functional brain imaging, CereScan's technology can see what traditional imaging like MRI often misses. By looking at how the brain functions through qSPECT brain imaging, CereScan provides indispensable information so survivors can receive a more targeted treatment plan and optimize rehabilitation outcomes. I did not learn of CereScan until 2017, when auspiciously I met John Kelley, CereScan's chairman and chief executive, at an Invisible Disabilities gala in Denver, Colorado.

N-Acetylcysteine (NAC)

A 2014 study, "Efficacy of N-Acetyl Cysteine in Traumatic Brain Injury"[40] by Katharine Eakin and a team of researchers, reported that early post-injury treatment with NAC significantly reversed behavioral deficits associated with TBI. According to Eakin et al., NAC likely works on a number of levels and clearly has antioxidant activity. The research team found that repeated single doses of NAC beginning at thirty to sixty minutes after an injury are expected to be most effective. In a setting of concussion from blunt trauma, a rodent model study clearly documented the positive benefits of NAC for preventing moderate TBI. The study suggested duplication of the protocol used in their clinical trial: specifically research that would use NAC in blast-induced mTBI in a battlefield setting. Eakin et al. urged continued research to develop effective NAC treatments in humans.

The *New York Times* published Barry Meier and Danielle Ivory's 2015 article, "Effective Concussion Treatment Remains Frustratingly Elusive, Despite a Booming Industry,"[77] reporting that a concussion expert with the Mayo Clinic, Dr. David W. Dodick, believes a cheap nutritional, antioxidant supplement, N-Acetyl Cysteine, "could help treat concussion symptoms" and that he hopes to study it. NAC is a very strong over-the-counter antioxidant and anti-inflammatory medicine. (Dr. William White tells me significant oxidation occurs during TBI, which means an antioxidizing agent such as NAC could provide much-

---

[77] https://www.nytimes.com/2015/07/05/business/effective-concussion-treatment-remains-frustratingly-elusive-despite-a-booming-industry.html.

needed electrons to repair/prevent the inherent oxidative damage caused by the inflammation/restricted blood flow associated with brain injury.) NAC is on the World Health Organization's list of essential medicines and, again, is not very expensive. Dr. Dodick reports that the US military was researching the benefits of NAC in treating Iraqi soldiers who had been concussed and found promising results. However, an associated study was soon caught up in controversy. Disputes regarding the trial prevented clarity about a possible breakthrough. Dr. Dodick still maintains, however, that NAC may be a valuable post-brain-injury "tool." He firmly believes in it and advises, "Every coach and parent could be carrying N-Acetyl Cysteine on the sidelines."

Barry J. Hoffer and a team of researchers wrote a 2017 review, titled "Repositioning Drugs for Traumatic Brain Injury—N-Acetyl Cysteine and Phenserine," [41] that focused on those two drugs, both with the potential to alleviate significant pathologies associated with TBI. They noted in their abstract that both drugs have been studied in human trials for other conditions without side effects, paving the way for application with TBI. In their review, Hoffer et al. explored literature that lends creditability to the assertion that NAC and Phenserine may be useful therapeutic approaches for TBI, "for which there are no currently approved drugs."

Hyperbaric Oxygen

Additionally, Barry Meier and Danielle Ivory (2015) highlight Paul G. Harch, a New Orleans physician who is a true believer in the benefits of hyperbaric oxygen. Harch's book *The Oxygen Revolution, Third Edition*,[42] Meier and Ivory report, sighted claims that hyperbaric oxygen treatment helps treat not only post-concussion syndrome but also autism and Alzheimer's disease. "Dr. Harch acknowledges that he is in the minority –'My generation of doctors thinks this is a fraudulent theory.'" One major professional medical group, the Undersea and Hyperbaric Medical Society, has said there is no evidence showing the technique is effective in resolving concussion symptoms; the same benefits, they say, were found in the placebo group. Hyperbaric oxygen proponents, however, are arguing with lawmakers that the Undersea and Hyperbaric Medical Society study's conclusions were misleading because patients who had received "placebo procedures" *were also getting the treatment* – though at a lower dose.

Dr. Harch and the International Hyperbaric Medical Association continue lobbying to get coverage for the treatment. They point to other studies with positive findings and claim the government does not want to pay for hyperbaric oxygen because of its cost. Dr. Harch estimates that, depending on location, the price of a series of forty "dives" typically ranges from $5,000 to $12,000. That, however, is scarcely "a drop in the bucket" by comparison with the financial ocean of what life with a severe brain injury can cost – $3 million.[78] It is, in fact, less than 0.003 percent of the total cost of a lifetime with severe TBI, so it is hard to believe that cost is what is standing in the way of prescribing hyperbaric oxygen therapy and making it more available to survivors.

Therapeutic Hypothermia

I would like to include in this chapter what I feel to be an important element of concussion treatment—immediate cold therapy (i.e., therapeutic hypothermia [TH], together with targeted temperature management [TTM]). Here is why: For seventy-two to ninety-six hours after a brain injury, our bodies dump a large number of hormones and chemicals into the brain, causing inflammation as well as a metabolic hurricane that terminates the life of hundreds of thousands of neurons and neuronal synaptic connections that leads to long-term negative consequences. Cold therapy, at this initial critical juncture, could possibly prevent/inhibit that metabolic hurricane—the death of hundreds of thousands of neurons—just as it preserves brain integrity *in a cold water/winter "drowning."* I read about the efficacy of such therapy

---

[78]   braininjuryrecoveryfoundation.org.

with brain injury once but since have been able neither to find where I saw it nor to run down much additional research on TH/TTM.

Doctors have explored therapeutic hypothermia for many years because of the obvious protective features associated with a cold water drowning. If someone drowned in freezing water and has not been breathing for hours can be resuscitated and return to a normal life without BI sequelae or other significant negative consequences, why wouldn't therapeutic hypothermia significantly reduce the negative consequences associated with ordinary brain injury? On the basis of such reasoning, patients have been experimentally anesthetized (put into induced comas) and submerged into cold water chambers days and weeks *after* their injury, in the hope that even belated TH will alleviate or reduce the brain damage they have suffered. However, the *New England Journal of Medicine* December 17, 2015, article titled "Hypothermia for Intracranial Hypertension after Traumatic Brain Injury"[79] reported that belated application of TH produced outcomes that were worse than standard care alone. (The group given TH showed no clinically important differences in effect on intracranial pressure, mean arterial pressure, and cerebral perfusion pressure from the control group. In fact, the addition of therapeutic hypothermia to standard care was responsible for considerable negative side effects, including but not limited to bleeding, cardiovascular instability, thermal burns, and pneumonia.)

I maintain, however, that the salvific component of TH in a cold water drowning is the *immediacy* with which it is applied. If the *immediate* therapeutic hypothermia involved in some winter drowning incidents can preserve a brain deprived of oxygen as it does, perhaps opportune, early, targeted, topical cold therapy can also preserve a brain exposed to the inflammatory, metabolic hurricane associated with traumatic brain injury. In a *Neurology* May 30, 2017, editorial, authors Gregory Kapinos, MD, MS, and Lance B. Becker, MD, declare, "The American Academy of Neurology affirms the revival of cooling for

---

[79]   https://www.nejm.org/doi/full/10.1056/NEJMoa1507581.

the revived"[80] in treating revived cardiac arrest patients. The doctor's declaration encourages me to maintain that immediate therapeutic hypothermia should be added to the emergency medical care protocol, then continued over the first seven days of hospital care for brain injury survivors until it is proved to be of no significant benefit.

Tapping Solution

In 2020, Dr. Roger Callahan, a traditionally trained psychologist who was working with a client in 1979 confounded with a phobia since she was a child. After treating his client with multiple conventional methods and very little success for over twelve months, Dr. Callahan looked to other interventions. He studied Chinese medicine's acupuncture meridians—energy channels that conduct chi, the vital life force, throughout the body. Each meridian and its corresponding energy channel have a specific location on the body that can "turn on/turn off" and balance the flow of energy either with acupuncture needles or by touching (acupressure). When his client said thinking about her phobia caused a terrible feeling in a certain part of her body, Dr. Callahan made the connection that tapping on that body part's meridian might relieve his client's terrible sensation and asked her to tap that spot with her fingertips. To their astonishment and delight, a single session of tapping relieved the phobia, and it did not reoccur. Dr. Callahan eagerly developed several patterns of tapping to address different issues. His student Gary Craig simplified the procedure with a single effective tapping pattern; he termed the intervention EFT (Emotional Freedom Techniques). However, during the following thirty years, with great EFT success, Western medicine and science could not explain or understand why or how it worked.

In his 2013 book *The Tapping Solution: A Revolutionary System for Stress-Free Living*,[43] Nick Ortner wrote, "What tapping does, with amazing efficiency, is halt the fight-or-flight response and reprogram

---

[80]   www.n.neurology.org/content/88/22/2076/tab-article-info.

the brain and body to act—and react—differently" (p. 4). "The Proof: Research at Harvard Medical School over the past decade has shown that stimulation of selected meridian acupoints decreases activity in the amygdala (the stress response begins in the amygdala), hippocampus (another part of the limbic system), and other parts of the brain associated with fear" (p. 5). In medical brain scans, when acupoints are stimulated, one can watch the amygdala's "red alert" being shut down. "Research on energy psychology compares favorably to standards set by the Society of Clinical Psychology" (p. 6). "Dozens of studies have now demonstrated the effectiveness of tapping for a variety of disorders and issues" (p. 7).[81]

I was compelled to include a reference to the remarkable success of EFT in providing a "change in perspective" to those dealing with PTSD, depression, anxiety, feelings of being overwhelmed, and the pressure of modern life—all common BI symptoms.

Meier and Ivory, cited early in this chapter, reported, "Effective Concussion Treatment Remains Frustratingly Elusive, Despite a Booming Industry," tell of a new business model has sprung up in response to the Silent Epidemic. Entrepreneurs of all kinds are now busy looking for ways to diagnose, prevent, or rehabilitate brain injury. Since 2005, the NFL, General Electric, and several other companies/ organizations have invested over twenty million dollars on head injury research. The military has put over $800 million into the same field. The amount of both public and private investment is respectable and to be applauded, considering the far-reaching negative consequences of brain injury. Nonetheless, medical experts fear this burgeoning business is riddled with nonscientific protocols, beliefs being promoted without facts to support them, and claims of breakthrough that prove hollow shortly after they are heralded. Meier and Ivory argue, though, that even if the growing BI industry is clouded with "sketchy claims," it is

---

81   www.thetappingsolution.com/research.

essential to examine every potential breakthrough with an open mind so as not to overlook the truly valid "detectors/preventers/therapies."

Had I known in the early years after my accident the truly valid detectors and proactive therapies I now know of—therapies that, rather than being proved "hollow," turned out to be both efficacious and medically necessary—I certainly would have made *better* progress at that time and would have done so *sooner*. Had I had the indispensable diagnostic information provided from a CereScan in hand and been able to employ the effective, synergistic therapies and support systems I have been describing, not only could I have made better progress sooner but I also could have avoided the secondary disabling consequences I experienced because of brain injury.

The late doctor Brucker told me in December of 2007, three months before he passed, that of all his patients in any of his clinics around the world, I had gotten "the best results." I have never met a more positive person in my life than Dr. Brucker. He always wore a smile, looked directly into your eyes as he firmly shook your hand, and spoke encouraging words with his reassuring deep, steady voice. I shared with him my dream of opening a satellite Brucker biofeedback center in Denver, Colorado, and he assured me in the presence of his staff that he would do whatever was necessary to make sure that that would happen. To date, the Brucker biofeedback center has had experience with over ten thousand cases and achieved a 98 percent success rate of restoring at least one level of function.

In 2009 when I was back in the Brucker biofeedback center for continued therapy, I again improved on all my previous neuromuscular recruitment/differentiation records and made the biggest increase ever (from one series of sessions to the next) in my left hand. In 2010, I achieved the biggest increase ever in the dorsiflexion of my left foot. Both gains took place more than twenty-eight years after my accident, making it obvious that I had not reached my maximum medical improvement when I was originally told, two years after my accident, that I had. Furthermore, in 2016, after undergoing a series of MAT sessions, I was able to generate a greater neuromuscular signal in my left leg than in my right leg while receiving the Brucker method of therapy. Then in 2018, after three months of daily enhanced microcirculation therapy combined with weekly MAT therapy, in my second biannual therapy sessions, I broke all those records in the Brucker Biofeedback Laboratory and have never been so happy since my accident in 1981.

In 2018, I had an epiphany of sorts after hearing Dr. Mark Hyman say in his Broken Brain series that it is not any one single therapy or support system that rehabilitates a damaged brain; it is the *combination* of a number of specific, effective therapies and approaches that restores a concussed brain to full function. Garrett Bussiere also taught me that it was *combining* superfoods, a nutritious and organic diet, and adequate quantity and frequency of specific exercise with taking "control of his thought process" that had the synergistic effect of restoring his vitality after he had been brain-injured many years prior.

Although I had rightfully and eagerly been promoting for a while the synergistic effect of combining Brucker biofeedback therapy with MAT sessions and enhanced microcirculation, I should promote a combination of *all* the therapies and approaches that have helped me—plus those I was unaware of but have helped others. Additionally, Garrett Bussiere told me that the medical advice to "go home and rest, and return only after he was no longer symptomatic" did not help him, for he indefinitely "remained symptomatic." Dr. Jeffrey J. Bazarian also maintains that the advice "Go home and rest" alone is not helpful and no longer acceptable because 20 percent of the concussed do not return to normal no matter how much they rest. With their admonition clearly in mind and building on the REAP protocol, which is foundational, I have myself now developed a new paradigm, a new protocol, that I call the CHAMP BRANDISE protocol (see next page)—it may well take brain injury rehabilitation to heights never before thought possible.

CHAMP BRANDISE PROTOCOL

C *Cold therapy, CereScan, Cocoa and Communication skills*: Cold therapy applied immediately and continued for the first seven days; CereScan as soon as a survivor is stabilized and before a rehabilitation program is developed, then repeated as necessary to monitor progress; daily unsweetened non-alkalized cocoa smoothies; communication skills training within the first two years then continued for life

H *Hyperbaric oxygen therapy*: thirty-plus sessions of hyperbaric oxygen therapy scheduled as soon as survivor is stabilized

A *The anti-inflammatory amino acid N-Acetyl Cysteine (NAC)* taken as directed

M *Microcirculation enhancement, Muscle Activation Techniques (MAT), and MojoFeet* orthotics: European PEMF* microcirculation eight minute sessions twice daily, both pre-injury (ideally) and post-injury, then continued for life; as soon as survivor is stabilized, weekly MAT sessions, followed by reduced MAT maintenance schedule to be continued for life; MojoFeet's custom-made orthotics created within the first year then replaced as needed

P *Prayer, Power, Penmanship, and Pace*: On the part of all concerned, earnestly pray to your higher power for healing, direction, and medical/therapeutic/financial provision; Whole Brain Power's Perfect Penmanship program; pacing the student athlete back to learning, activity—assessing while gradually increasing demand—before returning to practice and competition; vocationally pacing a survivor/employee back to a modified part-time work schedule before attempting to handle more responsibilities or work longer hours – with practical accommodations in place

* or any PEMF device that has been scientifically proven to significantly increase blood circulation throughout the microcapillaries of the body and brain for twelve to eighteen hours after a single eight-minute session

B   *Brucker biofeedback therapy and FocusBand*: Two years post-injury, scheduling regular Brucker Biofeedback sessions until survivor plateaus in progress and then a lifetime of annual/biannual maintenance sessions as needed; FocusBand pursue two years post-injury to optimize mental health and then continue using as needed

R   *Reduce and Relate*: Reduce physical, cognitive, and mental demands, especially throughout the first six to twelve months; Relationships are foundational to good health and great recoveries – find a way to cherish and develop quality relationships – use Dr. Rick Parente's mnemonics to positively affect behaviors between family and friends in addition to employing the Communication Game

A   *Accommodate*: The student athlete academically, the employee vocationally, and the family member socially as needed

N   *Neuro-optometric rehabilitation and Nutrition*: Fitting with Deborah Zelinsky's custom eyeglasses; nutritious and organic diet, including superfoods

D   *Designs for Strong Minds*: Training with Dr. Donalee Markus's brain-training program

I   *Infrared light therapy*: with Vigen** far-infrared light equipment (or near-infrared light equipment of equal effectiveness) within the first month, then continued for life

S   *Integrated Listening System and Tapping Solution*: iLs to optimize brain function, achieve personal goals and reach full potential; Tapping Solution for reprograming the brain and body to act differently in response to PTSD, depression, and anxiety

E   *Educate*: The survivor as well as families, teachers, coaches, employers, and medical professionals regarding brain injury, prevention measures, Dr. Robert Cantu's 26 symptom checklist, effective rehabilitation protocols and accommodation strategies

**   or any infrared light device that has been scientifically proven to emit 98.6 percent units of FIR light

This "masterpiece protocol"—if I may call it that—is my first attempt at constructing an evidence-based brain injury rehabilitation protocol. If one of the elements is found not to contribute significantly to positive outcomes in your case or in that of your survivor, simply eliminate it—but certainly do not throw out the entire protocol. The CHAMP BRANDISE protocol gives moderate and severe brain injury survivors a great opportunity to regain more of their normal selves. It is a pathway that may well enable them to replicate or surpass the success I myself have experienced after coping with a severe brain injury for over forty years. Granted, I am not 100 percent my pre-injury self; yet without question, I am closer than I have been since the 1981 car accident, and I believe I will improve further as I continue with the protocol.

The CHAMP BRANDISE protocol has been developed in an unfolding, exploratory manner—through my personal experience. Without trying to prove any preconceived ideas, my motivation is to shine a light beyond the current bleak expectation for survivors, to encourage seeing past the current grim Silent Epidemic hopelessness to the possibility of something much greater—that a satisfying life, a "near normal life," is possible for survivors like myself. I do not claim to have provided indisputable proof that the CHAMP BRANDISE protocol will work for everyone. (No medical paradigm has ever worked for everyone.) I do believe, however, that there are sufficient indicators to imply strongly that the identified therapies will benefit most survivors.

Arthur Schopenhauer said, "All truth passes through three stages. First, it is ridiculed. Second, it is violently opposed. Third, it is accepted as being self-evident."[82] I have been ridiculed by my rehabilitation counseling professors who were working to revoke my graduate degree and by different doctors who conducted their skewed IMEs all concluding that I had reached my MMI and that no further rehabilitation therapy was necessary. I have been opposed by my insurance company, who continues to refuse repayment for much of

---

[82]   https://medium.com/@alan_46156/the-three-stages-of-truth-eddd98151f0a

the CHAMP BRANDISE protocol. Regarding further publicizing my protocol, I can only hope that today or soon it will become self-evident to all involved that it is medically necessary to: reduce inflammation, prevent oxidation, optimize microcirculation, get the most precise brain diagnostic available, activate lost neuromuscular connections, once reestablished re-educate those connections, optimize gut health, eat nutritious brain super-foods; foster quality/reciprocal relationships, and continue with effective therapies to both achieve and maintain functional gains—for a lifetime, all while saving everyone money. Then when they recognize the CHAMP BRANDISE protocol is true by necessity or virtue of its logical form, it will become a tautology in the medical field, promoted to all our citizens and made available via insurance benefits. Please examine the potential breakthroughs of the CHAMP BRANDISE protocol with an open mind so as not to overlook its truly valid and efficacious therapy-based components.

10a.   Dr. Bernard Brucker was the founder and director of the Brucker biofeedback center at the University of Miami Miller School of Medicine/Miami Jewish Home and Hospital. He was also an aircraft commander for the US Coast Guard Auxiliary; a member of the Department of Homeland Security; an associate professor in the Departments of Psychiatry and Behavioral Sciences, Orthopedics and Rehabilitation, and Radiology at UM's Miller School of Medicine; chairman of the Brain and Spinal Cord Injury Advisory Council for the state of Florida; president of the Academy of Rehabilitation Psychology; and president of the Florida Brain Injury Association. He received the Gill Moss Award from the National Spinal Cord Injury Association for outstanding scientific and clinical contributions to spinal cord injury; the Lifetime Achievement Award from the Miami-Dade County Chapter of the Florida Psychological Association; and the Karl F. Heiser Presidential Award from the American Psychological Association. In addition, Dr. Brucker was one of the founders and the original codirector of the Miami Project to Cure Paralysis. An innovative clinician and developer of the world-renowned Brucker method, he found that his greatest passion in life was caring for the patients who came to him from all around the world—little ones and adults alike—all seeking restored mobility and function. Beyond the treatment he offered, Dr. Brucker provided the gift of hope and compassion as well. I have never met a more dynamic, encouraging, and positively capable person in my life. When he died in 2008 from a massive heart attack, the leadership and administration of the Miami Jewish Home and Hospital along with thousands around the world profoundly mourned the sudden and devastating loss. Dr. Brucker is survived by Dr. Rita Gugel, his wife of thirty-five years; his brother, Daniel Brucker; and his sister-in-law, Margaret Jarmolych. In a very real sense, he is also survived by a multitude of colleagues, friends, and patients who carry him in their hearts and minds. May his memory be eternal and his life and mission be lived and carried out by his family and those associated with him.

The Brucker Biofeedback Department of Miami Jewish Health Systems utilizes neuromuscular behavioral procedures and microprocessor technology to restore function to those with paralysis from central nervous system damage. Through strategic use of neurological and visual cues, the Brucker biofeedback method trains patients to use secondary muscles and viable, previously inactive nerves to restore function. The technique has had tremendous success for people facing permanent paralysis caused by trauma, central nervous system damage, and diseases such as

- Bell's palsy/facial palsy,
- brain injury,
- brain stem injury,
- brain tumors,
- central nervous system damage,
- cerebral palsy,
- certain neurological diseases,
- encephalitis,
- multiple sclerosis,
- myelitis,
- spina bifida,
- spinal cord injury,
- spinal stenosis,
- strokes,

The center works with children and adults from around the world and has received enthusiastic feedback from many on how the treatment has enriched their lives. Here are two examples:

I am from South Africa and have cerebral palsy with spastic quadriplegia. I've been coming here since I was five years old. Today

I'm seventeen, and thanks to the Brucker biofeedback, I'm more independent than I could have ever hoped for. (Kimberly)

I'm confined to a wheelchair for the rest of my life. So I started the Brucker biofeedback program in 2006. How has it helped me so far? I can ride a stationary bike for thirty minutes. I can walk with braces and a walker. I used to fall over and lose my balance in the car, but now my back muscles are strong enough to keep me from falling over. (Jennifer)

REACARE Magazine's article, Reactivating Paralysed Muscles: Examination of the Therapeutic Success of the Brucker Biofeedback Method*, reported, "The Brucker Biofeedback method has proved successful in the treatment of pareses attributable to brain damage. Under the direction of Head Physician Dr. Peter Bernius, the Paediatric and Neuro Orthopaedic Centre of Schön Klink München Harlaching has been a European center for the Brucker Biofeedback method since 2002 and has recently presented an evaluation of the treatment results in patients suffering from infantile or acquired cerebral palsy. This method seems to be successful, especially from the patients' perspective: they report a substantially improved arm function and better mobility."

I was disheartened to learn in 2020 that Miami Jewish Health suspended all of their outpatient rehabilitation services, including Brucker Biofeedback and Rosomoff Centers due to the COVID-19 virus lockdown. Following a logical approach to protect the most vulnerable, Florida placed great restrictions on campuses that house the elderly. Additionally, with the majority of Brucker Biofeedback therapy clientele coming from Europe, Miami Jewish Health was unable to re-open the Center in 2021. Sadly there are no plans to reopen the Miami Jewish Health Centers at this time. Consequently the future of Brucker Biofeedback therapy in America remains uncertain.

10b. Emilia Cabrera, AP, DAOM, NCCAOM, born in Cuba, from an early age was recognized by her family and neighbors as having the gift of healing in her hands and an unprecedented ability to "see" disease or injury inside a person. Repeatedly, people would come to her, and she would heal them of ailments and injuries. Emilia became a devout believer in the innate healing powers of the human body and pursued the healing/medical profession. After she earned a master's degree at the University of Havana in Cuba, she worked several years as a psychologist, which currently serves her in coaching patients and providing counsel to help them live vibrantly in mind, body, and spirit. Dr. Cabrera is a board-certified physician with the National Certification Commission for Acupuncture and Oriental Medicine and holds a doctorate degree in Oriental Medicine from Atlantic University. Over the years, Dr. Cabrera focused on treating complex conditions (cancer, neurological disorders, mental health issues, liver disorders, gastrointestinal and metabolic conditions, as well as pain) and strengthening the immune system. She accomplishes her healing work by affecting the patient's cells on an energetic and biochemical level. Through holistic medicine and complementary practices (acupuncture, counseling, far-infrared therapy, cupping, and ozone therapy), Dr. Cabrera individualizes a treatment plan for every patient—she treats men, women, and children. Dr. Cabrera strives to provide her patients at the Holistic Care Solutions in Bal Harbour Islands, Florida, with the most natural and comprehensive care available, combining Western science with the art of Eastern medicine. To learn more, visit www.holisticcaresolutions.com.

10c. Li Xin Zhang, Dipl. Ac., L. Ac., began his medical training at the age of nine, as he is the tenth generation heir to his family's medical lineage. He graduated at the top of his class at Heilongjiang Medical School and eventually became the Chief Doctor of the Acupuncture Department at Beijing's acclaimed Red Cross Hospital. There he administered inpatient and outpatient care throughout the 1,000-bed hospital, acted as a senior supervisor, and participated in the training and overseeing of hundreds of medical doctors in acupuncture. A number of

Dr. Zhang's medical research studies were published during the 1990s, and in 1993, he was appointed national consultant to the Chinese Family Doctors Association. Distinguished in his field, Dr. Zhang has been featured in both the Chinese national press and Chinese television.

Acupuncture treats regular health problems and chronic conditions for which drug therapy and surgery have not been effective. Dr. Zhang specializes in treating brain injury/neuropathological conditions that include but are not limited to seizures, stroke, Bell's palsy, MS, numbness, peripheral neuropathy, dizziness, migraine, and tinnitus. Lixin Acupuncture Clinics were founded to bring quality acupuncture and traditional Chinese medicine to the American public by Dr. Zhang from China and his family tradition. Acupuncture is the foundation of traditional Chinese medicine that originated in China over five thousand years ago. The intent of acupuncture therapy is to promote health and alleviate pain and suffering. The method by which this is accomplished, though it may seem strange and mysterious to many, has been time tested over thousands of years and continues to be validated today. Dr. Zhang and his personally trained staff believe in well-being, in challenging the status quo, and that true medicine should not only cover the symptoms but also *cure* the causes. Learn more at https://www.lixinacupuncture.com/acupuncture.

10d. What is far-infrared light, and how does it work? FIR wavelengths fall just below (that's what *infra* means) visible red light in the electromagnetic spectrum. At the molecular level, far-infrared light exerts strong rotational and vibrational effects that are biologically beneficial. Although the wavelengths of FIR light are too long to be perceived by the naked eye, we experience its energy as gentle, radiant heat that can penetrate up to 3.5 inches beneath the skin. According to the book *Alternative Medicine*, among FIR's healing benefits is its ability to stimulate the healing of injuries and other conditions. Far-infrared light is capable of expanding capillaries, thereby improving blood circulation, enhancing white blood cell function, and increasing immune response. It contributes by these means to the elimination of foreign pathogens and cellular waste products throughout the body.

Additional benefits of FIR include its ability to (1) stimulate the hypothalamus, which controls the production of the neurochemicals that are involved in such biological processes such as sleep, mood, pain sensations, and blood pressure; (2) enhance the delivery of oxygen and nutrients to the body's soft tissue areas; and (3) enhance the removal of accumulated toxins by improving lymph circulation. FIR also promotes the rebuilding of injured tissue through its positive effect on the growth of cells, DNA synthesis, and protein synthesis and thus on the growth of fibroblasts (the connective tissue cells involved in the repair of injury). It, therefore, is excellent for healing burns and scar tissue and for other skin problems. Further, far-infrared light can relieve nervous tension and relax auto-neuro muscles, thereby helping the body make the most of its natural healing abilities. In addition to all these benefits, FIR can reduce muscle spasms and soreness on nerve endings. The American Medical Association (AMA) has recognized FIR light as an effective physical therapy treatment.

Vigen's far-infrared light heat projectors are covered with a substance called Hygiea. Hygiea (hu-gee-a) is a material developed by Vigen Medical combining nineteen different minerals and metals. Hygiea has been shown to produce a maximum level of FIR output compared with other minerals, including jade—the most effective conductor of far-infrared light found in nature. Hygiea emits 14 percent more FIR light than jade, 98.6 percent compared with 84.3 percent. FIR and heat are the essential elements used in the Vigen healing process. Heat produces a moxibustion biological effect that compliments FIR, and together, they are especially useful in detoxifying the body.

Going back to the principles of Eastern medicine, clean blood and proper blood circulation are essential for well-being. Heat and FIR rays literally wash out cholesterol and toxins in the blood. The unwanted material is first dissolved and then flushed from the body. Vigen's FIR rays also help generate blood production from the bone marrow, which is important especially for weak immune systems. Additionally, FIR rays have the very important ability to shrink swollen tissues. If there is any infection or inflammation, FIR rays go to work to restore the body's natural health. FIR combined with heat has been called "twenty-first-century medicine" because together they help a body's healing process without the use of invasive surgery or the negative side effects caused by prescription drugs. Learn more at https://vigenmedicalusa.com.

10e. Bradley Bosick, DC, learned his technique through enduring adversities of his own. In high school football practice, he sustained a low back injury that put him in a metal brace covering half the length of his body for two years, and he was never able to play high school sports again. Nor could anyone relieve the pain his injury caused him for more than an hour, although he continued to seek medical doctors and health practitioners for the next twelve years. One day in college, however, a friend came up to him and said enthusiastically, "You need to go see my husband. He's a chiropractor. I know he can help you."

With the first adjustment from his friend's chiropractor—Bradley found twelve years of pain instantaneously gone. He knew then and there exactly what he himself was going to do for the rest of his life—help others the same way this man had helped him. Bradley became a doctor of chiropractic and even got back into sports. Dr. Bosick is eternally grateful for the people who referred him to chiropractic treatments that changed his life forever.

Throughout his life, Dr. Bosick fashioned orthotics for himself to improve his gait until he was introduced to MojoFeet orthotics. What separates MojoFeet orthotics from every other orthotic is (1) they are custom molded to each person's unique foot structure, and (2) they provide full-contact support with a one-of-a-kind material (in its density-to-flexibility ratio) that delivers a "functional orthotic." MojoFeet believes the basis for foot health is to have strong, mobile feet that are supported well when they are spending time on man made surfaces. Learn more at https://mojofeet.com.

10f.   William White, MD, FACEP, is a licensed physician and business executive with over thirty years of experience providing patient care services and managing organizations. Dr. White is a graduate of Stanford University and the University of Southern California School of Medicine. He completed postgraduate training in internal medicine at the University of Southern California Medical Center, in addition to a residency program in emergency medicine at the University of Arizona. Dr. White is a fellow of the American College of Emergency Physicians (FACEP) and founder and CEO of the Emergency Medicine Physicians (EMP, www.emp.com)—a physician-owned and physician-managed, multistate organization contracting with major hospitals to make available over eight hundred high-quality physicians. He has been recognized as Entrepreneur of the Year by both Ernst & Young and the NASDAQ stock market. Additionally, Dr. White is an accomplished medical instructor/lecturer and an author of many medical publications and has conducted extensive research throughout his career.

10f1. https://www.hopkinsmedicine.org/news/media/releases/how_dark_chocolate_may_guard_against_brain_injury_from_stroke

10g.   Michael J. Lavery—a modern-day Renaissance man—suffered a serious, life-changing event while playing varsity football as a sophomore in 1974. Lavery sustained a compound fracture of his left femur that hospitalized him for about three months with complications that resulted in additional surgeries to repair the severe damage. The operations were successful and enabled him to again participate in competitive sports—baseball, hockey, and football. It was during this "convalescent period" that Lavery fully embraced the arts and music and the awakening of his brain's right hemisphere. Interestingly enough, when he returned to his sporting endeavors, his hand-to-eye coordination was significantly elevated from the fine motor control training involved in painting, sculpting, and playing the guitar. Lavery is absolutely convinced that this was the point that he began tapping into brain plasticity, which he currently espouses in his coaching business called Whole Brain Power.

Lavery made a tremendous comeback in his sports career, and after graduating from Exeter Academy, he matriculated to Amherst College. He majored in fine art, and it was at Amherst that he earned the nickname "the Renaissance Man." He also lettered in four varsity sports, including baseball, football, hockey, and squash. He graduated in 1982 and was drafted to play professional baseball by the Toronto Blue Jays. He played one year in their organization before the lure of his creative pursuits persuaded him to immerse himself in the arts as a career. It was when he moved from Boston to Southern California, and he settled into the art colony of Laguna Beach. His skills at landscape and seascape painting offered him an opportunity to open up an art gallery in 1986. He developed a love for the game of tennis and quickly developed as a competitive tournament player.

It was when he expanded his brain training by learning to play tennis ambidextrously. At age twenty-nine, he made a total dedication to becoming ambidextrous at the sport. This opened up his investigation of neuroscience and its relevance to his determination to play dual-handed tennis in tournament action. With the growing body of scientific evidence from the neurological community that the brain has tremendous capacity to rewire itself, Lavery began an across-the-board brain training regimen that centered on ambidextrous gross and fine motor controls, including mirror image penmanship. He also developed creative and imagination memory exercises that tap into the integration of the left and right hemispheres of the brain. Currently,

Lavery is developing his Communication Game and feels it may be the crown jewel of his Whole Brain Power program. To learn more, visit https://wbp.io.

10h.　How does one get his or her body into ketosis and have his or her brain experience "neuroprotective benefits"? Eat less than 20g net carbs per day and eat enough sea salt. *The fewer carbs, the more effective the diet.* This means you'll need to completely avoid sweet, sugary foods, plus starchy foods like bread, pasta, rice, and potatoes. Basically, follow the guidelines for a strict low-carb diet; and remember, it's supposed to be high in fat, not high in protein. A rough guideline is 10 percent energy from carbohydrates (the fewer carbs, the more effective), 15 to 25 percent from protein (the lower end is more effective), and 70 to 90 percent from fat. Seek out the expert knowledge found at www.dietdoctor.com/low-carb/keto. There are free newsletter for exclusive advice, mouthwatering recipes, and extra motivation to succeed with your keto diet journey at www.ruled.me. For recipes to appease your sweet tooth while on the keto diet, visit www.amazon.com/Sweet-Savory-Fat-Bombs-Delicious/dp/1592337287.

10h1.　Maciej Gasior, Michael A. Rogawski, and Adam L. Hartman, "Neuroprotective and Disease-Modifying Effects of the Ketogenic Diet," *Behavioral Pharmacology* 17, nos. 5–6 (September 2006): 431–39, www.ncbi.nlm.nih.gov/pmc/articles/PMC2367001/.

10h2.　John Erdman, Maria Oria, and Laura Pillsbury, eds., *Nutrition and Traumatic Brain Injury: Improving Acute and Subacute Health Outcomes in Military Personnel* (Washington, DC: The National Academies Press, 2011), doi:10.17226/13121, PubMed/Medline, US National Library of Medicine National Institutes of Health, https://www.ncbi.nlm.nih.gov/pubmed/24983072.

10h3.   Eric H. Kossoff, MD, "The Ketogenic Diet: It's about 'Time'" (March 18, 2009), www.onlinelibrary.wiley.com/doi/full/10.1111/j.1469-8749.2009.03280.x.

10h4.   Mayumi Prins, "Diet, Ketones, and Neurotrauma," *Epilepsia* 49, no. s8 (November 2008): 111–13, www.ncbi.nlm.nih.gov/pmc/articles/PMC2652873/.

10i.   Garrett Bussiere, in 2006, had just finished his third year competing in college baseball's Pacific-10 Conference at the University of California, Berkeley, when he was drafted by the Saint Louis Cardinals to play professional baseball. The Cardinals began paying Bussiere to compete with their organization's farm team in Tennessee. With a supportive family, a great girlfriend, three-quarters of his undergraduate education at Cal Berkeley under his belt, a Major League Baseball contract, and money in the bank, life couldn't get much better for him or any other twenty-year-old American male. Then one day during an ordinary game, an unusual play resulted in a ninety-five-mile-per-hour baseball hitting Bussiere in the left side of his head, and he has never again been able to play the game. Bussiere's TBI devastated not only his professional baseball career but also his academic performance (for the first time in his life, he began failing classes upon his return to UC Berkeley) and his relationships with friends and family members (which were strained considerably and only resuscitated several years after the incident).

The medical community let down Bussiere as it has let down millions upon millions of other American survivors. He explained that, unfortunately, "[t]he first doctor simply recommended I rest and return only after I was no longer symptomatic—however my symptoms persisted. The second said the same, adding that I should reduce my activity and exercise levels. I did as told, but to no avail. Then came the weekly meetings with the neuropsychologist and neuropsychiatrist, the additional brain scans (all of which came back 'unremarkable'), the testing, the monitoring, and the futile redundancy of being thrown back and forth between different professional medical fields—each not fully knowing what the solution to post-concussion syndrome is." None of the professionals Bussiere worked with told him which "hazards exacerbate concussion symptoms, and which remedies clear them"—something that he very much wanted to know. So begun his self-directed journey of understanding his brain injury with only one urgent, burning question, "How do I get back to normal after a moderate traumatic brain injury?"

Like myself, Bussiere developed his own rehabilitation program and has also, in fact, surpassed all predictions made by the doctors involved in his case. I strongly recommend Garrett's book, *Concussion Healing Solution: Clarity Amid the Confusion*,[38] and his website, www.healingyourhead.com, to all survivors everywhere to help them recover the absolute best brain/body function as possible.

We met one afternoon at the Wynkoop Brewing Company in Downtown Denver when we were shooting pool on adjacent tables in the upstairs billiards hall that has more than twenty tables. After a while, we shot a game against each other and learned of our brain injuries, plus that Garrett knew my boss Gavin Attwood, CereScan's John Kelley, and Dr. Robert Cantu. We both feel that it was Providence that brought us in contact with each other. I am truly indebted to Garrett for adding his important contribution to my book and for his work on behalf of all survivors—via his website.

10i1.   Giza and Hovda, "The Neurometabolic Cascade of Concussion," *Journal of Athletic Training* (July–September 2001).

10i2.   A. L. Petraglia, E. A. Winkler, and J. E. Bailes, "Stuck at the Bench: Potential Natural Neuroprotective Compounds for Concussion," *Surgical Neurology International* 2 (2011).

10i3.   F. Gomez-Pinilla, F. 2011. "The Combined Effects of Exercise and Foods in Preventing Neurological and Cognitive Disorders," *Preventive Medicine* 52 (2011): S75–S80.

10i4.   A. Wu, Z. Ying, and F. Gomez-Pinilla, "Dietary Omega-3 Fatty Acids Normalize BDNF Levels, Reduce Oxidative Damage, and Counteract Learning Disability after Traumatic Brain Injury in Rats," *Journal of Neurotrauma* 21, no. 10 (2004): 1457–67.

Curcumin: www.ncbi.nlm.nih.gov/pmc/articles/PMC3918523/.
Avocadoes and Tomatoes: www.ncbi.nlm.nih.gov/pmc/articles/PMC4093981/.
Brewed   Cacao: www.bmcnutr.biomedcentral.com/articles/10.1186/s40795-016-0117-z.

10j.   Greg Roskopf, author of *The Roskopf Principle* and developer of MAT, also created a curriculum for MAT that has been taught to over two thousand students across the world. Mr. Roskopf's Muscle Activation Techniques Jumpstart and Specialist programs are now taught as a part of one American college's curriculum and is approved by National Academy of Sports Medicine (NASM) and Board of Certification (BOC) for Continuing Education Credits (CECs). MAT has proved effective with professional athletes. Over the years, Roskopf has been contracted to treat Peyton Manning and the whole Denver Bronco football team, the whole Denver Nuggets basketball team, Carson Palmer, injured swimmer Amy Van Dyken, and others. Manning reportedly had received the MAT sessions in Indianapolis with the Colts football team for six years before he joined the Denver Broncos in 2012. Before Manning came to the Broncos, he flew Roskopf to Indianapolis, Indiana, regularly for Greg to perform the MAT sessions on him. In a 2012 *Sports Illustrated* article, Manning affirmed it was MAT that helped prolong his football career.

Thankfully for the rest of us, MAT is not just for the pros. MAT works with clients at all physical capability levels who are looking to address challenges they experience due to injury, stress, or trauma to their neuromuscular system. When Mr. Roskopf was introduced to the concepts of Transforming Techniques Incorporated (TTI), he immediately informed Mr. Condon that he and his team at Muscle Activation Techniques will work in earnest to help recruit, develop, and train MAT practitioners for TTI's rehabilitation centers. Roskopf has been aware for a time that MAT success with professional and high-level athletes also will be effective with physically disabled people. Roskopf believes Transforming Techniques Incorporated can be an excellent avenue to bring MAT to the disabled public who are in great need of functional neuromuscular rehabilitation. Learn more at https://muscleactivation.com.

10k.   The PEMF device's working mechanism is a biorhythmically defined physical stimulus consisting of a unique multidimensionally configured signal (waveform) transmitted into the body via an electromagnetic field. Note that it is the rhythm of the multidimensionally configured signal—that is, the selection and order of wave frequencies with vascular specific allocations—and not the electromagnetic field that acts as the agent responsible for the positive benefits to the body—complementary, therapeutic physical stimulation of the smaller blood vessel's autorhythmic self-pumping action. Further, it has been verified that this PEMF device's specific, temporary, multidimensional signal order and structure, combined with the low flux density electromagnetic field, is paramount for effectively stimulating the mechanism for improving/regulating blood circulation.

The basic PEMF device's therapy plan is carried out for eight minutes twice a day (ideally every twelve hours), using the whole-body application module either in a professional setting or at home. The positive effects of PEMF device's therapy last for a long period compared with all other types of applied impulses. The average user can expect the benefits of a single eight-minute session of the multidimensionally configured signal application to last half a day or more. However, overall benefits from this PEMF device's enhanced microcirculation depend fundamentally on the user's diet, water purity/consumption, indoor air quality, lifestyle, and geographical residence.

101.   Dr. Clark Elliott, a professor of artificial intelligence at DePaul University, holds BM and MM teaching certificates in music, as well as an MS degree in computer science and a PhD with an emphasis on computer simulations of human emotion from Northwestern University's Institute for Learning Sciences. On September 27, 1999, he was in a car accident, waiting at an intersection when a Jeep Cherokee rear-ended him. Momentarily, he blacked out and was shaken up but didn't think anything serious happened to him. When the paramedics got there, they asked his name; Elliott had difficulty answering and could not understand why. The next morning, while he was not paralyzed, Elliott could not stand up or move his arms and had language-processing difficulties. Soon thereafter, he realized something serious had, without question, happened to him—his inability to understand conversations and wearing his shoes on the wrong feet made it obvious, yet disbelief caused him to question how there could be something so terribly wrong when he didn't even get hurt.

Days later in the hospital, the doctor asked Elliott the same question about his name. Elliott could not speak for a while and then just mumbled. After a host of standard testing, when they were ready to discharge him, the doctor assured Elliott there was nothing to worry about. Elliott asked him what the cause of his problems was, why he was having such difficulties, and why he felt so out of sorts. Before leaving the room, the examining doctor said he had a bad concussion and told Elliott that, after he got dressed back in his clothes, he could go home. The hospital staff gave Elliott some handout instructions and pills that he could not read or understand how to take. He recalled how much better it would have been were he given information that explained brain injury and its consequences and symptoms with recommended therapies and accommodations.

Elliott went on to recover remarkably well and write his amazing book, which he dedicated "[t]o the millions who suffer head injuries each year"—with the encouragement "There is hope." The book, according to Norman Doidge, MD (*New York Times* best-selling author of *The Brain That Changes Itself* and *The Brain's Way of Healing*), is the "most meticulous and informative account I have ever read of the effects of a traumatic brain injury on a single mind. It should be mined for years to come by all who care about the subject." The book, according to *Publishers Weekly*, "[d]elivers a harrowing account of a 13-year-long recovery from a disabling concussion that changed his life, and celebrates the science that came to his rescue." The book, according to Michael Sandler, host of the *Inspire Nation Show*, is "[a]n incredibly powerful book . . . one of my most important reads of the last year, maybe of ever" (www.clarkelliott.com). Dr. Elliott currently lives with his wife and daughter in Evanston, Illinois. He has raised four other children, studies Tai Chi and music every day, and continues as a casual marathon runner. To learn more, visit www.clarkelliott.com/ClarkElliottBioA.html.

10m. Dr. Donalee Markus worked with Ameritech, Los Alamos National Laboratories, and NASA. NASA asked Dr. Markus to design a new program for them because the current programs available covered only structured and semistructured problem-solving. NASA's Critical Thinking Skills Project chose Dr. Markus's Designs for Strong Minds because it is the only critical-thinking course specifically designed to enhance brain function for high-functioning adults. Designs for Strong Minds is an innovative program of exercises that uses gamelike, content-free exercises to filter out emotional influences, allowing the participants to work solely on skills. It also includes unstructured problem-solving that teaches people to effectively analyze and define problems and issues. Dr. Markus has designed programs for children, adolescents, professionals, and aging adults; plus, she has had tremendous success working with people who have suffered traumatic brain injuries. Since 1983, Dr. Markus and her Designs for Strong Minds associates have been maximizing intelligence for survivors, individuals, and corporations throughout the United States.

Dr. Markus's practice was 20 percent brain injury before 2015. Since the publication of *The Ghost in My Brain*, over 80 percent of her practice is devoted to rehabilitating brain-injured patients. Dr. Markus's Designs for Strong Minds exercises allow survivors to hold more information, sort and organize information in innovative ways, and collect information from a broader base. These skills then help participants enhance their communication skills, improve their analytical ability, understand their thought processes, and gain insight into their problem-solving strategies, plus offers the opportunity to identify and habituate new processing behaviors. Be sure to check out the two excellent iOS apps for BI survivors, Strong Mind Puzzles and Strong Mind Treasure Hunt. Learn more by visiting www.designsforstrongminds.com.

10n. Deborah Zelinsky, OD, is an optometrist noted worldwide for her work in neuro-optometric rehabilitation. She founded the Mind-Eye Connection almost thirty years ago to emphasize the pivotal role of integrating signals from auditory and visual systems by using eyeglasses to alter listening ability. Now known as the Mind-Eye Institute, the mission has expanded to teach Mind-Eye optometrists how to prescribe for the often overlooked peripheral retina using unique patented mind-eye techniques and to conduct research on brain mapping and other neuro-optometric techniques. One of Zelinsky's goals is to update the current eye examinations to include the visual skills necessary for the changing technology people use—to leave "20/20 testing behind in the 20th Century."

The retina is composed of brain tissue and is part of the central nervous system. As a result, individually customized eyeglasses affecting the frequency and direction of light dispersed on the retina can be used to selectively influence brain signals. Eyesight is one small part of vision;

there are many visual systems often not addressed during routine eye exams, such as the ability to internally visualize a picture while reading. Each of the systems develops in a hierarchy, linking with one another's development. For instance, motor skills and visual skills combine for good hand-eye coordination, or visual and auditory skills combine for reading.

In addition to her work with the Mind-Eye Institute, Dr. Zelinsky is a fellow in both the College of Optometrists in Vision Development and the Neuro-Optometric Rehabilitation Association, a community leader for the Society of Neuroscience, and a board member of the Society for Brain Mapping. Learn more at www.mindeye.com.

10o.   Graham Boulton grew up in Australia with a unique passion to assist with mental health issues—worldwide. However, he graduated from the university's Department of Civil Aviation as an electronics engineer in 1972. As an experienced chief executive officer with a demonstrated history of managing innovative companies, he launched several of his own successful companies—the last one showing on the Australian Stock Exchange in 1997. Boulton is credited with designing and building the world's first touch screen point-of-sale equipment in 1991 and then disrupting the cash register industry by introducing the forty-character receipt printers, replacing the twelve-character nondescriptive shopping receipts. His true passion caused his career path to boomerang and bring him back, with his extensive technology background, to digitize the current one-to-one mental health therapy protocol—allowing therapists to reach twenty times the number of people suffering from mental issues. His recent development and release of NeuroSelf Care—powered by FocusBand—is the IoT tool to gather data from a remote user to collate on Microsoft's Azure ML and AI with their bot providing the user interface automation.

10p. CereScan's "functional imaging" provides doctors with critical information and data on how the brain and its tissues are actually *functioning*—unlike X-ray, CT, and MRI scans, which can only show the anatomy of a brain. For example, PET brain imaging measures important body functions such as oxygen use, blood flow, and glucose (sugar) metabolism. Coupling PET measurements with CereScan's software enables one to clearly display the absolute metabolic rate in up to 120 regions of the brain, revealing areas that are potentially damaged and not utilizing as much glucose (energy) as they should. Electroencephalography, referred to as "brain mapping," is the measurement of electrical patterns on the surface of the scalp that reflect cortical activity beneath the skull (brain waves). A quantitative EEG (qEEG) is the analysis of the digitized EEG and shows how brain cells are actually communicating with one another and the body. SPECT imaging measures blood flow (perfusion) and can pinpoint problem areas below the cortex. In conjunction with PET brain imaging, qEEG, and qSPECT, CereScan's technology provides the most complete information about brain function and brain damage in 120 regions of the brain. The information CereScan provides can be used to develop more effective, targeted treatment plans and better track rehabilitation progress. The path to better brain health starts with better data, and CereScan assures me that they are committed to making innovation in neuroimaging accessible to brain injury survivors and their doctors. Learn more by visiting https://cerescan.com.

35   R. Kelley, "The Writing on the Wall," *Newsweek* 150, no. 20 (November 12, 2007): 69, https://www.questia.com/magazine/1G1-170830860/the-writing-on-the-wall.

36   D. Snowdon, *Aging with Grace: What the Nun Study Teaches Us about Leading Longer, Healthier, and More Meaningful Lives*, unabridged (April 30, 2002), https://www.amazon.com/Aging-Grace-Teaches-Healthier-Meaningful/dp/0553380923.

37   S. C. Anderson; J. F. Cryan, PhD; T. Dinan, MD, PhD., *Psychobiotic Revolution: Mood, Food, and the New Science of the Gut-Brain Connection* (Washington, DC: National Geographic Partners, 2017), https://www.amazon.com/Psychobiotic-Revolution-Science-Gut-Brain-Connection/dp/142621846X.

38   Garrett R. Bussiere, *The Concussion Healing Solution: Clarity Amid the Confusion* (2017), https://www.amazon.com/Concussion-Healing-Solution-Clarity-Confusion-ebook/dp/B06XCDFGVD.

39   Kenneth S. Kosik, "Outsmarting Alzheimer's: What You Can Do to Reduce Your Risk" (The Reader's Digest Association, Inc., 2015), https://boulder.flatironslibrary.org/GroupedWork/fccb67bb-99d7-3567-6eec-747fc779d869/Home.

40   K. Eakin et al., "Efficacy of N-Acetyl Cysteine in Traumatic Brain Injury," *PLOS One*, www.journals.plos.org/plosone/article/file?id=10.1371/journal.pone.0090617&type=printable

41   B. J. Hoffer et al., "Repositioning Drugs for Traumatic Brain Injury—N-Acetyl Cysteine and Phenserine," *Journal of Biomedical Science* 24, no. 1 (September 9, 2017): 71, https://www.ncbi.nlm.nih.gov/pubmed/28886718.

42   P. D. Harch and V. McCullough, *The Oxygen Revolution: Hyperbaric Oxygen Therapy: The New Treatment for Post Traumatic Stress Disorder (PTSD), Traumatic Brain Injury, Stroke, Autism, and More* (Hatherleigh Press, 2016), https://www.amazon.com/Oxygen-Revolution-Third-Hyperbaric-Definitive/dp/1578266270/.

43   N. Ortner, *The Tapping Solution: A Revolutionary System For Stress-Free Living* (Hay House, Inc., 2013), https://www.amazon.com/Tapping-Solution-Weight-Loss-Confidence/dp/1401945139.

11

MY CATHARSIS TO A NEW NORMAL

Having gained understanding of the limitations I experience because of my brain damage, I have grown to *better* accept them. After twenty-five years of rehabilitating, I was again able to respect myself. In the early years post-brain-injury, however, I was only an apparition, a cruel caricature of my former self—in a real sense, I was not all there. With my own determined persistence, my participation in specific therapies, financing via the Michigan Catastrophic Claims Association, the help of my support circle and by God's grace, I gradually fleshed out who I am today. I better recognize my disability now, and I continue working to accommodate my permanent losses. I graduated with a master of rehabilitation counseling degree seventeen years after my brain injury. A year later, I passed the national licensed professional counselor exam and then continued my graduate studies to become a certified school counselor. I worked in the Denver Public Schools (DPS) for a number of years as a school counselor in the Safe and Drug-Free Schools Department, serving students with a variety of needs.

And wonder of wonders, I began a relationship with the beautiful and brilliant doctor Lydia Prado, a clinical psychologist who at the time was a CEO with the Mental Health Center of Denver (MHCD); and after half a year, we became engaged. Lydia said yes to my marriage proposal. We met when we were both working, along with a number of other staff members from both DPS and MHCD, on a project for the children in our school district. Although we broke off the engagement after about a year, several months later, Lydia delivered our child—Lia Salome Prado-Condon—a beautiful and amazing daughter, who is the best thing in my life. The day she was born, coming into the world with big bright eyes looking all around and without crying at all—not one bit—I carried her to the waiting room to show the entire family. In awe, her brother Emilio said when he first saw baby Lia, "She is so beautiful!" Everyone agreed and could not stop looking at her face and into her bright eyes. Lydia and I live near each other, are mutually respectful and cordial toward one another, share custody of our daughter without any court orders, and have positive relationships with each other's extended families. We co-parent Lia, watching our child grow into an amazing young woman. Lia has brought such joy into my life and the lives of others; she is incomparable.

Today I work part time for the Brain Injury Alliance of Colorado[11a] (as their statewide support group coordinator and national speaker) and part time for my own 501(c)(3) company, Transforming Techniques Incorporated, with the mission of (1) advocating for the recognition and prevention of brain injury; (2) working to help rehabilitate survivors by selling effective therapy equipment, plus developing TTI clinics; and (3) urging ever-wider adoption of the CHAMP BRANDISE protocol as the best practice standard in brain injury rehabilitation.

The Brain Injury Alliance of Colorado had its beginnings in 1980, when it was called the Colorado Head Injury Foundation (CHIF). It has since developed into one of the nation's leading brain injury organizations. The efforts of its current staff have enabled BIAC to make great progress in supporting survivors and their families, as well as in positively affecting legislation in the state of Colorado. They currently have a staff of more than twenty five professionals offering a smorgasbord of programs, the foundation of which is Resource Navigation. In 2019, BIAC partnered with the city of Denver in breaking ground for a seventy-two-unit housing complex with complimentary offices offering rehabilitation services to disadvantaged citizens with brain injuries, to be completed in 2023. It gives me pride that BIAC's director, Mr. Gavin Attwood, told my parents, "Mark is an invaluable part of BIAC's team."

Master's degree, professional licensure, and BIAC recognition aside, I am every bit as proud of some hard-fought, mundane abilities I have regained over the years—and also for interpersonal growth I have experienced along the way. After ten years of not being able to tuck my shirt into my pants with my left hand, for example, I regained that ability. For twelve years, I could not brush my teeth with my left hand either; and then at a certain point, once again, I could. After sixteen years of not being able to snap my left fingers, I am proud to be able to do that again too. I am also proud that I was able to keep my grocery-sacking job as long as I did (five years). Ongoing psychological/social/spiritual growth has allowed me to accept the reality that I will never compete in hockey or rugby again. (In high school, I played a lot of hockey; and in college, I was the captain and coach of Northern Michigan University's rugby club.) I am now okay with the fact that all my competitive athletic performance is in the past; I have found other satisfying ways to remain physically active. And with the help of Coach Lavery in 2019, my communication skills are now better than at any time since my injury in 1981.

It was only after deeply grieving my losses that I became truly able to accept my disabled self. Grieving for me was not a once-and-done sort of thing, but after that remarkable, cathartic night of crying with my family (see the end of chapter 2, *THE FIRST DECADE OF MY BRAIN-INJURED LIFE*), we all made significant internal progress. Once I began to regain self-respect through acceptance of my new "normal," I stopped insisting that people call me "Mark John." I was happy to be "Mark" again, the real Mark. It again felt right to me and to my family, who had indulged me by calling me "Mark John" for more than twenty years. Then again, if the friends I made while I was calling myself Mark John still want to call me Mark John, that is fine too. I have simply stopped *insisting* I be called either one name or the other; that works better for all of us.

Looking back, I am even proud of the times when I was so ashamed because, even at those times, I never quit. I will never quit. Some have asked me how my determination has been possible in the face of the terrible loss and discouragement I have experienced. Others have suggested that I am a perfect example of the resilience required to overcome a life-altering tragedy. *Merriam-Webster* defines *resilience* as "an ability to recover from or adjust easily to misfortune or change." I certainly am not a perfect example of resilience because, one month, I am focused and making the most of my rehabilitation program, and then the next month, I am off track and regressing. None of it has ever been *easy* for me. If another way of expressing resilience is "an ability, with great effort and commitment, to gradually overcome misfortune after decades of continual adjustment," then maybe I am resilient. Formerly, experts thought resilience was an innate quality that some people were born with and others not. I attribute much of my never-quit character to my parents, who have worked so hard for everything they have achieved (including everything they have helped me achieve after brain injury) and who have passed on this ethic to all their children.

Along with other people with high levels of resilience, after my tragedy, I simply never asked, "Why me?" But instead, I asked, "What next?" In my case, it was, "How can I relearn to walk better? How can I relearn to talk better?" Despite the forlornness I experienced at different times, underneath it all was and still is an abiding hope and faith in God. My relationship of love with God is what strengthens and sustains me. Through it all, I—along with every other survivor—remain fully human. Despite our diminished ability, we never lose one whit of our humanity: That realization was the key God used to unlock my psychological prison door and I began believing that I am normal. I am the real Mark John Condon, and I am dealing with my brain-damaged life and circumstances the best I can. With determination, the support of others, and God's help, we can all develop the resilience necessary to overcome even the greatest of life's challenges.

God, my parents, my family, and my circle of support deserve the credit for my excellent adjustment. My brother Dan left his job in Alaska and stayed with me the entire time I was hospitalized. My sister,

Kathy, quit her job, sold her house, and moved to Lansing, Michigan, to take care of me after my discharge from the hospital. My great friend Tom Higley was with my family and me every day at the hospital. Kevin Hall, my best friend at Sacred Heart Academy High School in Mount Pleasant, Michigan, whom I had not seen since my family moved out of town six years before the accident, came to see me in the hospital. (Unfortunately, I cannot remember his visit or anything else from the months surrounding the TBI.) Doug Strachan and the members of his Fort Collins brain injury support group encouraged and persuaded me to pursue professional counseling as a career. Elsha Westhoff, who became as if my second mother, supported and worked with me for more than three years to get me on track and through graduate school.

Dr. Brucker pioneered the therapy that has so greatly helped me both physically and (indirectly) psychologically. Diana Diaz, Dr. Brucker's chief therapist, applied his technology in a unique way that helped me continue making progress from 2007 to 2012. Maria Varela, the current chief Brucker biofeedback therapist, has worked with me since 2012 and has been a part of my significant progress to date. Shaun Corbett, MD, medical director of rehabilitation services with Miami Jewish Health Systems, has been involved with my program since 2015 and has helped me greatly. Without Dr. Gerald McIntosh's oversight of my medical care (1990–2014), I would never have been able to participate either in Dr. Brucker's therapy or in the various supplemental therapies that complement and enhance the Brucker Method. Greg Roskopf developed and refined the Muscle Activation Technique treatment system that surpassed all physical therapy I had previously participated in. The European entity invented the PEMF device that has helped me in unbelievable ways—more than thirty-five years after my injury. Michael Lavery made the connections between brain hemispheres and the opposite sides of the body to develop his Whole Brain Power program, Perfect Penmanship, and later the Communication Game that, together, may well facilitate the neurogenesis survivors need to make it to the next level in their rehabilitation journey.

At the University of Northern Colorado, my professor Dr. Bonnie Drumwright[11b] recognized something in me and asked me to speak to one of her classes about my experience with disability. Without Dr. Drumwright's encouragement, I perhaps would never have begun to speak publicly or written this book. Dave DeLay and Sue Richardson at Bayaud Enterprises[83] worked with me during my graduate school internship. They also contributed greatly to my success. Logan Colter became my best friend in Fort Collins, Colorado; Christian Smith from England became my best friend in graduate school. John Colvin and Jay and Labinia McGee are my best friends in Denver. Elizabeth Rhoden and Tim Campion gave me a place to stay in Denver when I was homeless. Della Mason cuts my hair better than anyone ever has. Keith and Dr. Adelisa Shwayder[11c] read the very first draft of this book and greatly helped me with its wording, presentation, and the appeal of my story. Jane Kopp, PhD, the mother of a TBI survivor and a sometime professional editor among other things, read my third edition, got involved, and—working phenomenal numbers of hours on a completely volunteer basis—elevated my writing a hundredfold, resulting in the book *The Silent Epidemic: What Everyone Should Know About Brain Injury* in its present form. (Other commitments prevented her from checking the final draft and galley proofs, and she will thank me, I am sure, for acknowledging here that I have not always adopted her recommendations. She was not in a position to know or ensure that due acknowledgment was made to sources I have consulted and quoted—I myself am also solely responsible for the compliance of the book with APA Style and with all legal quotation restrictions and citation requirements. I have tried my best to comply with all requirements but cannot remember everything I have come across over the years and am indebted to the great authors whose publications have helped me understand and frame many of the concepts in this book.)

In 2007 when the insurance company refused to do so, Dr. William White paid for my Brucker biofeedback therapy sessions. (Without that financial help from Dr. White, I would not have been able to continue

---

83   www.bayaudenterprises.org.

making rehabilitation progress nor have had the chance to hear Dr. Brucker attest—before he passed—to my extraordinary progress and to his commitment to helping me open a Brucker biofeedback center in Denver.) The magnanimous Dan Puuri paid for my therapy in 2012, when the insurance company, again, had closed my case and refused to pay. Henry Canham with Automotive Search, Inc., in Denver, Colorado, has encouraged and helped me in a number of ways. Fr. Lou Christopulos of Saint Catherine's Greek Orthodox Church, the most Christlike man I have ever met whose faithful example has transformed our church, raising it to an altogether higher level, has also greatly helped me. Without my family, these amazing friends, these professionals, and the many others whom I may somehow have failed to mention (please forgive me), I could not have achieved what I have been able to achieve so far, and I would not be able to accomplish what I am going to accomplish in the future. I cannot begin to thank these people enough. Many, many thanks to all of you—including my uncle Martin.[84]

---

[84] Uncle Martin Domitrovich, my mother's youngest brother, my "favorite uncle" when I was a boy, was such an inspiration to me that I wanted to be just like him. A star running back in high school and college, he even had a chance to play professional football, but he decided to go into business instead and managed to build a financial empire of sorts with Cutco Cutlery. Uncle Martin always encouraged me to play football and would have me start as quarterback in our annual family "Christmas Snow Bowl" on Grandpa Domitrovich's farm in Ontonagon, Michigan. After my brain injury, he remained one of my strongest cheerleaders. The year after my TBI, even though I could barely run, he had me play quarterback in the Snow Bowl, calling me "the Comeback Kid."
Uncle Martin's encouragement and fighting spirit were invaluable to me as I pursued rehabilitation over the years: They still are, even to this day. After my injury, I followed in his footsteps for a time and won a nationwide Cutco Cutlery selling contest working for the Brekmar Company (distributors of Cutco Cutlery). This inspiring man helped many others as well—so many I cannot even begin to count them. (He was key to founding the Equestrian Connection.[11d])
Uncle Martin battled pancreatic cancer for a long time, remarkably beating the terrible odds again and again. It was a great loss for me, and more than three hundred others, when he died from that disease on October 29, 2007.

For the long process of recovery from brain injury then, my own determination has not been enough; I have needed God, along with everyone mentioned and unmentioned in my story here, to achieve what I have achieved. I have had to walk the whole walk, and I still do, but it was and will be others who have opened the doors for me to walk through. I have never lost faith in God, have never quit the rehabilitation routines I developed for myself, and have never stopped seeking feedback on my performance. I feel it is all worth it. I am thankful for who I have become through this disabled, brain injury journey.

Of course, I wish my brain injury had never happened—I suppose that must be how every survivor feels—but we cannot undo brain damage or deny its consequences. Not one of us were released from the hospital, returned home for a recovery phase, and then went back to life as normal. Unlike illness and bodily injury, it is impossible to recover from a brain injury as we commonly think of "recovery." When people get "better" from an illness or bodily injury, they are back to normal; when a survivor gets better, it is better than last month or last year but never "better" as we commonly think of the word—never back to normal as before the BI. David Hovda, director of the UCLA Brain Injury Research Center, explained that the concept of cure—as we think of it—does not apply to brain injury. He declares, "Traumatic brain injury is not an event that you recover from, it's an event that you live with for the rest of your life." CTE is an incurable and ultimately fatal neurodegenerative disease. What we survivors *can do* is decide what to do with the abilities we have post-injury, how best to accommodate our disabilities for the rest of our lives, and to keep working toward self-respect and life satisfaction.

Being able to accept, accommodate, and accentuate life after a traumatic disaster of any kind requires resilience. Over time it has become more apparent to researchers that a survivor's internal fortitude and personal characteristics before his or her BI significantly influence long-term outcomes (Rabinowitz and Arnett, 2018; Richardson, 2002).

Higher resilience has been associated with decreased rates of depression and anxiety and increased life satisfaction after TBI (Marwitz et al., 2018). Resilience has also been associated with healthy, regular social involvement (Marwitz et al., 2018; Wardlaw et al., 2018) and a reduction in depression (Wardlaw et al., 2018). Currently, mental health experts are of the opinion that resilience is multidimensional, not just an innate quality, something that without question is partially inherited but something that can also be developed and enhanced over a lifetime. The documentation of increased resilience in survivors via "behavioral interventions" strongly suggests incorporating "resilience training" into brain injury rehabilitation programs. Resilience is greatly needed after a BI, and survivors are encouraged to learn it. However, after a BI, it is so much more arduous to learn anything if your reference points for coping with tough life changes have been eliminated. No matter how difficult, I know each survivor can develop degrees of resilience—as we struggle to learn who we have become after brain injury and give ourselves the space and time to learn how we now best fit into the world.

It has taken me all these years to get to where I am today, and it should be clear that I do not recommend this journey of long-suffering to anyone. Some have suggested that the success I have achieved is a trophy in its own right. To me, however, it is a pyrrhic victory (a victory won at too great a cost to have been worthwhile for the victor). If possible, avoid every kind of brain injury. However, if your brain has been injured, take care to surround yourself with loving, positive people. The support of loving people is a central ingredient in all the best recoveries as it has been and is in mine.

I have been blessed to have a close family, one willing to sacrifice much time and effort on my behalf, and I am grateful that doctors and nurses treating me have commented many times about how caring and close we are. Cary, the physical therapist at Sparrow Hospital in Lansing, Michigan, remarked that I have a great family and should be proud of them. Physicians in the BI department there told my family that patients who do not have the love and support of their families do not make good medical improvement. My story, in contrast, is in many ways a story about how love heals.

If you cannot find loving people, I strongly recommend that you seek to bring the ultimate, loving higher power into your life. Seek out the love of God—there is nothing better. Gratitude is foundational in response to the higher power of most major religions and spiritual disciplines. Even the secular world recognizes that gratitude is a key part of a satisfying, quality life. People who decide to be grateful experience more positive emotions, better physical health, more consistent quality sleep, and a reduction in stress hormones. I would encourage you to begin saying "thank you" to God for helping you survive what would have been certain death in the past and for helping you today. Then start thanking your optimistic, patient, hardworking family members, friends, and caregivers. A gratitude attitude strengthens relationships, releases the feel-good hormone dopamine, and motivates people to meet their goals. Next, find valid, effective concussion/BI therapies, keep at your program, do not overdo it, modify it when necessary, build your communication skills, develop your relationships, and be careful not to subject yourself to a second head injury. The journey is worth it; *you are worth it.*

In the adorable movie *Finding Dory*, the title character has severe short-term memory loss. After becoming separated from her parents, she forgets them. Then in a flashback, she suddenly remembers everything. As she labors to get back to them, she keeps reminding herself, "Just keep swimming. Just keep swimming." In the movie *Catch Me If You Can*, Frank Abagnale Sr. tells his son Frank Jr., "Two little mice fell in a bucket of cream. The first mouse quickly gave up and drowned. The second mouse wouldn't quit. He struggled so hard that eventually he churned that cream into butter and crawled out."

Dabo Swinney, Clemson University's football head coach reminded his number one ranked team after losing their quarterback Trevor Lawrence (the 2019 National Collage Championship Game's MVP and two-time ACC Player of the Year, who tested positive for COVID-19 in 2020), that they "[h]ave to embrace 'the suck.'" Clemson's football team would have to find a way to compete in Lawrence's absence, the same way they embraced "the suck" and faced different trials over the years. The next game was played with the freshman quarterback, D.J. Uiagalelei, who led the team to score over forty points and forced the game against Notre Dame into overtime. Emphatically, brain injury sucks more than losing a starting quarterback and there is no bypassing that, nonetheless survivors have to find a way to continue getting through it—continue embracing it—as it persists for life.

Even more grounding is Winston Churchill's real-life admonition "If you're going through hell, keep going." I have been through hell myself, "brain injury hell," and the encouragement to "keep going" has helped me along the way—as it will you. I am Frank Abagnale Sr.'s second little mouse, and you too can be it. I have managed to crawl out of the brain injury bucket, and the next thing I intend to do is walk onstage in front of people in different states across our great nation to tell my story. I am not done yet and never will be; like Dory, I won't stop "swimming" and struggling. I keep diligently working to make improvements in my mind, body, and spirit no matter how slow the progress. I encourage survivors to just keep swimming, keep treading water if necessary, until he or she find the supports needed to take the next step up the brain injury rehabilitation stairway.

Always remember that no person on the face of the earth is the "same" person in every respect after a significant brain injury. With the help of others, conduct an honest inventory of the consequences of your brain injury and its associated ramifications (the broader effects that fan out into your world from the brain injury) and then do what you have to do to compensate for those changes in your life.

I keep in place my strategies and routines to accommodate for residual disabilities and to stay on track. The regimen does not work 100 percent of the time, but established routines make it easier to get back in the saddle when I fall off my rehabilitation horse. Like every survivor of a severe brain injury, I will never be out of the woods as far as brain injury goes; it complicates life, work, and relationships either a lot or a little—for a lifetime. But today I am a proud father who earns a small income, receives social security disability insurance benefits, and has solid relationships. I continue to work on personal improvement, and I am respecting myself more—all the time. What I hope fellow survivors and their families will take away from my experience is an awareness that you are not destined to be only a chimera (a thing that is hoped or wished for but in fact is illusory or impossible to achieve) of your former self. Rather, a fulfilling, satisfying life is possible when brain injury consequences are accepted, normalized, rehabilitated and accommodated.

I am intent on making it known to every survivor that my company, Transforming Techniques Incorporated, works with, the therapies and strategies I myself have employed to overcome the dim prognosis originally given to me and to improve my abilities year after year over the decades. I urge advocacy on behalf of every survivor for a change in insurance company policies. Coverage needs to expand treatment across the continuum of care that realistically is greater than twenty years. (Survivors who start from the onset of BI with what I have put together in this book have a good chance of making better progress than I have in much less time.)

As to the satellite Brucker Biofeedback/Transforming Techniques center that I want to open in Denver, Colorado: Before COVID-19 I was in communication with Dr. Rita Gugel (Dr. Brucker's surviving spouse and the present owner of the Brucker biofeedback therapy franchise), as well as with other management staff at Miami Jewish Family Home and Hospital (owners of the Brucker biofeedback center franchise)— developing plans to make that satellite a reality. Post-COVID the future is uncertain, the task is enormous and beyond my resources to carry out alone. P. T. Barnum of the Barnum & Bailey Circus famously said, "Without promotion, something terrible happens . . . nothing." I need other key players to help me promote our business plan/mission statement and to join me in raising capital, making appropriate land acquisitions, pouring the foundation, laying the bricks, purchasing/developing the equipment, and hiring/training staff to fill the center(s). The potential of this venture is tremendous and its benefits as far reaching as reducing the divorce rate of survivors, doubling their employment rate, improving the quality of life for their families, and contributing to the safety of nearly every other family in our country.

James P. Kelley, who I first met in 1998, was again the presenter for the Brain Injury Alliance of Colorado's annual professional conference in Denver, this time in 2015 where the subject of his speech was the National Intrepid Center of Excellence at Walter Reed National Military Medical Center. This center is a model of holistic, interdisciplinary evaluation and treatment in a family-focused, collaborative environment that promotes the physical, psychological, and spiritual healing of service members diagnosed with complex, comorbid TBI and psychological health (PH) conditions. (This is just the kind of facility I have in mind for Denver, one that brings together a variety of medical and mental health professions in a collaborative effort for the benefit of survivors.) In every detail from the wood paneling on the walls, the floor covering, the shape of the hallways, the treatment rooms down even to the upholstery and arrangement of seating, the National Intrepid Center of Excellence is designed to promote healing. It is no surprise that positive rehabilitation outcomes for survivors/families treated in this facility are reported to be exponentially greater than those obtained in any other setting. In addition to its work of diagnosing and treating survivors, the center is dedicated to advancing our understanding of TBI and PH conditions by conducting focused research and exporting knowledge and practices to improve TBI and PH outcomes for service members and their families throughout the Military Health System (MHS). The center's vision—"to be the nation's institute for traumatic brain injury and psychological health dedicated to advancing science, enhancing understanding, maximizing health and relieving suffering"—is one that I and many others can and will support.

No matter how attractive new Intrepid Centers of Excellence/ Transforming Techniques centers may be, however, even if we were to build one with all the latest technologies and breakthrough therapies in every state, such centers would not be able to serve even one percent[85] of people dealing with TBI, acquired brain injury (ABI), and other forms of BI. Additionally because of lack of capacity and financial/insurance coverage or because of individual dispositions, more than half of the survivors will never participate in the programs such centers could offer (some survivors simply will not allow or ask for help). That became apparent to me from working with hundreds of survivors over the years and continually researching the subject. But it dawned on me in 2018 (when I broke all my former rehabilitation records by combining Brucker biofeedback therapy, MAT sessions, and enhanced microcirculation) that much of work I have done to actualize such "never-before-seen medical progress" was done at home. If we can bring those same medical devices *into the homes* of other survivors and populate the nation with MAT specialists and Transforming Techniques centers that house Brucker biofeedback therapy along with other therapies in the CHAMP BRANDISE protocol, we stand a good chance of making never-before-seen progress a common thing among survivors. When that happens, we will effectively increase survivors' life satisfaction fourfold.*

In 2017 after I learned from Dr. Fredrick Parente that when survivors return to work, their two greatest problems are (1) poor social skills and (2) inability to solve problems or make decisions, I realized how far reaching those two problems are in every dimension of life. I also saw that the proposed Transforming Techniques centers need to expand their programs to address such problems. Survivors should be able to learn in our centers not only how to walk and talk again but also how to eloquently communicate, how to make better decisions or solve problems, and how to live in harmonious relationship with significant others again. If our centers can include linguistic proficiency

---

[85]   * "One percent" was derived by calculating the disproportion between the more than ten million survivors and the projected fifty rehabilitation hospitals/centers serving a projected 52,000 survivors a year.

with social skill building, perhaps mimicking the effectiveness of an institution started by my daughter Lia's amazing mother, Dr. Lydia M. Prado, namely, the Dahlia Campus for Health and Well-Being,[86] we will have done just that. When Dr. Prado was vice president of child and family services at the Mental Health Center of Denver, she directed the development of the Dahlia Campus for Health and Well-Being, which provides a place for community members to connect with their neighbors, learn practical skills, and find other needed supports to improve their lives.

With a mission of *"Enriching Lives and Minds by* Focusing on Strengths and Well-Being," the Dahlia Campus for Health and Well-Being is founded on the philosophy that treatment works—that people can and do recover from mental illness. (They provide child and family services, teen and young adult services, and adult services and provide a number of classes and programs such as the Aquaponics Greenhouse, which grows fish and plants together in one integrated system; Chef Lindita's Cooking Class, which teaches how to make traditional food healthier and how to make enough but not too much for different numbers of diners; Trauma Informed Yoga; and Interactive Journaling.) With a different clientele in mind, a Transforming Techniques campus for BI survivors will specifically address, of course, the multifaceted pathologies associated with brain injury.

11a. One of the crowning achievements of BIAC occurred on March 29, 2011, when Colorado governor Hickenlooper signed into law a hard-won piece of legislation titled the Jake Snakenberg Youth Sports Concussion Act,[87] making Colorado one of the dozen or so states to enact such legislation. This bill requires that coaches receive education about concussion, that a student athlete be removed from the field of play if a concussion is suspected, and

---

[86] * Severe BI survivors are 400 percent more likely to express "low satisfaction with life." www.mhcd.org/dahlia-campus-for-health-well-being.

[87] https://www.cde.state.co.us/sites/default/files/documents/healthandwellness/download/brain%20injury/sb11-040.pdf

that that student be signed off by a health-care professional before returning to play. Jake's Concussion Act will keep Colorado's young athletes safer for years to come. It was a proud day for Jake's family, for BIAC, and for all stakeholders who had worked on the bill for over a year. Please note that it took a family with direct BI experience to bring about such a positive change in our community. In the fall of 2004, Jake Snakenberg—a freshman football player—took two typical hits in a game, collapsed on the field, and never regained consciousness. Jake passed away from second impact syndrome on September 19, 2004. May his memory be eternal.

Another substantial legislative achievement for BIAC was finalized in December 2008, when then governor Ritter signed an executive order on traumatic brain injury.[88] This executive order was nationally groundbreaking in that it required that executive directors from a wide variety of state agencies designate a member of their professional staff to represent their agency in developing a coordinated employment plan to address the needs of Colorado state government employees who have experienced a brain injury. I was honored to speak at the forum and to be seated at Governor Ritter's table for the signing of that order.

BIAC is involved in many programs. It facilitates more than seventy support groups across our state, which have the purpose of helping survivors share with and support one another for the mutual benefit of each participant as well as that of the entire group. In addition to the sharing of experiences, a support group can provide (1) knowledge about and understanding of brain injury and (2) an atmosphere where group members can develop their communication/social skills to express both positive and negative views without being judged or labeled. BIAC's nationally recognized outdoor camps afford an opportunity to build friendships, gain confidence, and likely have more fun than their participants might have thought. BIAC's outdoor camps welcome

---

88   www.denverpost.com/2008/12/08/ritter-orders-agencies-to-smooth-patients-paths-toward-recovery.

inquiries from participants and volunteers all across the United States. BIAC is also a member of the Colorado Brain Injury Collaborative, which is dedicated to improving the lives of more than one hundred thousand survivors in Colorado. Learn more at www.biacolorado.org.

11b. Regarding Dr. Drumwright's encouragement of me to speak publicly, it was based in part on the letter she had read in my application file at the university describing what life for me has been like since my brain injury and what I have learned from it. My application letter was based on still another letter I had written earlier to the perpetrator of my brain injury—the drunk driver. I wrote to that driver ten years after our fateful car crash, letting her know exactly what harm she had caused. My hope was that I might help her take responsibility and *prevent her from driving drunk again.* In case she was forever tormenting herself about the incident, I offered her my forgiveness while reflecting on my own shortcomings. I began the letter like this:

> You don't know who I am, but you do know my name. I don't believe you know what I look like? I have never seen you and have no idea what you look like. We have never spoken to each other and I have never gotten a note, a card, or a letter from you—no communication whatsoever, none. However, you have changed my life *completely!* No one else in the entire world; not a member of my close family; not my best buddy; not a girlfriend; nor anyone else—has changed my life like you have. My name is Mark John Condon, I am the person who was driving the car you crashed into on March 7, 1981. But I am not the same Mark John Condon I was before that night. I'd like you to know some things about me now. I want you to know what you did to me, because I don't think you know. I want you to know how your six-point reckless driving

violation has affected me. I'd like you to know how your
crime has completely changed my life…

I spared no detail in trying to communicate to her what she did, but I closed the letter forgiving her completely and wishing her a good life. The fact is I have never spent time resenting her or holding her in debt for what she did to me. Many have asked me why not. It never occurred to me, and I didn't have time for that. I was committed to working on recovery. Also, I had learned from my religious education, and later from my psychological training, that lack of forgiveness is one of the biggest obstacles to health and well-being. Not forgiving a person is like you taking poison then waiting for the other person to die. I encourage you to let go of any unforgiving attitude you may be holding on to. Think of it as an anchor weighing you down and compromising your rehabilitation because that is just what it does. I do not need anything that compromises my rehabilitation progress, and neither do you. I made sure my letter got to the drunk driver (having it hand-delivered by my attorney back in Michigan), but to date, I have never heard from her. May God bless her.

With Dr. Drumwright's encouragement, I have developed my letter of application to the University of Northern Colorado into a speech on traumatic brain injury, weaving my experience in with selected, relevant national statistics. I spoke to her class, Introduction to Rehabilitation 101, for an hour. Later in the semester, Dr. Drumwright told me that my speech had had the biggest impact on her class of any of the presenters she invited. One student in the class looked me up to tell me he had changed his declared major to rehabilitation counseling after hearing my speech. In 2003, at the request of the Brain Injury Association of Colorado, I copyrighted a later edition of that speech, calling it "The Silent Epidemic: What Everyone Should Know About Traumatic Brain Injury." When Dr. Randy Lennon, one of my professors in graduate school who now calls me his colleague, read my article, he wrote a recommendation for it and encouraged me to write an entire book. *The Silent Epidemic: What Everyone Should Know about Brain Injury* is the culmination of my efforts in that direction—it adds supporting evidence, new viewpoints, and additional chapters and further develops some original ideas.

11c.   While on vacation in 1999, Keith and Adelisa Shwayder's son—who was twenty-four years old at the time—went for a swim with his girlfriend in a remote river in Mexico, only to suffer grave consequences. The river turned out to be laden with an undetectable toxin. The girl who was with their son died, and he himself continues to have cognitive issues more than twenty-seven years later. In April 2015, a similar tragedy occurred when three members of a Delaware family were exposed to toxic chemicals during a vacation at a Virgin Islands resort. The Esmond family of Wilmington, Delaware, was staying at a Caribbean resort when their incident was reported nationally. According to the Associated Press, "The Esmonds were vacationing in St. John at an $800-per-night resort when a worker sprayed methyl bromide in the condo below theirs, according to EPA officials. Within days, the family was sick."[89] EPA's regional administrator, Judith Enck, said, "When you're on vacation, the last thing you're thinking about is if your hotel room is soaked in pesticide. You're at their mercy." At the time, the family spokesman, James Maron, along with the medical professionals, expressed hope of a full recovery. Unfortunately, both the Shwayders and I know that the boys will never "fully recover" if they do survive this unthinkable tragedy. Almost a year after the incident, the wife and mother, Dr. Theresa Devine, was able to get out of her wheelchair. Steve Esmond, the husband and father, and their two teen sons, Sean and Ryan, were all afflicted with severe neurological damage and remained paralyzed.

---

[89]   www.delawareonline.com/story/news/local/2015/11/29/pesticide-poisoned-delaware-family-still-use/76545738.

11d. Equestrian Connection[90] was founded in 2001 by Diana Schnell, a mother of disabled twins who felt that hippotherapy could benefit her twins in a way that traditional therapies had not. Ms. Schnell said, "We began with four horses and twenty clients using rented space in a hunter-jumper barn. Our focus was hippotherapy and therapeutic riding but we needed more space . . . Martin Domitrovich stepped forward and made our dream come true. He was instrumental in locating and buying a ten-acre site, including a three-acre spring-fed lake, upon which site we built a 26,000 square foot state-of-the-art facility. Our indoor arena, the 'Domitrovich Arena,' is named after Martin and his family. We are grateful that his family continues to support our cause and carry on his legacy." Chad and Crista Jeske of Eagan, Minnesota, wrote in his obituaries, "There are only a few people in my life that I can honestly say made such an impact on me with the passive class than Martin did. It is good to know that his morals, professionalism, beliefs, and spirit will continue on through everyone that has met him. He will be missed, but remembered as a true champion." At his funeral, many others expressed their respect and thanks for who Martin Domitrovich was to them and for what he had done for them. If I, or anyone, can help half as many people as Uncle Martin did, it will be a tremendous accomplishment. May his memory be eternal and his life lived out through his wife, children, and grandchildren. He was the hero of many, and I was blessed to have him on my "team" for many years.

---

[90] www.equestrianconnection.org.

12

INSURANCE—CATASTROPHIC CLAIMS ASSOCIATION

The American Medical Association maintains that brain injury survivors reach their maximum medical improvement in two years. As a result and sadly, many insurance companies stop paying benefits after two years. Trisha Meili, the New York Central Park jogger who was raped, bludgeoned, and left for dead with severe brain damage in 1989, has not, for one, found the supposed "24-month window of recovery, after which improvements plateaus" to be a reality. She said, "I built an amazing support system that helped me focus on what I could do, rather than on my deficits."[45] Meili has continued to improve over the years, breaking rehabilitation records—regaining abilities— and given the progress so far, she looks forward to discovering just how far recovery can go. The implications of her case, as well as that of mine and other survivors, are that *recovery can continue for many, many years beyond the purported two-year limit*. Although still disabled, I have made some of my most dramatic improvements ten, twenty, and even more than thirty years post-injury. Peradventure it was the insurance companies that persuaded the AMA to adopt its untenable "two-year MMI" position regarding BI rehabilitation to limit their long-term, continuum of care liability?

In the 2010 groundbreaking article "Traumatic Brain Injury: A Disease Process, Not an Event" by Brent E. Masel and Douglas S. DeWitt, TBI for the first time was revealed to the world as a "long-term chronic condition." While their pioneering work was not a revelation for survivors and their families, it was an appreciated confirmation of everyone's experience. However, Masel and DeWitt's seminal report generated a paradigm shift for BI medical professionals and insurance companies and payers who were responsible for survivors' long-term care. Their understanding expanded and connected with the truth when they began to see BI as a progressive, lifelong disease rather than an isolated, onetime event. According to the 2019 *Brain Injury Professional*, a quarterly publication produced jointly by the North American Brain Injury Society and HDI Publishers,[44] ongoing research describing TBI as a chronic condition since 2010 has gathered near universal acceptance, with multiple reports and publications supporting Masel and Dewitt's position.

Prolonged rehabilitation for a chronic brain injury condition is expensive—nearly every severe survivor needs a long-term continuum of care rehabilitation program—and nearly every insurance company refuses to pay for it. Even with Masel and DeWitt's undeniable, scientifically based 2010 revelation that TBI is a chronic disease process with long-term health-care needs and long-term health-care costs, the implications of that advent to date have not been fully realized.

My family and friends have been extraordinary in their patience, sacrifice, and generosity, yet we would never have been able to afford everything that has been prescribed and purchased for my rehabilitation program over the years had it not been for a unique automobile insurance policy. My insurance policy was written in Michigan, and Michigan, as far as I know, is the only state in the nation that provides auto insurance with unlimited personal injury protection benefits via the Michigan Catastrophic Claims Association (MCCA).[91] The MCCA—a private, nonprofit, unincorporated association—was created by Michigan state legislature in 1978, three years before my accident. Michigan's

[91] www.michigan.gov/documents/cis/MCCA_FAQ_2007_190996_7.pdf.

particular auto insurance no-fault law provides unlimited lifetime coverage for medical expenses that result from "catastrophic" auto accidents. The MCCA reimburses auto no-fault insurance companies for each personal injury protection (PIP) medical claim paid above a set amount. Currently, that amount is $580,000. That means that the insurance company pays the entire claim but is reimbursed by the MCCA for medical costs over $580,000. All auto insurance companies operating in Michigan are assessed to cover catastrophic medical claims occurring in the state. Those assessments are generally passed on to auto insurance policyholders. The 2019 assessment was $220 per vehicle (i.e., everyone licensing a car in Michigan each year pays an additional $220 on top of the normal insurance fees). Since 1979, more than 40,715 catastrophic claims have been reported to the MCCA. With current estimates, the total claims paid, including the future payments for the 17,751 remaining active claims, is expected to exceed $85 billion.

For many years, the valuable exclusive, unlimited benefits provided by the MCCA made it possible for me to afford extensive hospital and rehabilitation treatments. Because of the MCCA, my insurance company continued to pay for all medically necessary therapies and support systems prescribed for me until 2015, more than thirty-four years post-injury. *I could not have made the significant improvement I have made without the therapy treatments and rehabilitation equipment purchased through the MCCA.* I cannot help thinking, therefore, that every state in our country should have a similar policy. My position is supported by the American Speech-Language-Hearing Association (ASHA), which reported in 2011 that even worse than the increasing numbers of brain injuries in our country is the fact that "inadequate insurance coverage may be the biggest obstacle to optimal recovery." It simply seems obvious to me (and to my professional colleagues) that every state in our nation should have a catastrophic claims association.

According to the National Institute for Disability and Rehabilitation Research, at least two-thirds of TBI survivors discharged from rehabilitation hospitals after a typical stay of sixteen days get no further treatment. Most need further treatment, but neither the patients nor their families realize that additional rehabilitation services are available. "The fact is, a lot of people are not getting into rehab," says Rep. Bill Pascrell, D-NJ, cochairman of the Congressional Brain Injury Task Force. Brent Masel, director of the nonprofit Transitional Learning Center in Galveston, Texas, is reported to have said, "Insurance companies do not want people [survivors and their families] to know that there's another step after they leave the hospital."[92]

The Brain Injury Association of America's online article "Inpatient Acute Rehabilitation Hospital Bills and Costs"[93] reported the average rehabilitation charges per patient were almost $1,600 per day and about $46,000 total. Rehabilitation together with room and board services (which were more than $46,000 total) accounted for 90 percent of the hospital bill. The estimated lifetime monetary costs of brain injury are $85,000 for mild, $941,000 for moderate, and $3 million for severe head injuries.[94] How could any family or any insurance company afford such an expense without a catastrophic claims association?

Unfortunately, even with the MCCA policy backing me, my insurance company found a way in 2015 to get around it and stop paying for the very therapies that their expert, whom they had hired to evaluate me and my therapy program, had said were "medically necessary." As a part of my final legal settlement with Travelers Insurance Company, on May 29, 2015, they had a doctor with Colorado Rehabilitation and Occupational Medicine—one who regularly conducts IMEs for Craig Hospital—conduct an IME on me. (Craig Hospital, I explained earlier in this book, is a

---

[92]   https://www.google.com/search?client=safari&rls=en&q=www.
        kingfish1935.blogspot.com/2012/05/need-rehab-after-brain-injury-check.
        html&ie=UTF-8&oe=UTF-8.

[93]   www.biausa.org/professionals/research/tbi-model-systems/
        inpatient-acute-rehabilitation-hospital-bills-and-costs.

[94]   https://news.northwestern.edu/stories/2015/12/opinion-next-avenue-
        brain-injury/

The Silent Epidemic: 215

world-renowned rehabilitation hospital exclusively specializing in neuro-rehabilitation and research for patients with spinal cord injury or brain injury.) Initially, I counted myself fortunate that this doctor was to conduct my IME because he speaks with the authority of *the* Craig Hospital. I was crestfallen and confused to read his report, however. He recommended that Travelers Insurance take away from me some of the very therapies he *also said were necessary to emphasize* at this point in my recovery. My head was spinning—how could this respected doctor contradict himself? Why would he do that?

About the benefits of Brucker biofeedback therapy, what this doctor wrote was the following:

> What I observed was significant improvement in overall gait mechanics with reduction of the left lateral trunk lean and much more normal mechanics throughout the left lower extremity, most notably absence of toe drag, which was significant in the videotape footage in November 2014 and almost completely absent in subsequent videotape footage in December 2014 post treatment.

He said further, "The emphasis at this point in his recovery should clearly be on active therapy as opposed to passive therapies." The biofeedback and gait training received at the Brucker biofeedback center *is* an active therapy, one that includes objective measurement of functional improvements post therapy. Yet in the same paragraph, this same doctor recommended eliminating Brucker biofeedback therapy altogether after only two more series of treatments.

I want to point out here that Muscle Activation Technique (MAT) sessions, as its name implies, are even more "active" than the Brucker Method therapy. MAT was brought to this doctor's attention—it epitomizes what he recommended as medically necessary for me—yet no mention at all of MAT was made in the IME. MAT sessions are exactly what this doctor recommended as medically necessary for me—active therapies. However, it must be that he does not know of, or cannot perceive, *what continued* Brucker biofeedback therapy, *regular* Muscle Activation Technique sessions, and *daily* enhanced microcirculation are *able* to rehabilitate or does not understand *how* they do indeed rehabilitate "permanent" brain injury neuromuscular disabilities. If I might borrow from a story in the Hebrew Bible, when Moses came down from the mountain with the Ten Commandments, the glory of his countenance was so great that the children of Israel could not steadfastly behold it, and he had to veil his face. Can it be that, to the vision of excellent doctors like those at Colorado Rehabilitation & Occupational Medicine, there are "veils" over the great Brucker biofeedback method, the Muscle Activation Technique therapy, and the PEMF microcirculation enhancement device? These doctors apparently cannot steadfastly behold the undeniable truth that the simple, brilliant activities of these three modalities combined are more effective for restoring neuromuscular function than any other protocol currently available.

I was perplexed but not in despair when I read the IME report. I actually am thankful that Craig Hospital via Colorado Rehabilitation & Occupational Medicine recommended discontinuing my effective and valid (if so far misunderstood) therapy regime. I am thankful for this reason. If I can, nevertheless, somehow continue with that regime and in fact *surpass* my 2015 level of function—something which that Craig Hospital doctor and most doctors say I cannot do—then perhaps they will all change their minds about what is possible not just for me *but also for other brain injury survivors*. I trust that that doctor who speaks with the authority of Craig Hospital will then help change the minds of other doctors—and in doing so help half a million brain injury survivors living in Colorado and many millions more beyond our state's border.

As to "affording to continue with my current regime," in 2015, I was fortunate enough to learn of a national nonprofit, the mission of which is to support community-based fundraising for people with unmet medical and related expenses resulting from cell and organ transplants or catastrophic injuries and illnesses. That nonprofit's name is Help Hope Live.[95] What it does is bring together family, friends, and communities to organize tax-exempt fundraising efforts to help patients and families pay for medical bills and services as well as gain access to much-needed alternative treatments and therapies. Each person and his or her campaign is paired with a Help Hope Live fundraising coordinator who can offer expert fundraising support. Help Hope Live fundraising campaigns are eligible for corporate and foundation matching gifts, and all donations are tax deductible. Help Hope Live even awards an incentive grant to each campaign once it reaches its first fundraising goal. Funds raised are not counted as income or assets for patients, so if patients are on social security income or social security disability insurance, those benefits remain in place. Help Hope Live has an outstanding track record (more than thirty years long) of building successful fundraising campaigns.

Legislators and insurance companies in other states beyond Michigan who may be considering making catastrophic claims insurance mandatory should note that the estimated lifetime costs of traditional AMA medical approaches for a severe brain injury are $3 million. That is more than *three times the cost* of the CHAMP BRANDISE protocol I am proposing (see detailed figures in the appendix). Even if there were zero cost savings, the significantly better rehabilitation outcomes associated with the CHAMP BRANDISE protocol—the significantly greater level of personal/vocational independence, quality of life, expanse and depth of relationships, dignity, self-respect, and community "payback"— would alone be worth it.

The fact that our medical profession adamantly prescribes the current therapy protocol that has failed me and so many other survivors, and that costs survivor families along with our country so much money, is unconscionable. John Steele Gordon, author of *An Empire of Wealth:*

---

[95]   https://helphopelive.org.

The Epic History of American Economic Power,[96] helped me understand how this folly has been perpetuating itself. Gordon wrote in "A Short History of American Medical Insurance"—published September 2018 in volume 47, number 9 of *Imprimis,* a publication of Hillsdale College—that no matter how you look at hospital insurance plans, they are polar opposite from other insurance plans. The insurance business was founded on the proposition that companies would—in exchange for a premium—pay clients for great, unexpected, and infrequent catastrophes while in such instances clients first pay a deductible.[97] Contrary to this workable proposition, the first hospital insurance plans used an opposite formula—instead of protecting against large unforeseeable losses, they paid for everything up to a certain limit or "cap." The insurance industry would never have conjured up such an ill-conceived formula—but the hospitals did.

Reflecting the profitability plans of *businesses,* hospital insurance plans were designed to make money—by generating a continual stream of money paid for medical care, therapeutic services, prescriptions, and equipment. Hospital insurance policies only paid out if bills were from the hospital, ensuring that most every case would be handled by and in the hospital, which according to Gordon is "the most expensive form of medical care." This insurance structure worked against the convenient, less expensive, and sometimes more effective treatments available in outpatient medical care facilities. Gordon said, "Additionally hospital insurance did not provide indemnity coverage." (Indemnity coverage reimburses for medical emergency events rather than for specific services so the customer can apply funds as he or she chooses.) In lieu of indemnification, hospital insurance paid for any and all of the specific *services* included in the policy. Consequently, there was no impetus or

---

[96]   www.johnsteelegordon.com/books.html.

[97]   An insurance deductible is the amount of money you will pay in an insurance claim before the insurance coverage kicks in and the company starts paying you. Once you pay your deductible, the insurance company will pay you the rest of the claim value up to the policy limits and conditions as specified in the wording.

reason for policyholders to look for a lower cost or better value, and "patients quickly became relatively indifferent to the cost of medical care," which was exactly what the hospitals wanted—sick, injured, diseased, and frightened people giving them the green light to provide any and all forms of medical services.

Gordon offers economical, commonsense, practical solutions to the medical insurance debacle that currently is consuming 15 percent of the country's GDP. He recognizes, however, that there are powerful economic interests arrayed against his solutions. Gordon's article ends on a note of hope, however. "But at least we have one thing on our side—Stein's law, named after the famous economist Herbert Stein: 'If something cannot go on forever, it will stop.'" If public attention can be focused on the Silent Epidemic and if far reaching publicity can be given to the fact that more affordable and medically effective therapies are currently available, then the practice of continuing to prescribe expensive *inadequate* therapies will not continue forever; prescribing deficient therapies that are bankrupting millions of families and our country itself will stop.

45   T. Meili, *I Am the Central Park Jogger: A Story of Hope and Possibility* (2003), www.shape.com/lifestyle/mind-and-body/trisha-meili-central-park-jogger-how-running-helped-heal-interview.

13

HOW MANY SURVIVORS? HOW IMPORTANT?

According to the 2010 American Board of Professional Neuropsychology's *Handbook of Forensic Neuropsychology*, second edition,[46] edited by Arthur MacNeill Horton Jr., EdD, ABPP, ABPN, and Lawrence C. Hartlage, PhD, ABPP, ABPN, there are more than nine million new cases of brain injury each year. By the age of sixty, an average American will have suffered two significant head injuries, and three out of five people in America will have been considered seriously head-injured.

The *Journal of Head Trauma Rehabilitation*'s survey "Prevalence of Self-Reported Lifetime History of Traumatic Brain Injury and Associated Disability: A Statewide Population-Based Survey"[1] reported that only 10 percent of the people surviving a traumatic brain injury are admitted to a hospital, 30 percent of whom suffer from "long-term disability." Yet in Colorado, they note, over 40 percent of adult residents have had a TBI at some point, and nearly 25 percent suffered a "TBI with loss of consciousness (LOC)." Of Colorado survivors in the survey, only 27 percent were hospitalized. The survey corrected a Centers for Disease Control (CDC) estimate of the number of survivors—raising it to three times higher. This major adjustment was made in part because the CDC's disability prevalence estimate is derived solely from people hospitalized with TBI, a category that clearly *fails to capture the full extent and impact of brain injury*. Compared with people with no history of brain injury, survivors of mild TBIs with LOC have a 100 percent increased chance of "poor outcomes." Moderate TBIs have a 200 percent increased chance of "poor outcomes," and severe TBIs face a 300 percent increased chance of "poor outcomes" with a 400 percent increased chance of "low satisfaction with life." "While the proportion of people with disability after TBI was higher in those with more severe injuries," the authors say, "the absolute number of people reporting disability after TBI was higher in those with less severe injuries." Whiteneck et al. conclude this excellent work by identifying survivors as "a clear population in need of services and interventions." Higher percentages of negative outcomes were observed, they note, for injuries of similar severity that were treated in less intense settings. "This suggests that brain-injured people who receive inadequate medical attention or follow-along services experience more serious consequences." The situation for these survivors is all the more tragic in view of the fact that valid, effective, and affordable therapies that could restore much of their lost function and life enjoyment are currently available.

In view of the astronomical number of people who suffer a head injury each year in the United States, proclaiming brain injury a critical national epidemic with far-reaching, complicated consequences is being unequivocally realistic and forthright. Furthermore, failure to immediately treat and thoroughly rehabilitate each and every survivor of this epidemic is ensuring far-reaching negative *social* and financial consequences. "It is clear that research, advocacy, and policy efforts need to continue at unprecedented levels so that individuals with TBI can more universally gain access to the care they need, when they need it—even decades following the initial event" (p. 10).[98]

Given the ten million US citizens who are brain injury survivors with long-term disability, how important is it to get out the message that it is time to reduce the incidence of drunk or reckless driving, helmetless bike riding, headfirst techniques in sports, falling, and domestic abuse? Will over $8 billion of savings each year be important enough reason?

---

[98] *Brain Injury Professional* 16, no. 3. (*Brain Injury Professional* is a membership benefit of the North American Brain Injury Society and the International Brain Injury Association.)

Will personal independence for more than two million survivors each year be important enough? Will improving the lives of more than twenty million family members be important enough? Will saving the lives of fifty thousand people each year be important enough? Will reducing the millions of violent acts perpetrated on the abused by the abused each year be important enough? Will keeping over two hundred thousand taxpayers gainfully employed as contributing members of society and off public entitlements each year be important enough? Will addressing the brain injuries our soldier warriors are suffering from, reducing their suicide rate, and improving the quality of their family life be important enough?

Will preserving some of our nation's favorite sporting events and entertainment venues be enough? Will maintaining the mental capacity of over a hundred thousand athletes each year be important enough? Will stopping the caregiver-killing, degenerative, brain-injury tragic horrors be enough? Gladiators fought to their death in the "glory" days of Rome, but they knew the risk of their "sport." For them, personal safety was not an issue because they did not have much of a life, or a choice, outside the arena. For young high school athletes today, however, real life takes place outside of sports; yet because of their coaches' negligence, most are left unaware that in contact sports they are at great risk for brain injury. Still less do they understand that if, after suffering a brain injury, they continue to participate in contact sports, they are in danger of incurring the kind of cumulative brain injury—CTE—that will permanently impair their quality of life or even kill them.

As you learn of the possible bewildering alienation that awaits you if you become a survivor of brain injury, you will, I hope, be more cautious when you are driving or riding in or on automobiles, motorcycles, bicycles, or horses because the truth is *great brain injury danger is invariably associated with those activities*. According to the National Highway Traffic Safety Administration, drunk drivers kill more than 10,500 people a year in the United States. In addition, motor vehicle/traffic crashes cause more than 290,000 traumatic brain injuries each year. Our entire nation rightly felt horror at the loss of life when New York City's Twin Towers fell on September 11, 2001, killing 2,977 people, yet drunk drivers are responsible *each and every year* for the equivalent—in terms of lives lost—of *three* 9/11 World Trade Center disasters. (In drawing this comparison, it is certainly not my intention to detract from the sacred memory of the victims of 9/11 or from the grief of those who mourn them.) What I am saying is that loss of life, no matter where or how caused—whether by a terrorist, a drunk driver, a virus, or something else—should *not* be treated as an acceptable routine matter without consequence.

After the 9/11 World Trade Center disaster, America rightly focused on making our homeland safe from foreign terrorists. The Federal Aviation Administration has said it spent more than $4 billion to purchase high-tech bomb scanners for US airports. It was estimated that over the following two-year period, state and federal governments combined spent more than $25 billion to prevent any similar foreign terrorist tragedy, and they will continue spending more indefinitely.

The US secretary of Health and Human Services (HHS) declared a public health emergency on January 31, 2020, under section 319 of the Public Health Service Act (42 U.S.C. 247d), in response to COVID-19. The threat of this unknown worldwide virus rightly warranted such intervention. After the virus spread beyond containment here in our country, even with employing social distancing and face masks, it was expected to infect 40 to 50 percent of the population and with a probable mortality rate of 1 to 2 percent, kill 1.5 to 3.0 million citizens. According to the CDC, just before we go to print, the projected number of deaths in our country from COVID-19 cannot be determined – the actual number of deaths was just over 500,000. In February 2020, to save lives and "flatten the curve" (the virus outbreak curve), our government made available $58 billion to combat and contain COVID-19. In March the US Senate and Congress made $2 trillion available to assuage the associated economic repercussions of COVID-19. In March 2021 another $1.9 trillion was approved by our government's new administration via the COVID-19 Relief Bill. If the amount of money spent by our United States government for government for COVID-19 relief were apportioned directly to tax paying citizens, each would receive $42,000 ($41,870), and each couple $84,000. Spending a tiny fraction of that money each citizen could have obtained the repurposed, long-standing, safe medicines that have proven to be as much as ninety percent effective in completely eradicating the COVID-19 virus—instead they were given a $1,400 check and a $42,000 tax debt with no foreseeable way to pay for it.

In March, Illinois governor J. B. Pritzker issued Executive Order 2020-10 requiring all Illinoisans to stay home from work to prevent the further spread of COVID-19. Pritzker said, "If I can take steps to save lives during this pandemic[99]—then I have an obligation to take those steps—no matter how difficult." In April New York governor Andrew M. Cuomo said, "This virus is truly vicious, it is an invisible, insidious beast, and we all have an obligation to do what we can to protect each other—to protect the most vulnerable." In response to the widespread concern that the economic shutdown will have negative consequences that outweigh the consequences of the COVID-19 virus, Cuomo—fully aware that 24 million people had become unemployed and anticipating that number could soon double—said, "How can the cure be worse than the illness, if the illness is potential death?"

Juxtaposed with the following facts:

- six teens (16-19 year olds) die each day from motor vehicle crash injuries;
- eight people die each day from distracted driving;

---

[99] Pandemic: The word "pandemic" comes from the Greek "pan", "all" + "demos," "people or population" "pandemos" = "all the people." A pandemic affects all (nearly all) of the people—it is an epidemic (a sudden outbreak) that becomes very widespread and equally threatens all the people of a whole region, a continent, or the world. By definition, a true pandemic causes a high degree of mortality—this virus only has a 0.1% degree of mortality. Further, COVID-19 has never affected all of the people "equally." The CDC reported COVID-19 mortality rates for ages 0-19 at .003%, and ages 70+ at 5.4% (people 70 years of age and older are 1800 times more likely to die from COVID-19 than people 19 and younger).

- twenty nine people die each day from alcohol-impaired driving;
- 1,000 bicyclists die each year;
- 5,900 pedestrians die each year; and
- TBIs kill over 50,000 people each year

With the conflicting lack of money appropriated to prevent such vicious loss of life from any one of these causes—TBI in particular—one cannot help but second guess our elected officials. This glaring discrepancy calls into question their declared "obligation to take steps – no matter how difficult – to protect the most vulnerable and each other from death."

There are views on both sides of the benefits or harm from society-wide steps taken to control the COVID-19 virus outbreak. While this virus and its victims have become a political football kicked in different directions, I only want to use COVID-19 (with the greatest respect for the deceased and their memory) to contrast the disparity between the monetary funding, public awareness, and medical effort directed at treating people threatened or infected with the virus—and what's being done to prevent or rehabilitate brain injury.

The Centers for Disease Control and Prevention reports 2,028,000 people have died from brain injury since my accident in 1981.[100] Additionally, you are now aware that 10 million US citizen/survivors suffer personally and daily from negative long-term consequences—my book describes many of those terrible outcomes, along with the dire concomitant familial/societal ripple effects of brain injury. Twenty million more people—family members/caregivers—also suffer daily from BI consequences. However, in any two-year period, the United States will spend less than $1 billion to prevent drunk-driving tragedies—one of the leading causes of brain injury. This monetary contrast glaringly demonstrates how much more could be done to protect the public from deaths and brain injuries caused by drunk drivers. Law enforcement and legislatures need to streamline the process for getting drunk drivers off the road, and society owes it to itself

---

[100] http://www.ncdsv.org/images/CDC_GetStatsTBIintheUS.pdf.

to make drinking and driving socially unacceptable. If our country's governors and elected officials truly feel an obligation to save lives and "protect each other," they will eagerly take the necessary, commonsense, cost-effective steps outlined in this book—"no matter how difficult"— to relegate the Silent Epidemic to an "audible occurrence" and force the brain injury scourge to drastically decline—saving millions of lives and improving multiple millions of lives—all while conserving trillions of dollars.

The family of a woman named Marisa Rodriguez (see chapter 5 "The Extended Impact of Brain Injury") was reportedly awarded $7.5 million by the tire company responsible for an injury she suffered when her vehicle crashed due to tire failure.[14] People who drive under the influence of alcohol need to be held similarly responsible for the costs they cause in the way of loss of life and diminished quality of life.

The *New York Times* printed an article by Dan Barry on September 11, 2017,[101] reporting that the state of New York had agreed to pay $22 million to a boxer who sustained severe brain damage during a heavyweight bout at Madison Square Garden in 2013. The settlement was awarded to an up-and-coming but now former Russian heavyweight boxer, Magomed Abdusalamov, and his family. Abdusalamov—thirty-six, the married father of three girls—was left unable to walk or speak in complete sentences, according to his lawyer, Paul Edelstein, who said further, "This award means everything to them. Their lives have been incredibly limited and reliant on the help of others. This is going to help them give him care and as dignified an existence as possible." The greater sporting world, criminals, and drunk drivers who injure the brains of their opponents and victims need to be held similarly responsible for the millions of dollars in costs associated with the loss of life—the diminished quality of life—they allow or cause. The same should be required of the perpetrator of any brain injury—to afford as dignified an existence as possible for the survivor and his or her family.

---

101   https://www.nytimes.com/2017/09/11/sports/mago-boxer-settlement-new-york.html.

According to the *American Jurisprudence Desk Book* (used for proof of fact in the US legal system), many of the millions of Americans who sustain traumatic brain injury each year are never diagnosed; furthermore, fewer than one in twenty patients gets the rehabilitation he or she needs. "Even where the patient has a clearly documented loss of consciousness, trauma physicians missed the diagnosis in 72 percent of the cases and emergency room physicians missed it in 52 percent." Certainly, this is in part why nearly every article on brain injury mentions a need for further education of health-care professionals. The *American Jurisprudence Desk Book* acknowledges that "[u]ndiagnosed patients may be at increased risk for development of additional symptoms that they may not identify as related to their brain injury." Currently, millions of undiagnosed survivors with symptoms such as depression, cognitive difficulties, anger control issues, and personality changes have not been taught that such symptoms may be properly attributed to brain injury. Not knowing this, survivors themselves shoulder the "blame" for such symptoms, feeling all the more inadequate, all the more alienated and alone. It bears repeating for everyone's sake that *trauma physicians, emergency room physicians, and every other kind of physician and health-care professional must place more emphasis to diagnose brain injuries and rehabilitating survivors.* For that to happen, the implication is blatantly obvious—brain injury education must become a significant part of medical/health-care academic programs, required for degrees and also for continued medical recertification.

In 2005, top neuroscientists and physicians from across the United States and around the world produced a document titled "Report to Congress: Toward Successful Recovery from Traumatic Brain Injury," which reported that "little has been accomplished in improving brain injury diagnosis and survivor outcomes since 1998." *Neither, unfortunately, has much been accomplished since 2005.* In 2017, the Colorado Department of Human Services report "Brain Injury Program: Hard to Serve Study"[102] found the following:

---

[102]   www.tbicolorado.org/tbi/wp-content/uploads/2017/08/CO-DHS-Brain-Injury-Program-Hard-to-Serve-Report-080417-Final.pdf.

There is no standardized screening and identification protocol to identify brain injury. Brain Injury is under-diagnosed or misdiagnosed and therefore treatment is postponed. This is true across systems, especially behavioral health, education, and vocational service providers.

Providers need better training on the symptoms of brain injury to avoid differential diagnosis for individuals. Behaviors related to a brain injury are often misidentified; therefore, interventions do not consider the brain injury, making them less likely to be successful. For individuals with co-occurring needs there are no clear lines to distinguish which symptoms are associated with which behaviors or diagnoses. This can lead to diagnostic overshadowing where these symptoms are attributed to the more prominent disability and are left untreated.

Complexity associated with treating brain injury and co-occurring conditions creates access limitations. Providers indicate complex needs as their biggest constraint to serving more individuals with brain injury. There is limited expertise in brain injury available for educators and providers with which to consult.

Holistic care coordination generally does not exist for people with brain injury. People with brain injury tend to have many providers involved in their care but communication and information sharing isn't consistent. Communication and information sharing between providers is limited because of information technology constraints and broader system silo issues.

Transition to adulthood is a specific example of where improved care coordination could benefit people with brain injury. School services supporting transition to adulthood are not perceived as successful by students with brain injury or providers. The transition from school-based to adult systems is inconsistent. (all italics added)

For the sake of our enlisted and veteran military personnel, recreational and professional athletes, young and old US citizens alike who are brain injury survivors, and all their family members, we simply must transcend the dysfunctional yet negatively consequential status quo of our medical/health-care systems when it comes to brain injury— the fiascoes of "missing the diagnosis," the frustrating insurance disputes, the lack of state-run catastrophic claims associations, and the clearly untrue pronouncement that MMI is reached after a few years. We must, in fact, fast-track the opening of centers/campuses that provide: Brucker biofeedback therapy, Muscle Activation Technique therapy, Designs for Strong Minds programs, Mind-Eye Connection programs, Mojo Feet orthopedics, Whole Brain Power exercises, Communication Game coaches, enhanced microcirculation devices, Vigen far-infrared light therapy, FocusBand, and informed rehabilitation counseling; as well as other valid, emerging, therapeutic approaches that can be shown to significantly improve neuromuscular function, cognitive abilities, social skills, and/or psychological health in a way that saves lives and/or significantly improves quality of life.

Even before such centers are built, we must work to equip the home of each survivor with a European PEMF microcirculation device and with Vigen far-infrared light therapy equipment. We also need to provide him or her with Whole Brain Power/Communication Game routines, Strong Mind Puzzles and Strong Mind Treasure Hunt apps, and other valid BI rehab products or programs. Such a combined home/clinic approach could cut through the Gordian knot of brain injury rehabilitation, a field that to date, according to the world's top neuroscientists and physicians, has not substantially improved recovery outcomes.

Of course, when the medical industry can make over $2 million per severe BI (over the survivor's lifetime) by merely maintaining the status quo (Even if at the expense of: each severe BI survivor's well-being; his or her family's quality of life; the best interests of the community; insurance policyholders and taxpayers.), the status quo may well remain ensconced. Dr. Mark Hyman is of the opinion that the health-care industry and everyone involved with it hold on to outdated ideas and prescribe and pay for medical specialties or ineffective brain injury therapies because, in his words, "Abandoning these ideas or ways of doing things, threatens their economic viability and maybe even their existence." Barry J. Hoffer and colleagues, who together researched pathways considered important in TBI rehabilitation, had to ask, "Why many animals used as rehabilitation models benefit from candidate treatments for concussions—while again and again these promising drugs fail to meet regulatory requirements for approval for human use?"

I know many excellent doctors, and I believe most doctors in our country are doing an amazing job of treating a wide range of aliments, injuries, and diseases. I do appreciate and respect them. The majority of doctors are not themselves aware, however, of what truly does work affordably well to rehabilitate brain injury survivors. These same doctors simply accept the fact of ten million survivors with long-term disabilities of various degrees trudging around as "walking wounded." I have had clients whose doctors released them once they had improved by 50 percent. My god! How can 50 percent be called success or be called maximum medical improvement? To me, such a low expectation is inconceivable. I understand, however, that such an outcome may be all that can be expected as long as doctors utilize only the Sisyphean rehabilitation therapies they prescribe at present, those "verified" in their laboratories and clinics to do no harm, even though they do not significantly rehabilitate the brain injured. In the human court of appeals, I maintain that to accept ongoing dependency and only partial rehabilitation for even one brain injury survivor—when that survivor could be much more fully restored—is doing great harm on several different levels—not only to the survivor but also to many others in the community.

Abraham Lincoln once said, "To correct the evils, great and small, which spring from want of sympathy, and from positive enmity, among strangers, as nations, or as individuals, is one of the highest functions of civilization." Ninety-six percent of the American public thinks it is important to invest in research to prevent, treat, and cure disability, yet research in our nation on brain injury remains deficient. I believe everyone who does something to reduce the prevalence of brain injury in his or her community or to normalize and accommodate the consequences of BI in the lives of people with brain injuries is participating in one of the highest and most important functions of civilization.

Teddy Roosevelt said, "Far and away the best prize that life has to offer is the chance to work hard at work worth doing." So many brain injury survivors can no longer work hard or maintain gainful employment. In an ordinary instant, brain injury robbed them of one of the best prizes life has to offer—being satisfied after a day of productive work. Inspired by Roosevelt's reflection, I and others working hard on behalf of survivors are, again, participating in one of the highest functions of our civilization. And we are helping survivors who are working their way toward reclaiming the best prize life has to offer.

How many survivors? *Ten million and counting.* How important an issue? One of the top ten issues of our lifetime—personally, locally, and nationally.

46 A. MacNeill Horton Jr. and L. Hartlage, *Handbook of Forensic Neuropsychology*, 2d ed. (New York: Springer Publishing Company, 2003).

14

INTERNALIZING WHAT YOU SHOULD KNOW

According to a recent MetLife/Harris survey,[103] older Americans are now more concerned about losing their cognitive abilities than they are about cancer or heart disease (the two leading causes of death). What people don't know, however, is that the fastest way to lose cognitive ability is via brain injury. Americans don't hear much about that because the public *does not want to hear* about brain injury. Being informed that someone is cognitively disabled or confused or cannot remember what has just been said, people choose not to relate. They have no idea how to fix it, and they are reminded of the vulnerable nature of their own minds. Even though the general public is more aware today of Alzheimer's, Parkinson's disease, brain injury, dementia, stroke, and CTE than it was when I was injured in 1981, most people still would rather not consider the possibility of their *own* "inevitable" mental decline. The less willing you are to accept that you yourself could suddenly become mentally disabled, the less you want to know about those who have been so afflicted. You naturally want to hold on to the belief that you will never be inconvenienced with such a cognitive adversity as those other people. Unless you die young, however, the one sure thing is that you will live part of your life with a mind that no longer allows you to complete simple daily tasks you carry out now without a second thought.

Recapitulating now briefly what earlier parts of this book have detailed: If you become moderately/severely brain injured, you might be

---

[103]   https://www.metlife.com/content/dam/microsites/about/corporate-profile/alzheimers-2011.pdf.

vexed with perplexity, distractibility, fatigue, and short-term memory loss. You will likely suffer from degrading mental health consequences, chronic pain, and low life satisfaction. You might have to think to turn your foot out, swing your leg straight, strike your heel first, and not hyperextend your knee backward with every step you take. You might get lost in the local supermarket or not be able to find your way home. You might not be able to assemble a simple eight-piece puzzle.[14a] You might repeatedly forget you left a stove burner turned on or water running in the sink or where your keys are. You might forget how to be intimate with your spouse. You might have to think about everything you do before you do it, but because it will have become so difficult for your brain to think, each time you do think, the effort of it might further deplete your mental batteries, making it all the more difficult to do anything proficiently. You might never get a good night's sleep again. You might be fatigued throughout the day, every day of the week, and be unable to work or socialize. You might repeatedly forget what duty your boss said needs to be done first, second, and third on any given day of the week—and become unemployable. You might find yourself with a warped sense of time, clueless to its lapsing, and always late for appointments.

You might suffer from aphasia (an inability to locate words) or dysarthria (slurred speech); you might speak disconsonantly (fail to enunciate consonants) or lose your ability to recognize speech patterns altogether. You might only be able to manage small talk and not be able to engage in the more substantive conversations that happier people enjoy, or you might maunder. You might lose your ability to understand spoken language and your ability to communicate. You might not understand idiomatic expressions ever again. You might be unaware that you always interrupt the person you are talking to and, by so doing, push him or her away. You might not be able to help yourself from angrily confronting your family and friends whenever a decision needs to be made—and again, by so doing, push them away.

You are likely to be rejected by family and friends and coworkers—which will "infect" you with a psychological cancer and its associated loneliness. Healthy self-esteem might become impossible for you. You might laugh when you want to cry or cry when you want to laugh. You might be ostracized, unwanted, and rejected by others, which necessarily might push you toward greater social isolation. That, in turn, will likely obliterate your self-respect and your internal locus of control—having lost both, you truly will become "enslaved" and may experience absolute solitary confinement. In the end, if you were to give up on the effort required to self-regulate, you will find it impossible to maintain relationships and be "buried alive"—lost to the world and those who knew you.

You might, for the rest of your life, be clinically depressed. You might be worse off than if you are blind, deaf, or paralyzed. You might become confounded with ordinary life, baffled by social expectations, bewildered with unspoken etiquette rules that everyone else seems to follow without a second thought. Being jejune, you will be perplexed and confounded when you are bamboozled, hoodwinked, and taken advantage of by different people you thought were friends. If you become addlebrained, you will necessarily be flighty, nonsensical, and befuddled much of the time or oblivious to your faux pas. You *might not know that you do not know*, while everyone else will.

If you become mildly/moderately brain injured, chances are you will never be examined or diagnosed for brain injury. With no medical record of concussion and no way to account for related problems, such as mentioned, you will not have an informed way to address those problems. Every level of brain injury greatly increases the chance of low satisfaction with life—*and multiple brain injuries likely make that inescapable.*

Family and friends often can empathize with the visible consequences of a more severe brain injury such as hemiparesis, mobility issues, or language and word-finding difficulty. Without obvious physical manifestations, however, they simply will not excuse the invisible mild/moderate BI disabilities that inherently have far greater negative consequences. Invisible disabilities commonly associated with mild/moderate brain injury such as controlling impulsive/inappropriate behavior, making proper eye contact, controlling anger, listening to others while in conversation, making simple decisions, solving ordinary problems, remembering what was just spoken, or simply thinking—without being understood and accommodated—become a contagion that infects and kills relationships.

With a brain injury, every day you might feel compelled to kill yourself. With your ego depleted, you might, in fact, commit suicide—as too many survivors do—with the nearest available method—a gun, an oncoming truck, a gallon of antifreeze, or a bottle of pills. Or you might inflict violent injury on others. Influenced by normalcy bias, you might have difficulty reacting to your brain injury "disaster;" you likely will not be adequately prepared for the lifestyle change it demands, and you might tend to interpret permanent consequences in the most optimistic way possible—as merely temporary. Your family, with their own normalcy bias, might think you should just be able to stop being so *forgetful* all the time or stop *procrastinating* all the time (substitute the *italicized* words with any number of brain injury outcomes) because, in their minds, a "bump on the head" can't be that big a deal. Soon after being brain-injured, you might well find yourself more depressed more often than you ever have been in your life. In addition to all this, your family might lose their lifestyle and be strapped with a financial burden they cannot bear alone.

While the thought of being buried alive gives us a horrific image, the actual threat is miniscule unless we work underground in construction, in sewage, or as miners. Solitary confinement, on the other hand, is the dreadful consequence of the worst of crimes, and it has been thoroughly studied. I think it better parallels the negative consequence of some brain injuries than does the analogy of being buried alive. Solitary confinement has been reported to cause hypertension, headaches and migraines, profuse sweating, dizziness, and heart palpitations. Many inmates in solitary confinement also experience extreme weight loss due to digestion complications and abdominal pain. Such symptoms are due to intense anxiety and sensory deprivation. Solitary confinement can worsen both short- and long-term psychological and physical problems or make it more likely that such problems will develop. Extended solitary confinement can cause insanity. It is so likely to cause insanity that the federal government has imposed a moratorium of fifteen days on holding prisoners in solitary confinement (after a transition period, during which it is capped at twenty-one days). Such a dreadful temporary consequence may well be fitting for the perpetrators of violent assaults. Assault victims themselves with brain injuries, however, may actually face fifteen to twenty-one years or more in "solitary confinement" from the inherent personal rejection and social isolation too many survivors are subjected to—and this "punishment" is never acknowledged, capped, or compensated.

It is not any one symptom that causes survivors' lives to fall apart but the gestalt of brain injury. The full gamut of brain injury consequences is what is so formidable, so life robbing, so difficult to deal with for survivors, *their families, and their caregivers*. With a brain injury, you lose yourself to some definite degree, whether that is a little or almost completely. Frank Sinatra sang in his song "My Way," "What has [a man] got? If not himself, then he has naught." After a brain injury, you will unfortunately no longer *have* yourself—not *all* yourself.

As a survivor, because of limits on your insurance policy—that is, if your policy was written in a state that does not have a catastrophic claims association—you probably will not get the rehabilitation services that are medically necessary. If your brain injury is invisible, as so many are, society will not know what is "wrong" with you. Consequently, they will paint you with a mysterious otherness and may ostracize you from the inner circle of relationships. There is no publicly recognized category for BI survivors, no Special Olympics they can take part in, and no clear answers from rehabilitation professionals about how they can maximize progress while accommodating their newly disabled selves. If you were to become brain-injured, you—like so many others—might be as helpless and isolated from the normal world as if you were on another planet or alone on a wide, wide sea—alone, alone, all, all alone.

For you to better appreciate what life can be like after a brain injury, let me use an illustration. We have all heard the expression "He is not playing with a full deck" or "She's a few cards short of a full deck," in reference to someone who is "slow" or incompetent in some way. In a sense, after a brain injury, you really have lost cards, neurological cards, that you can never get back—not completely. After severe brain damage, you will certainly be slower, both physically and mentally, and you will have to live the rest of your life with certain blind spots (the neurological cards you lost). What is it like to live life with brain injury blind spots? Take a deck of cards and paint some black on both sides—let these represent your neurological blind spots. Then if life can be compared to driving a car, take the black cards, tape them over half of each rearview mirror and half the windshield, and then go for a drive. You can see clearly out all the other windows but only out of half the windshield and rearview mirrors. When you are looking behind backing out of your driveway and maybe driving around the block, you do OK; in fact, your driving may look "normal" to everyone who is watching. But as soon as you get out in city traffic, you're bound to have an accident, are you not? With blind spots from a brain injury, when you get out in the traffic of real life, you are bound to have a relational or a vocational conflict, to offend someone, to say something you did not want to say, to forget a work procedure, or forget a meeting, an event, or a commitment again and again. You're bound to burn food on the stove—even burn the pan itself (I have done that twice), you will leave your tennis shoes in the locker room, or not take your medicine occasionally or frequently.

When you're not engaged in some real-life activity, you won't have any trouble; you will look normal watching TV or listening to music. However, because people cannot see your blind spots and you look just like everyone else when you are behind the steering wheel "parked in the driveway," they naturally expect you to be able to "drive around town" just fine, to take part in *ordinary* life like everyone else. When you "crash"—and you will crash—they will not understand why. They'll ask you why you did not see the "social stop sign," but you will not have a good answer. Either you will not know why or you will not want to admit having a disability that you do not accept or fully understand and may never be able to adequately compensate for. (It can take a long time to fully realize and admit the extent of your brain injury disabilities.) Depending on the severity of a brain injury, people lose a range of neurological cards, from dozens to thousands of thousands. Many survivors have to "drive" through life without a full deck, with more than half their "windshield, mirrors, and windows" all blacked out. If you suffer from CTE, you may lose "the entire deck" and die young.

Rene Descartes (1596–1650) was an eminent scientist who postulated as much as anyone ever has about the about the duality of human existence. He generated an understanding of what came to be known in Western philosophy as "mind-body dualism." He reasoned that the psychic "space" inside one's head is infinite and metaphysical and therefore must be of a nature different from that of the rest of the body. Descartes said that he could imagine himself being without his body, floating, moving around like a ghost, watching the happenings of the day at home or in public, but he could not imagine being without his mind and having just his body at home or in public. How could his body experience life or comprehend the interactions of those around it without its mind? Impossible. Wouldn't you agree?

Perhaps you have heard of Descartes's famous proposition "Cogito, ergo sum." (I think, therefore I am.) I bring Descartes up to help you understand that he could not and you cannot imagine what it is like to be unable to imagine—to be unaware of social dynamics, to not know your normal self, to be unable to stop "the voices" in your head, to not know what needs to be rehabilitated (let alone how to rehabilitate it), or to not know that you do not know. It is as if the life of a survivor becomes a foreign language, but it is even more difficult than that, for this is a foreign language that no one speaks, a foreign language almost no one can understand or interpret. Only a few interpreters of this very foreign language have ever lived—the late Oliver Sacks was one; Dr. Robert Cantu is another. If severe brain injury has entered your life and if you have only the AMA's rehabilitation guidelines to go by, most likely, you and your family will be baffled by brain injury's confusing consequences, and all of you will have difficulty living your lives for the rest of your lives. Of course, you as a survivor cannot understand post-injury life expressed "in a foreign language" either; so naturally, you withdraw—with a brain injury or stroke that steals your language ability, you will likely withdraw far away from ordinary life.

This next illustration of what BI life compares to should better help you put yourself in the place of a survivor—to better empathize with BI survivors you may know. Why you "as a BI survivor" get stuck in procrastination, *why* you have persistent cognitive fatigue or depression, *why* you no longer have the executive function you once had, or *why* you can no longer control your anger is vastly different from why your family and friends have their failings. The difference between your experience of life as a survivor and theirs might be better understood by comparing looking over the edge of the Grand Canyon from behind a safety barrier with walking up to the bare edge to look straight down. From behind the safety barrier, you ooh and aah in appreciation of the astonishing immensity of nature, you breathe in the fresh air, you laugh together with your family or friends, you shout and listen for an echo, you look for hawks flying in the sky, and you take pictures. In complete contrast, if you are like me and most people, if ever your feet are on the sheer edge of a great cliff or skyscraper under construction without a safety barrier (without a reference point), your whole body tightens up; you get as low to the rock face or floor as you can—even on your belly—or reach for something secure to hang on to. You don't laugh, you don't notice the birds flying above, and you won't dare take your camera out because you cannot afford to be distracted. It is as if you are utterly alone. To "survive," so as not to fall, you abandon even the thought of any other activity.

As brain injury survivors struggle to deal with life (a fearful life that feels skewed, foreign, and unfamiliar), some feel not only that their safety barriers (their social or vocational reference points) have been taken away but also that they are alone on the edge of the cliff, fatigued and with a strong wind blowing: Devoid of memories and life-lessons learned, they have nothing to hold on to. In a survivor's confounded quest for that which no longer has dimension, where there is nothing he or she can lay hold of, neither place nor time, neither measure nor anything else our damaged brains can seize, many of us slip at every point, at every situation and every exchange that we cannot grasp— then, without a "handhold" become dizzy, lost, perplexed or defensive. No wonder we tighten up, withdraw, and shut down both in body and mind. Feeling awkward and isolated, such survivors don't know how to act or react. What they want to do is crawl away to safety. All too often, they simply avoid others or withdraw from many aspects of life, get stuck procrastinating, or develop "negative pacifier habits" to avoid such feelings.

I have compared here the feeling of life with a brain injury to the universal human fear factor because we all know how fear can seize us on the edge of a cliff, in front of a crowd, or near big growling dogs. We can walk with no problem balanced on a four-inch beam on the ground, maybe even with our eyes closed; but put it ten feet up in the air, and most people simply cannot do it. We understand easily how fear affects us but do not understand so easily how a brain injury can affect ourselves, our spouse, how it can "freeze" our children or friends in a similar fashion. People do not understand how a moderate concussion can prevent even an *intelligent* survivor from maintaining a regular schedule or an intimate relationship or doing a hundred other things. If fear can seize the average person, and it most certainly can, a brain injury can capture and confuse the average survivor in a similar manner. The next time you deal with a survivor (there are a lot of us in Colorado and across the country), I hope you can begin to grasp what that person may be dealing with. Please listen patiently, express yourself succinctly, be willing to clearly and slowly repeat what you have said, allow him or her to repeat his or her own words if necessary, and take the time to learn if there may be a way you can help.

Understandably, minor head injuries receive less attention than severe head injuries because they have less dramatic or observable consequences—initially. However, there is a definite risk of major complications occurring in a small percentage of people with minor head injuries. The sheer number of such people constitutes a significant public health problem. Prof. Sam Wang, who is associate professor of molecular biology and neuroscience at Princeton University and coauthor of the best-selling book *Welcome to Your Brain*,[47] has emphatically said that the common belief that we only use 10 percent of our brains is untrue. Professor Wang points to extensive research showing that, although we have one hundred billion neurons in our brains and we only directly engage ten billion during an average day, we need all one hundred billion of them active and available to function normally.

I noted in chapter 3 that Knox, Mehl, and Ludden found that damage to specific areas of the brain may render survivors unable to read or hear what is communicated through this or any other book. Brain researchers Marcel Just and Tom Mitchell at Carnegie Mellon University tell us that when different people read a sentence about people or animals doing things or watch the activity on a video, researchers with an MRI machine and a computer program can see that the same thought is occurring in the same volume element of the brain of each person. Whether watching the video or reading the sentence, at the conceptual level, it is the same brain activity—in the same location. Just and Mitchell have found a "universality of the alphabet of human thoughts" that has been called a "common language" of all people or the "innate language of thought," which has been recognized and researched for many years. They have expanded on this observation, maintaining that thought precedes and is directly tied to both spoken and written speech across all languages. They have observed that the brain clearly has a "vocabulary," and they are beginning to understand it. Unfortunately, in some survivors, there is a break in the conceptual level of understanding language that leaves them incapable of comprehending what written or spoken words mean. For them, the "alphabet of human thoughts" is mixed up and cannot be understood. The work of such excellent people as Marcel Just, Tom Mitchell, Bernard Brucker, Robert Cantu, James Kelley, Oliver Sacks, Michael Lavery, Rainer Klopp, and Graham Boulton may eventually lead to universal solutions to communication difficulties, neuromuscular pathology, and psychological issues for survivors all around the world.

Addressing the causes of brain injury is one urgent priority; improving the record of accurate diagnosis and informed treatment is another. Gretchen Voss, author of "Women and Concussions" in *Dr. Oz the Good Life*,[31] tells the story of Lynn Staffa, who regrets not being more self-aware and persistent with her health-care providers after her car accident in December 2012. Although Staffa did go to the ER with a severe headache, the physician simply recommended ibuprofen and never mentioned or screened for the possibility of brain injury. Consequently, Staffa said, "The thought that I had a concussion never crossed my mind" (p. 49). Had the doctors knowledgeably diagnosed her concussion and at least recommended rest and recovery before returning to her normal work schedule, she said she would not have gone right back to her job as a social worker with demanding twelve-hour days.

Five months after her car accident, Staffa could not concentrate, her balance was unreliable, and she was plagued with "unexplained anxiety." The doctors were at a loss to account for her symptoms. Eight months after being rear-ended, a doctor suggested she might have had a minor brain injury and referred her to a "specialized clinic." By the time the referral was made, she could not drive a car or walk safely without accommodations. After months of therapies to correct her symptoms, her neurologist told her, "The symptoms would most likely continue for a long time. Perhaps forever" (p. 49).

It was once a widely held belief that people suffering a minor head injury recover "with no residuals." Sir Charles Symonds, KBE, CB,

DM Oxon., FRCP, an honorary consulting physician to the National Hospital, Queen Square, London, WC1, and consulting physician emeritus for nervous diseases at Guy's Hospital, has always disagreed with that assumption. Symonds has expressed his opinion in the article "Concussion and Its Sequelae,"[48] published in *the Lancet* magazine *"the best science for better lives."* He maintains that each injury to the brain is everlasting and intrinsically serious. Over the years, more doctors who treat survivors have developed the same opinion as Symonds. In 2011, medical research documented that about 20 percent of annual patients with "mild" head injury (1.2 million) continue to have persistent post-concussive syndrome symptoms. In light of such statistics, Symonds's declaration "It is hard to think of any brain injury as 'minor'" rings true.

People beleaguered with post-concussive syndrome have to live all or a part of their life with residual symptoms such as depression; constant headache; chronic fatigue; poor sleep; emotional lability (emotional instability, rapidly changing emotions); susceptibility to overstimulation (when overstimulated, the brain freezes and is unable to function even at its diminished capacity); difficulty handling stress and calming down; loss of executive functions; hypersensitivity to light, sound, motion, touch, and the like; pain in the neck or back; reduced range of motion in arms or legs; reduced flexibility and strength; numbness or tingling in hands, fingers, or arms when waking up; loss of grip strength; inability to perform job duties; diminished vocational earning capacity; incoordination; loss of fine finger dexterity; compromised immune system; irregular digestion and elimination; hormonal imbalance; compromised muscle activity/connective tissue/ skeletal system; neurometabolic cascade (neuronal dysfunction due to ionic shifts, altered metabolism, impaired connectivity, and changes in neurotransmission); chronic pain; difficulty in producing speech and communicating; inability to process auditory information or read printed words; inability to understand spoken language unless it is enunciated slowly and repeated once or twice; inability to produce eloquent communications or clear speech; inability to multitask or focus and concentrate on more than one thing at a time; inability to comprehend normal, everyday matters or to problem-solve; limited short-term memory capacity; tendency to abuse alcohol or drugs; inability to maintain intimate or personal relationships; great difficulty in decision-making; and a tendency toward psychological/mental health problems and social isolation. Survivors are often inept with relationships and lack the financial wherewithal to entertain friends, go out on the town or travel, causing further social isolation. If they are plagued with poor sleep and constant fatigue, any effort they make is likely to be desultory. Brain injury can also cause epilepsy and increases the risk for both Alzheimer's and Parkinson's diseases or other brain disorders associated with old age. Survivors alive twelve months after a TBI are 2.33 times more likely to die than normal non-brain-injured people and have a reduced life expectancy of nearly ten years (Brooks et al., 2013; Harrison-Felix et al., 2015). Teenagers and middle-aged survivors are especially at risk for death compared with their normal counterparts.

Given the vast number of people suffering a head injury each year in the United States, to respond to brain injury as anything less than a *major national epidemic with far-reaching, complicated negative consequences* would simply be less than rational.

14a.   I drew the brain-puzzle picture on the inside flap of the back cover twenty-two years after my accident. It vividly reminded my mother of the time when I could not put together a simple eight-piece puzzle in the hospital. (I did not know I was unable to assemble a puzzle in the hospital after my brain injury until the year I copyrighted the first edition of my book and my mother saw my brain-puzzle picture on the cover. Then she told me what happened in the hospital and that she thinks of it every time she sees the brain-puzzle picture.)

47 S. Aamodt and S. Wang, *Welcome to Your Brain: Why You Lose Your Car Keys but Never Forget How to Drive and Other Puzzles of Everyday Life* (New York, London, New Delhi, Sydney, 2008), https://www.bloomsbury.com/us/welcome-to-your-brain-9781596912830/.

48 C. Symonds, "Concussion and Its Sequelae," *Lancet* 279, no. 7219 (1962): 1–5, http://www.oalib.com/references/14262809.

15

CONCLUSION

Everyone needs to know about the prevalence, lifelong consequence, preventability, and treatability of brain injury. A brain injury may begin in a variety of everyday ways—as an acute medical injury from a slip and fall, from a car accident, from contact sports, from an infection, and the like—only to become a permanent chronic health condition with far-reaching complications that negatively affect not only the survivor but those closely associated with him or her as well. While a brain injury is likely to have significant negative consequences for a survivor's spouse and immediate family in particular, its ripple effect can extend far beyond, from reduced productivity in the workplace to increased violence in the extended community. Even when a survivor can adequately perform his or her old job, lingering BI symptoms will likely deprive him or her of the quality of life he or she had before being brain-injured. Over the years after a brain injury, a variety of symptoms and growing needs may gradually emerge and require the involvement of multiple service systems. A well-coordinated, functional, person-centered approach to rehabilitation and reintegration, however, can ensure that survivors get the medical and holistic care they need to achieve better health and life outcomes. A statewide catastrophic claims association (supplementing insurance policies) can be indispensable for accommodating the huge financial obligations of utilizing a variety of medical systems from different levels of health care for decades after brain injury.

The phrase "Silent Epidemic" was coined back in 1980 by Martin Spivack, MD, when his daughter Debbie became a brain injury survivor. Brain injury is not as "silent" as it once was—thanks to the work of

Debbie's mother, Marilyn Price Spivack; to Jake Snakenberg's family and the Youth Sports Concussion Act[104]; to the media's coverage of military TBI survivors returning from the Middle East; to the groundbreaking new hospital design of the Walter Reed National Military Medical Center and Dr. Kelly's work there; to the American Stroke Association; to Dr. Bennet Omalu, who discovered CTE, and Will Smith's spot-on portrayal of him in the movie *Concussion*[105]; to the tremendous efforts of educating the public by the King of Concussion, Dr. Robert Cantu; to the Brain Injury Association and Brain Injury Alliance of America; to sports commentators who are exposing the long-term effects of CTE in professional football players, boxers, volleyball and soccer players; and to Gale Whiteneck and her colleagues for giving us a more accurate assessment of the far-reaching extent of the Silent Epidemic. But the depth of the problem is still a far cry from being common knowledge. And tragically, the frequency of brain injury has not slowed but continues apace, affecting a disproportionately large number of people. *Brain injury is still epidemic.*

It is hard for me to believe, but since my accident more than thirty years ago, the incidence of TBI has not decreased. In fact, it has increased. The American Speech-Language-Hearing Association recently reported a "dramatic increase" in traumatic brain injuries among the civilian population nationwide. Currently, with every day that passes in our country, 22,000 more people have *unexpectedly* been head-injured, more than 153 of these have died, and more than 2,317 others have become permanently disabled. By next week, 110,000 more will have become brain injury survivors. It makes me cry that

---

104 https://www.cde.state.co.us/sites/default/files/documents/healthandwellness/download/brain%20injury/sb11-040.pdf

105 *Concussion* is a 2015 American biographical sports medical drama film directed and written by Peter Landesman based on the 2009 *GQ* exposé "Game Brain" by Jeanne Marie Laskas and starring Will Smith as Dr. Bennet Omalu, the forensic pathologist who fought against efforts by the National Football League to suppress his research on the brain damage suffered by professional football players. The film also stars Alec Baldwin, Gugu Mbatha-Raw, and Albert Brooks. Columbia Pictures released the film on December 25, 2015.

most of these terrible injuries/fatalities *could have been prevented* if only the perpetrators had followed existing laws or rules or if only the survivors had employed safety measures. Haven't we learned anything yet? What is it going to take for society to wake up and deal with this epidemic? All of us—including the powers that be in the sporting world who have disgracefully ignored the prevalence of brain injury and its life-diminishing, caregiver-killing long-term consequences—need to address this national epidemic *today*.

The neuropathological realities I have been trying to describe in this book are ineffable—beyond spoken or written words. Such realities transcend any possible "normal" life experience. Whether I compare life with a severe brain injury to driving a car with blind spots, reading a text without its schema, being on another planet, being in the worst quagmire, being all alone in the middle of a wide, wide sea, trying to understand a foreign language that no one speaks, walking on a narrow beam or tightrope up in the air or standing on the very edge of a cliff, the fact is that life with significant brain damage is beyond any comparison. Words *truly cannot* capture the experience. A brain injury can even prevent a person from being aware that there has been a drastic shift in his or her own cognition. What it is like to live with brain injury is beyond any human ability to imagine. Only great authors like Oliver Sacks and Dr. Cantu can help us approach what we cannot actually comprehend about brain damage. Quite simply, our non-injured counterparts in the general population *cannot* conceive what surviving a brain injury is like. Yet it has never been more necessary for us as a community to begin talking both locally and nationally about brain injury—strengthen our efforts to prevent brain injury and to more fully rehabilitate survivors when brain injury has occurred.

With open dialogue, the use of reasonable precautionary measures, and the proliferation of National Intrepid Centers of Excellence/ Transforming Technique campuses offering as axiomatic the effective therapies I have so far identified and those we will discover in the future, traumatic brain injury could cease to be the dreadful *Silent*

Epidemic that it now is. I have written this book, often using the personal pronoun *you* intentionally, to help each reader realize that he or she, without exception, is in the at-risk category for a brain injury. Brain injury happens all the time, a hundred times more frequently than AIDS infection and all other STDs combined. The need for precautionary measures against at-risk sexual behaviors is recognized and promoted without question, as it well should be. Not at all publicly understood, however, is *how much is at risk* in the case of brain injury nor how likely such injury is. Even more shocking, measures to *reduce* that risk are not promoted vigorously enough. Brain injury/brain health education is inadequate, the promotion of preventive, safety measures is lackadaisical, and effective rehabilitation protocols and campuses are woefully scarce.

With *The Silent Epidemic: What Everyone Should Know About Brain Injury*, I have done my best to awaken people to the imminent threat of brain injury and its far-reaching consequences, to offer insight into the mysterious otherness associated with it, and to inspire the over ten million survivors in our country with the hope that they can significantly improve their lives and their relationships if they face the fact of their brain injury's consequences and take measured, proactive step to accommodate such. Hope is a feeling of expectation and desire that a future positive event will materialize—even if it is unlikely. Health-care professionals now recognize that hope is linked to happiness, resilience, and better physical and psychological health. Doctors who treat patients with life-threatening illness have told me that hope can be as powerful as any prescription drug. While the medical odds are against BI survivors, following the CHAMP BRANDISE protocol may well make a positive future more likely than not—for all of us—I hope it does. The author James Baldwin said, "Not everything that is faced can be changed, but nothing can be changed until it is faced." Please, with courage face your life post-brain injury and put together a protocol that works for you.

◆

This book is a brief sketch of the traumatic brain injury experience in America. I know much more needs to be said, yet what I do manage to say here I dedicate to all who are experiencing disability because of—and who are attempting to grow through—brain injury. If you are a survivor, please do not use me and my story for purposes of comparison (everyone's brain injury and situation is different) but rather for encouragement, if it can be that for you. You will always be a normal human being, quintessentially a normal human being, although you may feel otherwise. Certainly, you are more like everyone else than you are different from everyone else, regardless of any changes that may have occurred in your mind or body. Perhaps now you will be able to see through all the charades and dishonesty that people hide behind when they separate themselves from "others"—other ethnicities, other religions, other social standings, other political parties, other XYZs. Carolyn Vash, in her book *Psychology of Disability*,[49] attempted to break down the barrier between the statistically normal population and others and wrote, "The fact is human beings are more alike than different, regardless of variances in their physical bodies, sensory capacities, or intellectual abilities." Not nearly enough people have read those words of Carolyn Vash, but I hope to make them more widely known. Every survivor is a normal person no matter what variance his or her mind or body manifests. The physical, cognitive, and psychological disorders that result from brain injury are the *normal* outcomes with that kind of injury.

The Hunchback of Notre Dame by Victor Hugo is the story of a person who was born deformed. His appearance was so different and unattractive in the eyes of most other people that they mocked and ridiculed him. Quasimodo was indeed born with an ugly twisted body, but his heart and soul, full of compassion and love, were beautiful, even though few around him sensed the inner beauty that was his. A contrasting character in the story, though appearing in priestly garb, had nothing like a priestly or even a naturally good nature. One of the lessons of the novel is that we cannot judge a person by his or her appearance or social status.

In the same way, a brain injury survivor may be badly misjudged because of his or her speech or behavior. A brain injury survivor may look "normal," but that person's broken brain may be anything but normal, and his or her behavior may be stuck in some "ugly" mode. It may remain stuck there for a time—like a broken record—yet "beautiful" functioning may again become possible for that survivor with the help of a loving family and a valid, effective long-term, continuum of care rehabilitation program.

I do not want any survivor to give up and be resigned to his or her current disabled status. I believe every survivor can make degrees of significant improvement by participating in specific therapies—in some cases a little progress, in others a lot. Victor Hugo acknowledges in his novel that fate plays a powerful role, but he implies that free will matters. Use your free will *survivor,* along with what remains of your brain's capacities to work toward improvement. Brain injury sucks! Embrace the suck. Be the second little mouse that Frank Abagnale Sr. told his son about, the mouse that with great effort managed to churn the cream into butter and crawl out of the bucket. (Warning: It is not simply effort that can benefit a survivor's rehabilitation progress; it is effort combined with supportive family members and friends, effective therapy programs, home-based rehabilitation equipment/programs, positive cognitive/ communication skill building, and available rehabilitation campuses. In fact, repeated effort with the wrong therapy programs and approaches can be counterproductive.)

I know with all my heart that if you can take one step forward with a brain injury, it is as if you have climbed a mountain. Do not expect others to acknowledge your accomplishment – your mountain. To them, it looks like just a small step, a molehill. So what? For you with a brain injury, it is not a small step; it is a gigantic step, even equivalent to reaching the summit of a great mountain. Being able to snap the fingers of my left hand was, for me, like having reached a mountaintop—it took me sixteen long years to be able to do that, but I did it. From that "mountaintop," I then looked for the next "small" step to take, for my next "mountain" to climb. Never forget that after a serious brain injury, a little progress is truly substantial progress (medically significant progress)—so please do not disparage yourself if you have to take "baby steps" for years like I did.

Actually, if you undertake the CHAMP BRANDISE protocol that has significantly rehabilitated me—and do so sooner that I did (thirty-plus years post-injury)—the chances are you will make even better progress sooner than I have. Importantly, keep in mind that the CHAMP BRANDISE protocol or any other protocol will not be a complete emancipation. While the CHAMP BRANDISE protocol helped me more than anything else had, it did not resolve all my brain injury consequences, for some of which I must continue to accommodate—as will you.

With renewed hope, rise to the task. Call on and develop the resilience required to assume more internal control of your life. Take responsibility for what you can manage and acknowledge what you cannot. Organize the maze-like chaos inherent with a brain-injured life and develop a greater sense of confidence in overcoming challenges both great and small. With a brain injury, every challenge is significant and counts as another chance to be resilient.

Meaningful relationships are important as well when it comes to developing and expanding your resilience. Work to improve your communication skills—skills that are foundational in personal relationships. Expand your resilience by exploring your interests and engaging in activities you enjoy, especially those likely to lead to new personal connections. Meeting people who are like-minded is most probable when you do what you enjoy. I greatly encourage support groups, volunteer work, religious fellowship, and charity connections, all of which can develop your social network in meaningful ways and be very rewarding. Belonging to a positive, proactive group builds resilience in each of the group's members.

And again, do guard against picking a grandiose goal the way we survivors are prone to. Instead, with trusted counsel, pick a realistic goal you can achieve sooner rather than later and make flexibility a foundational part of the equation. That said, ask yourself what simple and practical action now feels like a mountain to you. Make that your goal and pursue it with *Atomic Habits*. Give it your best effort, network with others who can help you in the process, revisit and modify your strategies (i.e., be flexible), develop your awareness, and hone your problem-solving ability along the way. Then when you reach that "summit"/achieve that goal (within the time limit or deadline you set), look for the next "mountain" to climb, the next step to take (again with a time limit), and take it with all your *proactive habits* working on your behalf. Keep your momentum moving forward, modify your program as needed, continue working your plan built on reasonable measures. Let Trisha Meili inspire you to keep going until you break through the limiting-rehabilitation forecasts pronounced over you. The ultimate survivor Anne Frank said, "Everyone has inside of him a piece of good news. The good news is that you don't know how great you can be! How much you can love! What you can accomplish! And what your potential is!" Who knows how far you will go? Gather all the fortitude and resilience you have for the journey before you set out—it will be needed—and then fix your focus, your determination, to that immovable place inside your soul and habitually employ the reasonable measures necessary that will get you closer to your goal, and you surely will make progress—gradual, consistent, *significant* progress.

Take "quick" out of your thinking altogether and instead put a picture of the tortoise on your rehab goal board. Be the tortoise who wins the race with persistent doggedness, with slow, deliberate, safe steps all the way—while avoiding another head injury. No matter what therapy regimen you follow, your success in establishing a satisfying life after brain injury depends completely on your ability each day to embrace new habits of accommodation; push yourself to practice rehabilitation exercises, ambidextrous penmanship, and movement patterns daily; increase your microcirculation; make sure you get plenty of rest; eat healthy, quality food, super foods, avoiding the opposite; take excellent nutritional supplements; enhance your communication skills; let go of resentment and retribution; forgive those who have harmed or offended you; and change any negative thoughts into positive thoughts.

In baseball's Major League it is so hard to hit a fastball, a curveball, or a slider that players who fail 7 out of 10 times are Hall of Famers. After a brain injury it is so hard to both relate socially and perform vocationally that you, your family and your boss, are all well advised—in light of your reduced abilities/awareness/energy—to adjust expectations for your behavior and performance, and to employ as well reasonable accommodations. Certainly, too, you can keep trying (as I have)—to improve. Consistent, incremental improvement is the secret to achieving the greatest feats in life. Strive to: be consistently courteous and "on base" with friends; "hit intimate homeruns" with your spouse; and keep working to "score wins" for your boss. Maybe someday, with BI education, they will recognize you too are a Hall of Famer even if you only get it right half the time.

The escape artist Harry Houdini said, "My brain is the key that sets me free." Unfortunately, millions of brain injury survivors are trapped in their damaged brains yet somehow have to use those very brains to *set themselves free*. Even though the average doctor maintains it is impossible to "escape" from the disabilities associated with severe brain damage, I and others are the proof that that is not true. A combination of therapies, nutrition, personal resilience, and prayers has made me more and more free from my disabilities—and it has continued to do so ten, twenty, and even more than forty year after my injury. I realize that I will never be "completely free" and accept that as fact, but these days, I am so much closer to being *my normal pre-injury self* that it is *fantastic*. We, as survivors, have to search beyond average doctors to find the exceptional doctors who, with knowledge, will prescribe effective therapies for us. We then have to pound on the doors of insurers to get them to pay for those therapies—which will, in fact, save them money. I want to work with as many survivors as possible to help them find the proactive, valid therapy combination that will help them be more and more free.

We have all heard motivational speakers talk of looking at a glass of milk as half full instead of half empty. With a brain injury, forget about that comparison altogether. Simply pour your milk into a smaller glass and see how full it is—without question, more than half full. Sure, it's a smaller glass; but for me and those I have worked with, it has always proved better to take a realistic approach to life after brain injury, to see our abilities and achievements as they really are—reduced and lesser but plenty admirable and worthy of respect. I believe such an approach will benefit you as well. I would love to see millions of survivors come to a point where they can agree with Dr. Seuss. "You are you. Now isn't that pleasant?" It is never too late to improve your life—there is always something you can do. I have heard it said, "You will never change your life until you change something you do daily." Use this sage advice to your advantage and work in some way every day to change your life for the better. Work to rehabilitate your mind, your brain-body connection, and your self-esteem; then in time, you will likely and rightly, honestly respect yourself.

◆

This book is also directed to families of those so injured. The family makes possible the greatest degree of improvement for a survivor. The family may also *experience* most of the life-changing consequences of a severe brain injury. Over the years when a survivor's family is necessarily working out a new lifestyle to accommodate their severely injured survivor, it is possible that each member may be able to increase the range of his or her values, de-emphasizing the physical and intellectual and find a deeper meaning to life. That will be nearly impossible, however, without learning something about brain injury. So, *family members*, please seek to educate yourselves about the condition—any one of the books cited in the references might be a good place to start. Then get out a notebook. You will need it to do a good job of record keeping and collaborating with medical professionals, teachers, schools, and employers to document the effect of different interventions and help your survivor reach his or her highest level of rehabilitation success.

Unfortunately, a family can also be the most negative component in rehabilitation program/quality of life for a survivor. The family is like a double-edged sword that can cut both ways—either positively through the Gordian knot of medical/insurance, academic/vocational, and social/relational issues or negatively to the very heart of the survivor by denying altogether the reality of his or her brain injury. Family denial can magnify the disabilities associated with brain injury and interfere with rehabilitation progress by adding undue stress. Too many of my clients report that their families tell them that all their problems are imagined. The same families refuse to learn anything about brain injury or best rehabilitation practices. They will not even read a pamphlet, let alone a book, that will alter their misconceptions. I have yet to find a way to open their eyes to see the light of day when it comes to life with a brain injury. I think we may have to start with updating the academic programs for medical professionals. Respected medical professionals—once BI educated—will understand better than me how best to rehabilitate injured brains while accommodating all the secondary cognitive and physical consequences. Then such doctors could reach out to resistant families and help them better understand the realities of what their survivor family member is going through— what they themselves will likely be going through if they have suffered a similar brain injury—plus, how best to support their survivor and help them regain as much of his or her life as possible.

Finally, I write to the rest of the population, to all readers who have not yet had any experience with brain injury, either by being injured themselves or by living with a brain-injured family member or friend. Please take every reasonable precaution to prevent yourself or a child from suffering this most complicated disease—from becoming a part of the Silent Epidemic.

I hope you have not experienced MEGO as you have been reading my book, especially the more medically detailed parts of it. (*MEGO* is old journalistic slang for "my eyes glaze over," referring to a reader's reaction to a story that is dull.) Please just remember that brain injury affects more than one in four people and is a bigger threat to everyone's wholeness and happiness than any other disease or injury. My aim is to leave you not with a bunch of facts but with a *conviction* in your heart so strong that it impels you to take *proactive measures* to prevent yourself and those you care for from being brain-injured—so that you may both continue to live life to the fullest.

◆

I hear it said again and again that our brain is what makes each of us who we are—that it makes you yourself. However, I maintain that the three pounds of flesh in our skull, with its universe of multiple trillions of neuronal connections, is what *allows us* to experience the world, perceive sensations from the environment, analyze and understand those sensations, relate to the people around us, work to provide for our needs and those of others, organize to reduce chaos, make ourselves safe, compare every encounter with past memories, use those memories as reference points to build upon, and express our uniqueness. *Who* we are, however, goes much deeper than all that. Who we are originates deep in our soul and our spirit, for the soul and spirit of a man or woman made in the image of God transcends both the brain and the body. Who we are is ever present, and we are fully human no matter how much brain capacity we lack. Our person is present even when our brain is unconscious or in a coma or when our body is completely paralyzed or disfigured. Nourish your soul, encourage it to grow more and more beautiful in relationship to the other souls around you. You are the only human being created with your DNA, your fingerprints, your eyes, your unique personality and skill set. Respect your brain as that which allows the unique being you are, to know and be known by others, to perceive the world around you, and to accomplish your goals. Protect your brain and the brains in your care; nurture them accordingly—for as long as you live.

The Greek philosopher Plutarch said, "The mind is not a vessel to be filled, but a fire to be kindled." I hope to have kindled your mind and to leave it now burning bright next to other minds alight with the same flame, the same enlightenment—namely, that the far-reaching implications of brain injury affect more people than any other health condition, that we have to act both locally, statewide and nationally to reduce the prevalence and rehabilitate the consequences, of brain injury—that you as an average person, you are more like survivors than you are different from us—and that we survivors are more like you than we are different from you. Survivors, be assured, we are more like the average person than we are different from him or her.

Antonio Damasio wrote in his book *The Feelings of What Happens*[9] that consciously knowing the feelings caused by emotions is "indispensable for the art of life." The full and lasting impact of feelings requires consciousness "because only along with a sense of self do feelings become known to the individual having them." Damasio believes that this precious and fragile neurological connection to life has not been properly appreciated. Being unaware of one's own emotional/feeling connection inherently renders him or her, while in communication, unable to understand the emotional/feeling connection to others—and necessarily pushes them away. Please begin to appreciate your sense of self, your power to develop thoughts, your awareness of the circumstances you find yourself in, your ability to perceive emotions and feelings—both your own and those of others—your ability to communicate fluently, and your ability to maintain intimate relationships. Please try to understand survivors who have lost that sense, that power, that awareness, and that ability. It is not possible for you to fully understand us, but it is important that you try. *Please try.*

49 C. Vash, *Psychology of Disability* (New York: Springer, 1981), https://www.amazon. com/Psychology-Disability-Second-SPRINGER-REHABILITATION/ dp/0826133428.

16

WHO IS MARK JOHN CONDON?

Jane Kopp, PhD

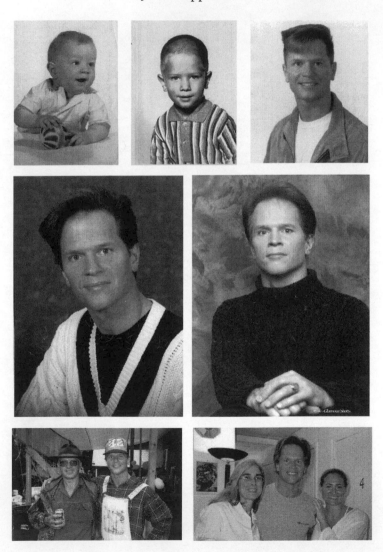

When I first had the opportunity to read Mark John Condon's third draft of his book, *The Silent Epidemic: What Everyone Should Know about Traumatic Brain Injury*, I was struck by its powerful account of the consequences of a brain injury—consequences that, to say the least, are not well understood by the general public. (In 2001, my own son, at the age of twenty-nine, was brain-injured. In spite of a high IQ and decidedly out-of-the-ordinary creative abilities, he has found himself facing some difficult challenges as a result.) I have been glad to volunteer to Mark my training as an editor in refining the prose style of what is now the fourth version of his manuscript, and I suggested to Mark that he add to his book this present chapter explaining more of who he is because I believe some people will want to know. If you do want to know more about Mark John Condon, the following pages will give you further details about his life.

(Note: Necessarily, Mark had to provide me with a draft of his background and history. I myself have not interviewed any of the people involved, so this is Mark's story the way he himself sees it and has compiled it. In what follows, however, the words of a number of people other than Mark are quoted, words that they themselves wrote in letters and other documents. Keeping to standard editorial practice, I have left untouched the wording, spelling, capitalization, and internal punctuation of all such direct quotations of others, except to break up long paragraphs into shorter ones.)

Mark John Condon was born in 1958 in Ontonagon, Michigan, the son of Tom and Dorothy Condon. His father, Tom, the son of John and Mary Condon, was raised in Hancock, Michigan; and his mother, Dorothy, the daughter of Frank and Mary Domitrovich, was raised fifty miles away in Ontonagon, Michigan. No one can understand Mark without knowing about the core of his existence, the close-knit, resilient family he grew up in.

Mark interacted more often with his mother's side of the family, which is now more than ten times bigger than his father's side. Specifically, he spent a considerable part of his early life either doing anything and everything there was to do on his grandpa Domitrovich's farm or in the woods under the supervision of his lumberjack uncles and with his cousins Jerry and Tom Domitrovich, who were of the same age as Mark and his elder brother Dan respectively.

Dorothy's father, Frank Domitrovich, was born on February 18, 1898, in the little village of Osojnik near Severin na Kupi, Yugoslavia. Frank was the first child of Anton Domitrovich and Dora Kramerich, who later gave birth to Frank's only sister, Marija. When he was three years old, Frank's father went to America to earn money for the family. Frank's mother did all the farmwork while Anton was gone. After three years, Anton came back to Yugoslavia, announcing he would go back yet again to America in a year or two, but it would then be to earn enough money to buy a farm and bring the entire family over with him. However, not long after Anton did return to America, he was in a terrible railroad train yard accident and died soon afterward. Frank was only eight years old when the family learned that his father had died.

Though all the family were crying together around the kitchen table, little Frank told his mama not to cry. When he grew up, he told her he himself would go to America, buy a farm, and bring her over to live with him. When Frank was fifteen years old, he was big and strong enough to work just as hard as any man, so he persuaded his mother to let him go to America. A month after that day, he was off to the "other world."

In America, young Frank Domitrovich worked long and hard wherever he could—first in the coal mines of Pittsburgh, Pennsylvania, carrying water for the miners, and then years later in Ontonagon, Michigan, where he bought three hundred acres of forest with a little farm in the middle of it. He became a citizen of the United States when he was twenty-five years old, and at twenty-six, he went back to Yugoslavia to get his mother—and a wife. Friends had been telling him of this or that woman back in the old country who they thought would make a good wife for him. Frank did, in fact, find a good woman while he was back in Yugoslavia. He wrote of her in his diary, "In Severin, on the way home one night we stopped at Strbenac where they had music playing and people dancing. I dance with Mary and I like it, my heart went jump and I ask her if she would marry me. I said, 'Don't tell me now, think it over few days then you can tell me.' I know she was going to say yes because I think she loves me just as much as I love her. Next time I saw her she said yes."

Frank and Mary went back to America as newlyweds along with Frank's mama, Dora, and they raised nine children on their farm. Today there are over 125 descendants of Frank and Mary Domitrovich, one being Mark John Condon. As he grew up, Mark admired his grandpa's strength and that of all his uncles, whom he would watch working as lumberjacks and farmers. He positively enjoyed working together with the uncles and aunts and all the cousins to get farm chores done—milking cows by hand, cleaning the barn, feeding the chickens, bailing hay, peeling the bark off the poplar logs his uncles cut before trucking them to the pulp mill in Ontonagon, and preparing food for everyone to eat at any given meal.

The great-grandfather of Mark's father, Tom, one Morris Condon, was born in Tipperary, Ireland, in 1835. Tom's father and Mark's grandfather, Joseph Condon, was born in the United States in 1902. When he was eighteen years old, Joseph married Tom's mother and Mark's grandmother, Clara Josephine Payn. James Payne (the *e* was dropped in the early 1800s), Clara's great-grandfather, was born in Devon, England, in 1729. In 1930, Joseph Condon was living in Iron River, Michigan, and working for the Atlas Powder Company packing dynamite sticks into wooden shipping boxes and then later as a sales manager for a retail electrical supply company. By 1940, he had moved to Hancock with Clara and their three children, Mary (thirteen), Tom (eight), and Jack (six). Mark's grandmother Clara Condon, whom he never had a chance to meet, worked as a saleslady at a dry goods store. She died in 1949 from multiple sclerosis. At the time of Clara's death, Tom—Mark's father—was nineteen years old. Mark's grandfather

Joseph Condon died in 1966 from congestive heart failure and cirrhosis of the liver when Mark was eight years old. Mark has fond memories of rocking in one of the several rocking chairs on Grandpa Condon's front porch overlooking the Portage Canal while Grandpa Condon told stories.

Mark was well grounded in the love and faith that his immediate and extended family shared at mealtimes, doing chores, traveling and camping, or going into town. His family has always been close, going every week to church, encouraging one another to be their best, and supporting one another however they need supporting. Mark maintains that, apart from his amazing family, his life as a child was unremarkable and average in every way. He was the middle child of a middle-class family of five kids, raised in the heartland of America with the common comforts that most American families of the time had.

Although he was born in Ontonagon, Michigan, where his extended family resided, he and his immediate family lived over eight hours away in Mount Pleasant, Michigan, where his father worked for Central Michigan University. Despite that distance, every year as Mark grew up, his immediate family would travel back twice a year (summer and winter vacations) to visit the relatives and work on the farm. Mark's fondest memories are of getting ready to go back to Grandpa Domitrovich's farm in Ontonagon—to play each summer with all his cousins, do chores, swim in the swimming hole on the farm or in Lake Superior (which most of the time was too cold for his liking), and spend Christmas each winter in all the snow of the Upper Peninsula of Michigan.

Mark started first grade when he was four years old. He continued to be the youngest in his grade until he graduated from high school. Every year his father would build a hockey rink in the backyard where they lived, and he taught Mark and his elder brother, Dan, how to play hockey. Dan and Mark grew up being the best hockey players in their grade (hockey was not a big sport in Mount Pleasant at the time), and they, in turn, taught some of their neighbors how to play the game. One neighbor the brothers taught was Pat Sheppard, Mark's best friend for many years, who went on to play semipro hockey. Pat always thanks Mark for teaching him the game of hockey. As for school, although Mark did fine academically, he never liked it. He always preferred to be outdoors doing something like hunting, canoeing, or playing hockey.

Early each morning before school started, in addition to their household chores, both Mark and his brother Dan, from seventh grade on through high school, had big paper routes, delivering newspapers to all Central Michigan University's dormitories. They would also set up newspaper wagons after church each Sunday morning and sell a hundred newspapers to the parishioners of Sacred Heart Catholic Church in Mount Pleasant. They earned enough money in these ways to buy shotguns and hunting rifles, ammunition, reloading equipment, and all kinds of hunting paraphernalia and were able to save some besides. With Dan, Mark went partridge and deer hunting whenever possible; and when he was a junior in high school, Mark bought an English setter hunting dog, a pointer that he trained to hunt pheasants. He named the dog Buckshot, and he and the dog together got the season's limit for pheasants the first year they hunted together.

In 1975, just before Mark's senior year in high school, his parents bought Paul's Supper Club and Bar in Silver City, Michigan, on the shores of Lake Superior just fourteen miles west of Ontonagon. Mark first worked in the restaurant as a dishwasher with his younger brothers, Tom and Jeff. Dan, who had cooking experience from Embers Famous Restaurant in Mount Pleasant, was trained to cook Paul's menu by Tiny Yaklovich, the former owner. Kathy, Mark's sister and eldest sibling, was one of the waitresses; his mother, Dorothy, worked as hostess; and his father, Tom, functioned as boss, head chef, manager, accountant, bartender, maintenance man, public relations specialist, human resources director, and anything else needed to run the place.

After the first year, in 1976, Dan left for Alaska to make a life for himself. After Dan's departure, although Mark was enrolled at

Northern Michigan University (NMU) in Marquette, he was taught by both Tiny and his father to replace Dan as the head chef. He worked in that capacity in between college semesters for over four years. Kathy stayed in Michigan, went on to college, and graduated as a registered nurse. She too would work in the restaurant between semesters. As Tom and Jeff went through college, they also worked in the restaurant just like everybody else and then afterward went on to become accomplished artists and designers. Mark's parents kept the restaurant for thirty years, each working over fifty hours a week. They even expanded the restaurant to include a three-story Best Western Hotel with 120 rooms, a swimming pool, and 45 employees.

In 2003, however, they finally sold the business, and both are now glad to have put all that work and struggle behind them. Tom and Dorothy Condon, both in their 90s, today still enjoy good health, and they love visiting all their grandchildren in Michigan, Colorado, Ohio, and Alaska.

During his senior year of high school in Silver City in the Upper Peninsula of Michigan, Mark made friends easily, played on White Pine High's football team, worked every day for his father, and hunted whenever he could. He was able with little effort to pass all his classes, and in 1976, he was accepted into Northern Michigan University. Since at the time he had never had adequate career counseling, Mark thought at first he would like to be a game warden so as to be able to work outdoors most of the time. Accordingly, he enrolled in classes that would prepare him for a profession of that kind. In his second year at NMU, however, he interviewed a game warden and was chagrined to learn that, in fact, game wardens spend most of their time behind a desk—and that furthermore most game wardens are former police officers. He began looking for a better career match to pursue academically. Meanwhile, he became a member of NMU's Lambda Chi Alpha Fraternity and lived in the chapter's house at 619 Fourth Street, where he made a number of great friends.

Mark rushed Lambda Chi Alpha with his high school friend Jon Nissen, who was his NMU roommate at the time, and with two friends they had made from their dorm floor, Joe Kulwicki and Richie Basala. Once a member of the fraternity, Mark also made great friends with Tom Bok, Charlie Noonan, Don Kromer, Joel Gregg, and many others. Don Kromer, the summer before Mark's second year in the fraternity, had a terrible accident. Diving into a shallow lake, he broke his neck and became a quadriplegic. In the aftermath of this shocking event, Mark promised Don and his family that he would make time available to Don so that Don could return to his studies at Northern Michigan University. That fall semester, they returned to school together, Don as a quadriplegic and Mark as his roommate/health-care provider. The whole fraternity became involved in accommodating Don's return to campus—modifying the bathroom, bedroom, driveway, entrance, and first floor of the frat house to make them all wheelchair accessible.

In addition to being a full-time student himself, Mark was Don's physical therapist, guiding him through his exercise routines and stretching his ligaments. He was Don's practical nurse as well, catheterizing him, bathing him, and administering his medicines, and he took Don to doctor's appointments as well as to class. Mark also did Don's laundry, helped him study, and listened to and encouraged him as often as he could. He continued to care for Don until the end of the school year, after which, as had been planned earlier, Mark transferred schools. Don told him that he never could have returned to school that fall semester had it not been for Mark. Don himself went on to be elected Lambda Chi Alpha's NMU chapter president and eventually graduate from NMU. He credits Mark's care and support for making it all possible.

Mark transferred to Michigan State University. This time, he was entering college with a changed worldview; he had become a born-again Christian. His conversion had come about in Marquette at NMU through the work of his brother Dan, Cathy Parker (a high school classmate who was also attending NMU), and NMU's InterVarsity

Christian Fellowship, in which Cathy Parker was involved. Finding himself now in East Lansing, where MSU was located, Mark became a member of the Work of Christ Community; and through involvement with that community, he continued to grow in faith over the years. In fact, the community surrounded him with love and prayers at the time of his own accident, and it helped his family as well in more ways than can be counted. To this day, even though many miles separate them, Mark still maintains relationships he made with faith-filled friends in the Work of Christ Community.

Piper Fountain was and is a long-standing member of the Work of Christ Community. She writes of her recollection of Mark:

> My earliest memory of Mark John was when he first lived with his sister, a couple houses down from us, after his accident. I would see Mark John out most days, walking with his sister for exercise down the sidewalk, very awkward and jerky, and seemingly oblivious of onlookers. I thought his sister, who must be a nurse, was one very smart and brave lady to know how to guide him! Since I did not know Mark John before the accident, my only knowledge of him was from that point on. He seemed to make fast progress and soon was walking and functioning much better.
>
> We had the practice of renting a room to single men and women in our community, and after a couple of years we invited Mark John to live with our family. We had four small children when he moved in, and he was a delight to have in our home for just over two years. I don't remember too much amiss with Mark, for I had no idea of the scope of his disabilities or struggles.
>
> One fond memory I have was when he decided to make some chocolate chip cookies. The recipe

said—after the ingredients were all added—to mix by hand. So he put the flour, eggs, etc. into the bowl and proceeded to stick his hands in and mix it all together! Of course the cookies were excellent and we all laughed later as we ate them together.

My husband remembers helping him do his exercises, mostly helping him stretch, pulling on his arms and legs, day in and day out. Mark John was very disciplined in this! He was always so cheerful, positively upbeat and funny! After he moved on, Mark John would sometimes come back to visit. Over the years we have kept up, and I've been very impressed with the extent of his growth in every area, not just as a brain injury survivor, but as a human being. He continues to live life fully and excels in more areas than most people. I still especially delight in his silly sense of humor and high energy!

Mark graduated from MSU in December 1982, twenty-one months after his car accident, with a degree in packaging design engineering. He worked on a contract as Forth module packaging design engineer for Oldsmobile of General Motors in Lansing, Michigan, where he was responsible for designing returnable containers for the Forth module's engine components. Mark showed great promise as a design engineer, but because of his brain injury (and associated executive function loss, short-term memory loss, walking/standing balance issues, communication skills, and the like), he had significant difficulty in working as a professional, so a shadow fell across his promise.

When he applied for a permanent position after the Forth module contract concluded, he had the recommendation of several key Oldsmobile employees. Thomas C. Brockway, PE, senior industrial engineer, wrote, "The first week Mark Condon began working with me, I asked him to design conversion parts to adapt the two door quarter panel rack to a four door quarter panel rack. He is a sharp individual and quickly came up with the design. We have tested the parts he designed and currently have them in production. Experiencing Mark's skill and knowing him personally I do not hesitate to recommend him with confidence to Oldsmobile."

Bobby Longmire, SPC trainer, center plant, wrote, "I really respect Mark Condon, I have seen him handle a number of tasks in trouble-shooting the Center Plant's defect problems. I also spent time discussing these problems with him and I am impressed with his insights. I give my strong recommendation to Oldsmobile to ask Mark Condon to work in our Quality Engineering." Several other employees who worked with him also gave their equally strong recommendation that Oldsmobile should hire Mark permanently.

However, Oldsmobile, which had no knowledge of how to accommodate a brain-injured engineer, thanked Mark for his accomplishments as their Forth module packaging design engineer but did not ask him to continue working for them. When he subsequently was released from another packaging design engineering job because the company knew he was likely to be seriously injured on the factory's heavy stamping equipment, his family and friends encouraged him instead to pursue rehabilitation counseling for a career.

The two vocational experiences and his family's feedback started Mark on a somewhat serpentine path to become a rehabilitation counselor. The process began with an application to Michigan State University's graduate school counseling program. Mark had glowing recommendations from professionals and colleagues. One recommendation from Richard L. Williams of the Williams Law Firm in East Lansing read,

> As a student of mine in the College of Business Law at Michigan State University, Mark exhibited an outstanding grasp of the material including, but not limited to: contracts, negotiable instruments, and business organizations in franchise law and marketing.

Mark is an exceptional student and has repeatedly expressed a keen interest in entering your program. . . . Aside from his academic and intellectual interests, Mark is also of superior character and spirit. From past experiences, Mark has shown remarkable ability to maintain and achieve goals in the face of the strictest adversity. . . . In my opinion, not only would Mark Condon benefit from your program, but will prove to be an asset to it.

Luis Posada, MD, wrote, "This letter is in reference to Mark Condon, who has been my patient since his automobile accident on March 7, 1981. Mark's fast rate of recovery has been amazing. I recommend him for any position where determination and optimism play a big role." Regardless of these and other recommendations, MSU did not accept Mark into their program.

A year later, he moved to Colorado after being accepted into the University of Northern Colorado's rehabilitation counseling master's degree program. For a while, he was living with various friends and working an assortment of jobs to establish Colorado residency so graduate school tuition would be more affordable. In one such job with Martin Luther Homes, Mark hoped to gain experience caring for the mentally retarded as a residential counselor in what he thought was a rehabilitation situation. It turned out, however, that the primary function of Martin Luther Homes was to do a wonderful job of maintaining and managing their clients rather than rehabilitating them to be able to live independently, which was what Mark had in mind for himself and his future clients. Mark's concept of rehabilitation was working with clients to improve their level of independence or their employability, and he wanted experience in a facility with the same mission.

At about this same time, Mark was also becoming an active participant in the bimonthly meetings of the Colorado Head Injury Foundation's Fort Collins support group. This support group was an excellent one. The members told one another the stories of how they had been brain-injured, lent understanding to one another, and shared with one another their frustrations and fears related to traumatic brain injury. Mark recognized the value of commiserating and empathizing with others in a similar situation, as well as the value to each member of being heard telling of his or her own traumatic brain injury, but he did not want to get stuck merely retelling/hearing—again and again, his and the others' stories. His experience of that particular CHIF support group was that telling and retelling their brain injury stories was all they ever did.

Mark's own goal was to move past his brain injury; strive for physical, psychological, and vocational improvement; and help others do the same. He wanted to get better, and he wanted to be involved with others so inclined. His combined experiences with Martin Luther Homes and CHIF's support group had caused Mark to mistakenly conclude that the field of rehabilitation was not for him. At the time, he would have put his misapprehension like this: "Rehabilitation counseling does not primarily help the disabled improve; rather, it simply tries to reconcile them to their 'fate.'" Mere resignation as a goal was at serious odds with his own belief that—while acceptance may be a primary step in the rehabilitation journey—many additional steps beyond acceptance are equally important. Further, while Mark knew that empathy and understanding had helped give him the strength to accept his disabled self, he also knew that he had moved on to work towards regaining as many of his lost vocational abilities as possible. He believed other survivors could and should do the same. Mark was all about self-improvement. He wanted to work in a field with the same philosophy and purpose. Because he had incorrectly concluded that rehabilitation counseling was not such a field, he tried to get back into engineering. To pay bills in the meantime, he began to work as a sacker in a grocery store and at assorted other jobs.

At this point, he came into contact with Rocky Mountain Neuropsychological Sciences in Fort Collins and got involved with their support group, in which people who had recently undergone closed head injuries shared their resulting confusion and fears. In this new group, Mark yet again shared his own experiences and discussed with other members the parallels between his experiences and theirs; but in this group, he took the further step of offering to other members insights about what to expect in the future and encouraging them to take the "next step on their journey." This support group changed his perspective on rehabilitation counseling—it *was* what he wanted to do.

Douglas E. Strachan, MS, CSP, the facilitator of this Rocky Mountain Neuropsychological Sciences support group, encouraged Mark to reapply to the University of Northern Colorado's graduate rehabilitation program. Mr. Strachan and various members of the support group as well wrote in support of his reapplication. One member, Deborah Correll, wrote,

> My own work towards recovery from a mild brain injury has been difficult for me. I have found Mark John's presence to be reassuring and his accomplishments in his own rehabilitation inspirational. Mark John acts naturally as one of the group's informal facilitators, offering intelligent, pertinent advice and sharing the valuable perspective of one who has dealt successfully with a severe head injury. His approach towards problems, with a combination of compassion and pragmatic attitude, has worked again and again to the benefit of group members and has well earned him their respect. Mark John has a wonderful knack for saying exactly the right thing at the right time, lending encouragement that has been as helpful to me as some of my professional counseling.

Chris Walker, MS, at the time a doctoral candidate in psychology and also a participant in the support group, wrote, "During our group sessions, Mark John shows himself to be a good leader. He consistently provides others with accurate insight regarding their problems/concerns. He displays an appropriate degree of empathy while also challenging people to embrace reality. Given his own determination to reach out for a life that many might have once considered an impossibility, I can see how Mark John could be particularly inspirational to others in similar circumstances."

Still another group member, Thomas Leonard, wrote, "Mark John has brought such a special contribution to our group collectively and to myself personally. In a sense, I consider him to be our 'senior' member on the long road of recovery, since his accident was 14 years ago. Therefore, Mark John brings with him a wealth of experience, insight, and wisdom, which those of us who are only one or two years post accident are just beginning to realize. He certainly has been a comfort and an inspiration to me in the aftermath of my own accident."

Douglas Strachan himself wrote to UNC in support of Mark's application, saying:

> In my capacity as facilitator of an ongoing brain-injury support and therapy group, I have had the occasion to observe Mr. Condon's considerable impacts on others in their adjustment and recovery from significant disruption in their lives secondary to the misfortune of head injury.
>
> The extensive treatment exposure and background, which Mark John brings to this situation enriches his contributions greatly. The gains that he has made through diligent personal efforts, serve as an inspiration to me as well as to his peers in the support group, and I see that these others draw strength and solace from his adaptive processing of the many issues of recovery. . . .
>
> A particular strength has been Mark John's ability to choose very constructive terminology and imagery

to explain and reframe his listener's confusion and concerns in a manner that helps them grasp ideas in new and therapeutic ways, sometimes allowing them to reach insights which are healing experiences. . . . In my professional judgment, Mr. Mark John Condon will make an excellent candidate for your program in Rehabilitation Counseling.

Strachan, who was a key influence in Mark's decision to resume pursuit of a master's degree, said in person to Mark, "Mark John, I could never learn in all my years of doctoral studies what you have learned through your brain injury experience. You have to bring what you know to the brain injury rehabilitation world."

Tom Higley, who was a lay pastor in the Work of Christ Community at Michigan State University when Mark was an undergraduate there and who was leading a group of men who were involved in campus ministry, also wrote a letter of personal recommendation in Mark's behalf. When Mark was in the hospital in 1981 after his accident, Higley had visited him every day; he had also encouraged Mark's family like no one else could. Mark's mother, Dorothy, does not think she or Mark's siblings could have made it through those trying times—the nights when Mark nearly died or all the days of his therapy—without Tom Higley's encouragement. Tom himself later went on to graduate from Harvard Law School and then become a "serial entrepreneur extraordinaire," with six start-ups to his credit after the onset of the dot-com gold rush, including Service Metrics and StillSecure. He now is also a prolific start-up mentor with Galvanize and Techstars and a serial angel investor. His latest project is 10.10.10, bringing ten CEOs together for ten days to cure ten massive headaches for various industries in the USA. Mark calls Tom his most Promethean friend. In 1995, however, when Mark was reapplying to UNC, Higley was working in Fort Collins for the Fischer, Brown, Huddleson & Gunn Law Firm. His recommendation letter reads:

Mark John and I have known each other since 1980. As his lay pastor, I worked closely with him and had an opportunity to observe his character, skills and experience. I regarded him then—as I do now—with great admiration and respect. In 1981, Mark John incurred a serious head injury. After substantial time in a coma, he regained consciousness and began the long, arduous process of re-acquiring many skills he once took for granted. He re-learned a host of things: speech, basic motor skills, social skills and all manner of related abilities. Throughout this recovery, he refused to become discouraged. Instead, he made continuing progress—beyond what his close friends or family could reasonably have anticipated. For a time after the accident, Mark John lived with my family. I was impressed with his ability to learn many social skills that were lost to him immediately after the accident. His progress has been nothing short of miraculous.

Today Mark John continues to amaze me. His most evident character qualities include boundless enthusiasm, unwavering commitment and self-sacrificing kindness. His skills include a remarkable creativity and intelligence, and I marvel at his ability to see new and better ways of accomplishing ordinary tasks. I am honored to know Mark John and eager to recommend him to you as a candidate for the master program.

Thanks in part to Higley's recommendation and to those of others, Mark was readmitted to UNC and began graduate studies in the fall of 1996.

Mark readily accommodated to campus life, living in the graduate students' apartment complex with three roommates, two who were foreign exchange students from Europe. He got into a disciplined study routine, earning a nearly 4.0 GPA, and not a single professor or administrator voiced any concern that the consequences of his brain injury would interfere with his academic or professional performance in any way. (This lack of understanding and acknowledgement on their part regarding brain injury was and is typical of the majority of medical/mental health/educational professionals.) However, Mark's "second mother," Elsha Westhoff, knew there would be situations in the real world after Mark's graduation when his particular circumstances would have to be accommodated if he was to perform well as a licensed professional counselor. She tried several times to bring her concerns up with UNC's faculty when Mark had completed his coursework and was pursuing an internship. They simply dismissed her, saying that Mark would do great, just as he had in the classroom. His professors said that Mark always asked the best questions in their classes, that he was exactly the type of person the rehabilitation counseling field ought to embrace, and that of all the students they had worked with, he was exceptional from many standpoints.

Mark quickly secured an internship with a Denver rehabilitation hospital under the supervision of a neuropsychologist. Mark was eager to learn from observing his supervisor how best to intervene with various kinds of disabled patients and their family members. Unfortunately, he never had that opportunity. Instead, the supervisor asked Mark to attend hospital staffing, hold family consultations, counsel various patients, and write regular reports updating patient files—all by himself. Mark rarely saw his supervisor except at the beginning and end of each day or when the supervisor would ask Mark to follow him outside for one of his cigarette breaks. While the neuropsychologist hurriedly smoked cigarettes outside, they would talk about the approach Mark was taking with this or that patient; and each time the supervisor would agree that Mark's approach was the right one, never mentioning particular considerations or offering a different view. This neuropsychologist would also sign his name on top of Mark's signature, completely obscuring it, each time Mark wrote a counseling session update in a patient's medical file.

He did allow Mark to attend a neuropsychological test he administered to one patient, and Mark was flabbergasted at his supervisor's technique. Mark had learned proper test administration technique at UNC. One of the first and most obvious principles to be followed in a neuropsychological test is to remain neutral when administering it (i.e., to make no indication about whether the person taking the test is answering correctly or incorrectly so as not to influence answers). Yet in this instance, as the test taker answered each of the first few questions correctly, right away, the neuropsychologist would enthusiastically say, "Yes, that's right!" "Again, that's right,!" "Good job, you're right,!" and so on, and the patient would become elated to be answering correctly. By the time the patient reached the tenth question, however, he had given wrong answers on each of the last four questions. After each wrong answer, the neuropsychologist showed a flat affect without any congratulations whatsoever—before quietly asking the next question. The patient realized he was answering incorrectly, became despondent, and clearly lost confidence. The neuropsychologist remained sober and neutral for the rest of the evaluation so as not to indicate whether the patient answered correctly. Never hearing another "attaboy" predictably, the patient put little thought into the rest of his answers. The way that test was administered completely invalidated the results. Nevertheless, the neuropsychologist entered those misleading results in the patient's file and went home early for the day.

During that internship, Mark was also asked to develop and run a family support group for families of the hospital's brain-injured patients. Some of these families were having a very difficult time dealing with the sudden change in their loved one and with the resulting changes in their family dynamics. On his own, with no involvement from either the neuropsychologist/supervisor or any other hospital staff member, Mark researched and wrote a fifty-page guideline to be followed in the support group he was going to lead. Mary Anne Catlin's son was one of the brain-injured; she herself worked at the hospital, attended the support group, and later wrote in a recommendation letter for Mark:

> I am the Director of Radiology at Sunrise Rehabilitation Hospital and the mother of a 28-year-old man who has suffered three episodes of minor brain injury as a child. I had the opportunity to attend the Family-Group Counseling Series developed and led by Mark John Condon here at the hospital. The Family Group was a revolving series of six independent sessions to benefit families of brain injury survivors: AVM's, CVA's, strokes, TBI's, tumors, etc.
>
> The purpose of the Family-Group was to provide a forum for family education on a variety of topics such as: The Nature of Head Injury; Getting to Know the New Person; and Factors in Long-Term Improvement. The "tool" of the series was the 50-page document, researched and written by Mr. Condon. There was ample opportunity for sharing fears and confusion, and for asking questions. Mr. Condon answered all the questions, acknowledged the position of each person, and proved to be a very capable mentor/counselor for the group.
>
> Many of our patient's family members told me what a great help this series has been in dealing with their grief, loss, expectations, and in establishing a new relationship with their brain injured loved ones. It has given me a much greater understanding of what the patients at Sunrise Rehabilitation are going through, and it has improved my relationship with my son.

Another time, Mark was "alone" (without his supervisor) in a family consultation meeting at the same hospital. All the other doctors and therapists were present as usual, talking with the family about their daughter, a head-injured teenager. The medical staff took turns, each specialist speaking to their area of expertise. When it was Mark's turn (in his supervisor's absence), he asked a couple of general neuropsychological questions and then about the girl's social life pre-injury and specifically about intimate relationships. He apologized for his frankness but pointed out that after a head injury, survivors often are left oblivious of other people's possible ulterior motives, then, unable to read people—easily manipulated. Consequently, survivors may become credulous and susceptible to sales gimmicks and hidden agendas, which not uncommonly results in survivors being taken advantage of both financially and sexually. Mark knew it would be unethical for him not to address this delicate subject, given numbers of reports in current literature of survivors being taken advantage of in such ways by both "friends and people of trust." The family, in this case, felt sure their daughter would not have any such issues because she had not really dated yet, was not sexually active before her injury, and had no plans of becoming so before marriage. They thanked Mark for bringing the subject up and said there was no reason for him to apologize.

As has been explained (and as was typical), the neuropsychologist who was Mark's supervisor was not present at this family consultation. Some of the other staff, lacking specific training in head injury sequelae, felt uncomfortable with Mark's line of questioning; even more than that, they felt it was inappropriate that the supervisor was not accompanying Mark at this and other family consultations/staffings. Word got back to the hospital administrator, who decided to lay the supervisor off for two weeks for failing to provide the supervision specified in Mark's internship agreement. The supervisor, in turn, told Mark (who had no idea know what had been going on behind the scenes) that he, the supervisor, was "going on vacation for two weeks" and that he had heard from the staff that Mark was inappropriate in family consultations. Mark asked how specifically he was inappropriate and in which consultation. The supervisor would not tell him. Mark pleaded to know how he was inappropriate and pointed out that this was exactly the purpose of his internship—helping him learn to perform at professional rehabilitation counseling standards—but the supervisor refused to say.

The next two weeks while the supervisor was "on vacation," Mark handled all the counseling work on three of the five different hospital wings. (The other two wings were a lockdown facility for violent patients and a drug/alcohol treatment facility for addicted patients.) Mark wrote letters to all the doctors and therapists he had worked with, explaining what his supervisor had told him (that they felt he was inappropriate in a family staffing) and asking them to let him know how he was inappropriate. Word got back to the hospital administrator, who felt that the shameful way the neuropsychologist had left Mark in the dark about what was judged to have been inappropriate—his failing to provide supervision—was the last straw. The whole incident prompted the administrator to gather other negative evidence about the supervisor's performance and move to force him to resign.

It turned out that the rehabilitation hospital had been looking for ways to terminate this particular neuropsychologist for over a year but was hesitant to do so because the neuropsychologist had been terminated from the hospital where he worked before—and was suing that other hospital for terminating him. For obvious reasons, the rehabilitation hospital did not want a legal mess on their hands. However, the neuropsychologist's unethical treatment of Mark prompted those in authority to move forward with termination. The rehabilitation hospital was able to force the neuropsychologist's "voluntary" resignation.

With just a month left before completing his internship, Mark was reassigned to the drug addict wing, and everything was back on track. The terminated neuropsychologist, however, recruited a friend of his who worked at the hospital to give false reports on Mark's job performance to his new supervisor. On the basis of those fabricated, negative reports, the new supervisor terminated Mark's internship.

UNC remained supportive of Mark and helped him find another internship. Together, they found an internship in the office of a neuropsychologist who specialized in brain injury. It looked like a perfect fit, but there were problems with this internship as well. There, Mark was first assigned to shadow a vocational evaluator in the office and do vocational evaluating. Considerable fine finger dexterity was needed to set up, take down, time, and record the vocational tests. Mark could not use his left hand in such a fashion; for that very reason, he had not specialized in vocational evaluation in graduate school but instead in counseling (i.e., he never intended to work as a vocational evaluator). He did, however, closely watch the vocational evaluator on site and asked thoughtful questions when the testing was completed and the client had left.

On one occasion, this new neuropsychologist had Mark sit in on a court deposition during which attorneys from both sides of a case were questioning both a client of the neuropsychologist and the neuropsychologist himself. Mark was observing the interaction of all the parties involved and following the line of questioning when, at one point, the neuropsychologist asked the client what his new job was post-TBI and after being treated by the neuropsychologist. The client said, "Cook." And the neuropsychologist moved on to other questions. Later, however, Mark revisited the job question. Having been a cook himself in the past, he explained what the different types of cooks are, what different levels of multitasking skills are inherent in each type or level of cooking. (Some cooks simply drop French fries in a fryer until a bell dings, others have to prepare seven different main dishes and fourteen side dishes for an order and time that preparation so that it is all done and ready to serve at the same time, and still others have to prepare banquet dishes from scratch, combine recipes from memory, follow inventory levels, order replacements, maintain working relationships with many suppliers, and so on.). Mark asked what *kind* of cook the client was since the ability to multitask is one of the best indicators of vocational level of ability/disability after brain injury. The client said he was a backup cook who prepared side dishes in a Wendy's Restaurant. Mark asked additional questions: The answers to which gave a much more complete picture of the client's vocational skills and performance levels.

After the deposition, the attorney working with the client on behalf of the neuropsychologist was having an informal chat with a group that included the neuropsychologist, a psychologist in training, the client, and Mark. The attorney felt that the proper information had come out and was now a part of public record, so it was a celebration of sorts. During this exchange, it was mentioned that Mark himself had suffered a severe TBI, after which he had been in a coma for thirty-two days, and that he had been pursuing rehabilitation for over seventeen years. When the attorney heard that, his face lost color and grew ashen; he did not speak for a minute. Then with all eyes on him, he said to Mark, "I cannot believe you were severely brain-injured. You followed everything, understood everything, and asked the best questions."

Then he turned to the neuropsychologist and said, "You cannot bring Mark John to court or ever let the opposing side know of him, *of his recovery,* because they will simply point to Mark John, explain how severely he was brain-injured, and then say we can expect our client, who was not injured as severely as Mr. Condon, to recover as well—or better."

Soon afterward, this neuropsychologist terminated Mark's internship and reported to UNC that Mark could never perform the duties of a professional rehabilitation counselor. One of the reasons given for his termination was that he did not take notes when observing their vocational evaluator conduct testing. The fact was Mark had not been *able* to take notes. (On account of severely compromised fine finger dexterity resulting from his brain injury, the Student Disability Department at UNC assigned Mark a notetaker for each of his graduate school classes.) Nor was it Mark's intention to be a vocational evaluator. Nevertheless, this so-called "rehabilitation professional" held it against Mark that he had not taken notes during his internship.

This time, UNC agreed with the neuropsychologist involved and completely terminated Mark's master's degree. Mark met with the chairperson of UNC's rehabilitation counseling department, Dr. Juliet Fried, to ask her if there were some additional classes he could take to address his deficiencies or develop compensating support systems for the disabilities associated with his brain injury. What happened next he could never have anticipated. Abruptly, she straightened up and said, "Absolutely not. As long as I am the chairperson of this department, you will never graduate." Mark's head was spinning in confusion from the transformation in his professor, in this "champion of the disabled," this chair of the Rehabilitation Department, this woman who had marked with her famous "red pen" every grammatical error, every unprofessional phrasing in Mark's vocational evaluations until he himself could write like a pro. How could she now be his enemy?

At this point, Tom Higley came back into the picture (he had never really left), functioning now in his capacity as a respected lawyer. He saw the need for legal representation in Mark's case, but he himself could not ethically enter a dual relationship with Mark; he could not himself represent him. Searching his professional network, Tom found that Diane King of King, Smith, Anderson LLC would be willing to represent Mark on a pro bono basis. (Mark had no financial means to hire an attorney.)

Ms. King did indeed take the case pro-bono, and she followed the procedures to file an appeal of Mark's termination. The first hearing was before the rehabilitation counseling department faculty, including Dr. Juliet Fried, the chair. Mark remembers the hearing: All the professors were seated around the table looking down on him like towering Easter Island statues. Some had their arms crossed the entire time and others would not look at him directly. Mark felt that when they did look at him they did not see a human being with abilities, they saw a brain damaged, handicapped individual—with **dis**abilities that **dis**qualified him from becoming a counselor. In effect, they "spread" his brain injury sequelae across his whole person, obliterating his strengths and unique insight, rendering him **dis**barred from entering their profession—the rehabilitation counseling profession. Their questions were all basic questions that Mark fully answered. Not one of the questions was directed at what accommodations would have to be in place in order to help Mark be successful. Although they regularly declared from the podium in classrooms and taught in their curriculum—that disabilities, properly accommodated, need not be obstacles to employment—no such possibility occurred to the professors when it came to Mark's invisible disabilities. The UNC rehabilitation counseling staff's discrimination against Mark became blatantly apparent to Ms. King and at the next stage of the appeal process in a one-on-one before the Dean of Human Rehabilitative Services—to Dr. Scalia as well.

His research since that time has informed Mark that the misunderstanding associated with brain injury and other invisible disabilities is rampant—spreading across educational, medical, psychological, vocational, and judicial fields. International Disability expert, Joni Eareckson Tada, explained it well when she told someone living with debilitating fatigue, "People have such high expectations of folks like you (with invisible disabilities), like, 'Come on, get your act together.' But they have such low expectations of folks like me in wheelchairs, as though the thought is that we can't do much" (https://invisibledisabilities.org/what-is-an-invisible-disability/). The majority of BI survivor's disabilities, like Mark's, are invisible and those in relationship with these survivors cannot help but dismiss them when they can see no reason why these survivors cannot get their act together.

This hearing did not, in fact, change the faculty's mind. Unfortunately, they became only more entrenched in their determination to terminate Mark's degree process. The next hearing then was with Vincent Scalia, EdD, UNC dean and professor emeritus of human rehabilitative services. Diane King told Mark what she remembered from that exchange, that he answered all Dr. Scallia's questions demonstrating great understanding and full comprehension of the rehabilitation counseling profession just as he did in the first hearing with the five professors. Then toward the end of the second hearing, when Dr. Scalia said he did not think that the Rehabilitation Counseling Department "intended" to discriminate against Mark: King clarified one point of the ADA—it does not measure intent of a perpetrator, rather the appearance of an action, and the professors actions toward Mark without question appeared discriminatory. Dr. Scalia got it and had no more questions—the meeting was ended.

In King's car on the way back to Denver, Mark asked how long before they would know the outcome. She said it should take no more than a week. However, while they were still en route, her cell phone rang, and it was Dr. Scalia, who said that he had reinstated Mark and that Mark would have the full support of the university in working to complete his master's degree.

Once Mark was exonerated and back in the rehabilitation counseling MA degree program, he quickly secured an internship with Bayaud Enterprises, a nonprofit corporation providing vocational assessment, vocational training services, and employment opportunities for disabled people. (Since 1969, Bayaud has served thousands of people in the Denver community.) Susan Richardson at Bayaud was going to be Mark's internship supervisor, and Dr. Fried attended an initial meeting with both Ms. Richardson and Mark before things got started. This time, Dr. Fried highlighted Mark's disabilities, made suggestions about how those disabilities might be compensated for, and before the meeting was finished assured Mark that she would do whatever might be needed to make him successful on this internship. He was reassured to find the Dr. Fried he had originally known back on his side in this way.

Mark successfully completed the internship at Bayaud Enterprises. Afterward, Ms. Richardson wrote a recommendation letter for him that read:

It is with pleasure that I write this recommendation
for Mark John Condon. I was his internship supervisor

during which he continually demonstrated excellence in advocacy situations and an unmatched ability for connecting one-to-one with clients. For instance while working with a 19 year old learning disabled client, who was about to be terminated because of non-involvement, Mark John was able to make a connection and helped him set realistic goals, thus greatly improving his involvement and personal life. Another day, with a young, violent/threatening autistic client who would not let anyone approach him and was determined to leave early, Mark John just sat near the client's workstation without saying a word. After some time and with a few words of acknowledgement from Mark John, the client de-escalated, displayed a calm countenance and stayed for the entire workday.

As a member of our rehabilitation team, Mark John demonstrated enthusiasm while participating in staff meetings, special task force meetings, staffings with referral sources and intakes with new clients. He became known for offering helpful suggestions and bringing a different perspective on the issues of discussion.

I recommended to Mark John that he avoid being stuck behind a desk in a "paper pushing" job. Rather, I feel he should find one that emphasizes the personal contact/counseling skill that he has a flair for. Mark John is enthusiastic, dedicated, hard working, and very resourceful. I feel certain that in the right position, with adequate support, Mark John will greatly benefit the agency and people he works for and with.

Bonnie Drumwright, PhD, CRC, who met Mark during his first year at UNC, left the university to join the faculty at California State University in Sacramento during Mark's second year. After his graduation, she wrote a recommendation letter for Mark that read in part as follows:

> Initially, I became aware of Mark John due to the power of his very positive personality. Long before I introduced myself, I had noted his interactions with colleagues in the Department and felt there was something extraordinary about him. Largely out of curiosity, I reviewed his entrance file and that is when I first learned about Mark John's personal experience with traumatic brain injury. This led to a conversation with him during which I requested that he address my class on his experience with traumatic brain injury; the class was *Introduction to Human Rehabilitation Services*.

> I had no idea what an impact Mark John would make with his speech upon me, and many of the students in my class. Of all the speakers who came to my class, Mark John made the greatest impression. He increased our understanding of the incredible disorientation and loss of self that can be the consequence of injury to the brain. I had many students indicate that his presentation was so moving, their perception of disability would never again be the same. Other students indicated that they decided to pursue a degree in rehabilitation as a result of Mark John's presentation!

> As an instructor, I was impressed with the amount of effort and energy Mark John invested in his presentation. I realized it was more than simply an opportunity to share insights he possessed but was in fact a mission he has chosen for his life's work. Mark John believes that his personal experiences afford him a unique insight into the needs of people with traumatic brain injury. His goal is to learn as much as he can about

this disability in order to better serve the rehabilitation needs of persons who sustain this type of injury. His personal reaction to his own traumatic brain injury is nothing short of inspirational. Mark John is an impressive human being and this is why he has such an impact on people.

Elsha Westhoff, Mark's "second mother," tells how she first met Mark a couple of years before he was in graduate school, when he was still working as a sacker at Steele's Grocery Store in Fort Collins, Colorado, where she shopped. Elsha noticed Mark was always working with a smile, and he packed her groceries better than anyone else, so she would make sure he was her sacker each time she shopped. Elsha had emigrated from Holland to the United States with her husband, Odi in 1958. Since half of Mark's family came from Yugoslavia, when the two of them became acquainted with each other in 1992, they would talk about the then current crisis in Yugoslavia, and Elsha would bring in articles on that topic. Elsha says, "Eventually Mark John learned that I lost my only daughter when she was 22, and my husband seven years before I met Mark John. . . . Mark John was such a capable individual despite his disability, and his conversation was so well informed, that when he said he was considering returning to graduate school, I strongly encouraged him to do so, in fact I said that I would do whatever I could do make that happen." Mark did apply and got accepted.

When his graduate school housing arrangements fell through, Elsha said he could use the spare bedroom in her house; so the summer before his first semester at UNC, he moved in with her. At first, he was spending time out with friends—late at night—but that had to stop if he was going to continue living with Elsha. They made an agreement— to get him through grad school. The condition was he had to put his best effort into that goal. As time went by, Elsha became more familiar with Mark's susceptibilities and his strengths. He could only focus on one thing at a time, so Elsha began to take care of other things for him like washing clothes and preparing meals to free him to concentrate on his studies. She learned to see when fatigue diminished his awareness/presence by a few or many degrees, depending on how tired he was. They became a true family, including Mark's parents, who became some of Elsha's best friends and remain so to this day.

In 1996, Elsha wrote to Mark John's parents in reflection:

> When I think back to the first day when Mark John came to stay with me I can hardly believe how he has changed. After a year there is not much left of the darling little boy that we call Markie Mark, in fact Markie Mark has not been around for a long time. . . . Let me tell you about his lecture in October at UNC. Mark John was facing an amphitheater with 60–70 kids of whom he knew not one, only the teacher and me he knew. He was very good with his presentation, having little gestures, showing the fingers of his left hand and how difficult it is for him to move them, showing the trouble he has walking with his left leg and foot, while he kept moving from the left to the right in front of the class, facing up or down, referring to the notes and looking at each person. He surely had them; there was communication between him and the students, not one was fidgeting or looking off somewhere! Off and on I would look around and what I saw was an audience that was spell bound. It was his own experience that he gave them, with some figures and remarks in general thrown in, nothing in a victim kind of way, he was more objective than that but it was still a personal lived experience and the students recognized it. He had on what I call his engineers-face, he was very focused and motivated, and he was the 37 year-old man who had something to teach them.

One woman whose daughter had brain damage from a car accident hung on his lips and was so moved that she started talking about it with me at the end. Afterwards you should have seen the people that wanted to talk to Mark John, standing neatly in a row waiting for him. That was when the professor, Dr. Drumwright, a very positive, friendly and simple woman came over to me and we said at the same time, "I am so proud of him!" to each other. Of course Mark John was exhausted afterwards, he went to bed in his dorm room at 4:00pm that Thursday, then slept late in the mornings on Saturday and Sunday in his room at my house—he was very tired from this great big event. Later I told him: now you are out of the victim cage; these people will never see you as a victim, but instead as a teacher, and they have great respect for you. He is very happy with that idea. He wants to do more talks for different audiences, and I am inclined to say: yes do that!

I had a wonderful life before Mark John came into it, and it did not change, I still have a marvelous life. The Lord has always taken care of me, when I was a teenager in World War II, and when Odi and I immigrated to the United States, when we had our child Nella, and also afterwards when she died and then when he died, always has He been there. Then one day He decided that there was still something that needed to be done, and that I was the person who could do it with His help, and that was when Mark John came in my life. I thank God every day, and ask Him for wisdom and guidance, and He has helped me. Mark John is also wonderful to me, he is considerate and helpful and makes me laugh, calls me by my Dutch name that nobody has used for 40 years.

Elsha added, "I was so happy when the internship problem got worked out. I tried to tell UNC before the problem arose that he would need supports, but they were certain that he would not, and told me not to worry." Her own life, Elsha now feels, improved in several ways from working along with Mark and seeing him graduate with a master's degree. It was quite an accomplishment for both of them. "I did not mind typing all his papers, I enjoyed reading what he had written," she says. The two continue their relationship to this day, just as any family would, and look forward to their times together.

Another good friend of Mark's from those days, Mike in Fort Collins, recounts an incident when he and Mark were roommates, and Mark was working at Steele's Grocery Store. "Mark John came home for lunch one day, which was unusual, and he was more shook up than I had ever seen him. I asked him what was wrong and he told me that one cashier and a sacker at the grocery store were mocking him, laughing at him, right to his face, and imitating his broken gait and constricted left arm." Their mindless cruelty had caused Mark to begin thinking of how difficult his recovery had been and of all that he still could not do. All that negative material had suddenly flooded and all but overwhelmed him. Mike did what he could to console Mark and help him work through it, but the psychological pain involved was intense. After some difficult moments had passed, Mark finally regained his composure enough to go back and try to finish his workday at the grocery store. As he was leaving, Mike asked him who that checker was.

Later that afternoon, Mike went into the store, made sure he knew which one the offending cashier was, went through the right checkout line, and when he got up to the cashier said, "I know what you did. It is despicable and cowardly." He then proceeded to leave the store, but the cashier followed and stopped him before he got outside. He demanded to know what Mike was talking about. Mike explained that he knew the cashier had ridiculed Mark John and laughed in his face. The two men then had a heated exchange. Mike forcefully told the cashier how much he had hurt Mark John, pointed out that the cashier couldn't even imagine how difficult life was for Mark John after brain injury, *and* made it clear that if he ever humiliated Mark John again, it would be his mistake (implying that Mike would give the cashier a knuckle sandwich). Their confrontation drew the attention of the store manager. Over the next ten days, the owners of the store themselves, Robert Steele and Russ Kates, investigated the matter, interviewed everyone involved, and in the end fired the cashier, who it turned out had some other negative job performance issues. Mike was glad to have helped vindicate Mark John.

One of Mark's friends John Colvin, who knew Mark both before and after his brain injury, writes:

> I had the pleasure of meeting Mark John Condon in 1978 during my freshman year at Northern Michigan University. He would come to campus ministry events, always with a contagious sense of humor, being a very popular man about campus involved in the Greek fraternity system. We both transferred to Michigan State University for different reasons, Mark a year earlier than I, and we became roommates on campus. During my first year at MSU, I came back from my Father's second wedding and heard that Mark had been in a serious accident. I was stunned. Since I was involved in a faith community, we prayed for Mark's life and his recovery, fully aware that he was in a coma and near death.
>
> Once he got out of the hospital and was struggling to manage life, Mark could have become, a "victim" and indulged in self-pity, with a sense of entitlement because of the injustice served him by a drunk driver. I say most assuredly that he did not. He asserted a "can-do" attitude related to his recovery and pressed on to accomplish whatever he could despite the horrible accident. This accident did not define him, instead he

chose to use his experience to help others that have been brain injured, and work to prevent TBIs as much as possible, any way possible.

Knowing Mark prior to his injury, he could have lived a very comfortable life with his good looks, intelligence, sense of humor, and athleticism. Certainly that fateful night changed the course of his life. However I have found Mark does not dwell on this. He looks for opportunities, not excuses. He is grateful and not bitter. He is thankful for every gift he has. He enjoys the time he shares with his delightful daughter Lia and he has a tremendous circle of friends that I am glad to be a part of. In 2012 I remember hearing Mark give the keynote address at the first Cathleen's Cause Gala Event Fundraiser for a Cathleen Herzog who suffered a traumatic brain injury, and there was not a dry eye in the beautiful ballroom of more than 200 well-heeled Denverites. He demonstrated how much he cared. Mark shared how much he worked on his own cognitive health and recovery. He wore his heart and concern on his sleeve. He showed how he dedicated the remaining days of his life to research, encouragement and advocacy for those sustaining brain injuries. I am privileged to count Mark John Condon as one of my best friends for more than 30 years.

Tom Steinen, a first cousin of Mark on his father's side of the family, wrote:

I remember getting the phone call from my mother telling me of the terrible accident Mark was in. My wife and I were shocked. After a couple of weeks, while Mark was still in a coma, we made plans with other family members to travel from different parts of the country to go see him in the hospital. It was overwhelming to see him so skinny with all the tubes coming out of him, lying there, not moving at all. We kept in touch daily from home and were so thankful for his progress. Years later Mark called us in Arkansas and said he needed to buy an inexpensive used car with limited resources and wanted to come to our place where the winters were kinder to car bodies than Michigan was. He asked if it would be OK with us. We said it would be fine and Mark scheduled the trip. Actually we were struggling with some issues in our marriage and it was not a good time for us—or so we thought.

When the day came for Mark to arrive we went to the bus station to pick him up. This was a few years after his accident and his condition was still greatly compromised. We imagined the bus trip would be very hard on Mark, but he got off the bus with a big smile on his face and shared how wonderful the trip was—he had the opportunity to talk to various passengers seated next to him. As we spent the next few days helping Mark find a car we could not help but notice that he had something we did not have. It was a peace—a peace that enveloped Mark—a peace with God and with himself.

When we waved goodbye as Mark drove off in his "new used car," my wife Kathy and I looked at each other and said, "What is it that Mark has?" It was a peace with God and we realized that we did not have it. God used Mark's little trip to Arkansas to demonstrate what this personal relationship God wants with each of us looks like. I have since pursued working in Christian ministry and became a pastor of a small Church in Arkansas. Our walk with our Lord has been amazing and we thank Him that He loved us so much that He would send people like Mark into our life at just the right time to help us in our journey with God. Thank you Mark for being who you are, for being the light in our life when we needed to see it.

Mark's brother Jeff, who was in his first year of college when Mark was hospitalized, put things this way:

> Before the accident my brother Mark was a charismatic man that wanted to see the best in those around him. In 1980 I was in high school and Mark was home for the summer, he helped me train for a halfback position on the High School football team— running, throwing, catching all summer to improve my skill level. He also was involved in a summer bible study with several other young people, their joy drew me in and eventually led me to a personal relationship with Jesus Christ. At MSU, Mark was a leader in the Christian group that my brother Tom and I became a part of. Mark was jovial and well liked in the group. He was a no nonsense kind of guy with a great sense of humor—lots of laughs.

> When Mark had his accident and was laying in the ICU, the severity of his condition could not be perceived, for he had no visible damage to his body other than his broken ribs which were not obvious. Then as the weeks wore on with the unknown future looming in the hospital room, it was devastating to see his body withering away, the brain injury sucking the life out of him and our hope and joy along with it. When Mark first opened one eye, his entire family celebrated. But we had no idea that years and years of recovery lay ahead for him. We were scared, I was scared, and I think I failed most of my classes that semester.

Years of small steps of growth for Mark followed: social skills, motor skills, regaining knowledge, what is OK and not OK relationship wise, learning to live life all over again. Small steps from an outsider's point of view, but each was a huge, huge step for Mark. Relearning the social norms of society was really difficult for him to relearn as a brain injured adult—I saw how those around Mark reacted if he asked an odd question, or did something out of the norm—it was awkward. From my point of view, his youngest brother's point of view, this Mark was not the same Mark—but I was never more proud of him. He was so determined to be the best he could be. Currently, I can still see improvements from year to year, whenever we are together. More and more of his "original" personality returns each time. After years of recovery, Mark still has his great sense of humor. My kids love him and his laugh. Mark is extremely disciplined in the areas he chooses, loving his daughter Lia, being the best Dad to her.

Mark's brother Tom says:

Mark is a few years older than me so growing up I knew him as the fun older brother that had lots of friends and lots to do. He had a wild side that seemed to only fuel his popularity among his friends and fascination from his little brother. Then everything exploded as I answered the phone late at night in my dorm room at Michigan State University—Mom and Dad passed the phone between them as they described what had happened then urged me to find my younger brother Jeff and for both of us rush to Mark's bedside at the hospital soon as possible—BEFORE HE DIES! We did just that and watched and prayed as Mark fought for his life.

The years that followed were full of physical and emotional struggles that none of us can really know. Mark's determination and will to continue on comes from *his* inner strength and is supported by God's unfailing love. I'm sure there are more situations of despair than I know, but I saw him dejected at different times after working so hard only to experience another set-back, and I saw him rejoice after regaining a simple function that the rest of us take for granted—like snapping his left fingers. How many of us have lost the abilities that "define" who we are, the abilities that allowed us to operate in the world, and then have to work like crazy to reestablish those abilities—then only be able to get half of them back? How many of us have had to deal with hurtful statements like, "You embarrass me." or "I don't want you around my friends."? It must be so difficult to be on top of the world and then to have to start all over with relearning and doing so much. Mark gives credit to lots of friends and family but it wouldn't happen without Mark making it happen.

Mark's elder brother, Dan, is a retired Fairbanks, Alaska, Fire Department captain and paramedic. He currently is a critical care flight paramedic with LifeMed Alaska. Dan married Cathy thirty years ago. He is the father of four and the grandfather of five and lives on a small farm in Fairbanks, where dog mushing is one of his hobbies. Dan writes:

I'm 16 months older than my brother Mark. We were close brothers growing up, playing together and getting into mischief—once, catching on fire the little field behind our house, and another time covering one side of our house with mud—later, going into the woods with my uncles while they logged, fishing with my dad or cousins, and playing hockey after school in Mt. Pleasant, Michigan. We were good Catholic boys, with good parents who taught us to be honest and kind. As we grew up we had some friends in common and some friends unique to each of us, and this was more so as we grew older. In middle school and high school, Mark had some friends that could be a little on the meaner side, maybe more apt to get in trouble. I remember walking home from school one afternoon and sort of admonishing Mark not to follow their example, but to be kind and good. I don't remember my words or Mark's response exactly, he didn't say much at the time, yet he was not dismissive or defensive. Several years later he thanked me for those simple words. Apparently they were good words, spoken at the right time, to a heart that wanted the truth.

In the spring of 1975 our family moved to Silver City. I worked full time in our parent's restaurant, Mark had one more year of high school, and worked part time in the restaurant. He made friends easily and our lives were quite different at that time. A year later I moved to Alaska where I worked and attended The University of Alaska (UA) in Fairbanks.

It was there the following spring that I heard God speak to me a very simple but pointed question. I grew up with a love and respect for God but my lifestyle over the last couple years had in many ways betrayed that love. Very clearly God asked me, "Who are you living to please, Me or yourself?" I immediately knew the answer was myself and I immediately knew that is not what I wanted, that was not my heart. This led me, along with a couple friends, on a quest, reading the Bible and any other religious material we could find. One night on my bed in UA's Moore Hall I prayed, "God I want the truth, I want Your Holy Spirit, I want to be born of Your Spirit and to know the Truth and to walk with You." Something happened, something happened inside of me, I got up off the bed and suddenly it was as if someone turned the lights on—I could see! I could see my faults and sins and it was joyful and wonderful because I knew that God was alive in me and I was washed of all guilt and condemnation. The joy and freedom I experienced was amazing, I knew my life would never be the same.

I'm a quiet person, I don't usually talk a lot. Silence is fine with me much of the time. That summer I returned to Michigan for a visit for the first time. Though part of me wanted to tell everyone what had happened to me, I shared it only with my brother Mark. He was attending Northern Michigan University that fall. Mark did not say much at the time—again he was not dismissive or defensive. The following Christmas I went home again for a while. We had a very memorable family time that Christmas Day. I wanted to share with my whole family what had happened to me since I invited Christ into my life, plus the importance of seeking the Lord and reading the Bible. Guess what the best surprise was that Christmas? Mark too had been born again (John 3:3) that fall at NMU! We shared our faith together. It sort of became an *Us vs. Them* lively discussion: Mark and I engaging Mom and Dad with Tom, Jeff And Kathy mostly listening. Our parents were aghast—they thought we had abandoned the faith because we no longer attended Catholic Church and hoped it was only some odd religious phase. My sister and my younger brothers listened. As the emotional conversation wound down—the most intense conversation we had ever had, or ever would have, my dad asked our siblings what they thought. I clearly remember brother Tom's response;

"I don't know, but whatever they have, I want." What a day!

So Mark and I were both changed men, we lived different but similar lives, our hearts were the same. Mark moved to Lansing and found fellowship with a vibrant group of disciples. Then there was the accident. I got the phone call from Mom, they were on their way to Lansing, Mark was in a coma and may not live. I was able to travel to Michigan a day or two later. We stayed at his bedside as much as we were allowed to, we prayed as much as we could. I stayed at the Work of Christ's Brothers House, a group of young men who desired to be true disciples. Tom Higley was a true friend and host, coming to the hospital every day, praying and spending time with Mark and our family members from out of town. Friends like that are invaluable and rare. During the first two weeks the doctors were not at all optimistic for recovery but in the third week there were signs of Mark starting to come out of the coma. Back then I thought people would come out of a coma like waking up in the morning and be better. Not so, it is more like taking weeks or months to wake up, gradually. One of the things the hospital warned us of was that many people, especially men, would be vulgar and maybe even vile when they awoke and were waking up from a coma. The first time Mark opened one eye he did not say anything. Then a few days later Mark spoke his first words, "Praise God, we have the victory!" That was Mark! A couple weeks later he was doing physical and occupational therapy. I was with him one day when the therapist asked him, "What is your number one pet peeve?" Mark kind of shrugged and said he didn't have one. She persisted and asked well what really frustrates you, what makes you mad? He thought another minute then replied, "When young men don't seek God, and make Jesus Christ their Lord, that's what bothers me most."

It would be normal to observe what had happened to Mark and say, one day he was in an accident and a month later he woke up a different person. But there is a lot going on inside of a man, in the deepest most eternal place, and that doesn't stop because the brain is injured. This was apparent as we watched Mark in the worst days of his injury and during his recovery. Badly injured and unable to function outwardly the same way he did before, Mark was the same person: like a person who loses the use of their legs due to a traumatic accident, they are, and he was, still the same person. Our brain is an organ that allows us to do the amazing things that people can do, but there is so much more to us than an assembly of organs and neurons and muscle systems. When we die our brain will be done yet our soul will live on, as will our spirit. A few weeks after Mark came out of his coma I returned to my life in Alaska and Mark continued in his recovery—badly injured but going strong, moving forward, and growing, he truly is an amazing man. A couple years later Mark wrote me a card and signed it "Your brother eternal"—what truth could be more treasured?!

Mark's sister, Kathy, writes:

I was leaving work and had a sense that I should pray come over me. Driving home the sense became an urge that pressed down and I knew I had to stop. I stopped at a church and sat and prayed. I didn't know who I was praying for or why but asked the Lord to hear my prayers.

Later that evening the call came from my parents. My brother Mark was in a car accident and the doctors didn't know if he would survive the night. Weeping I told my parents I would be in Lansing as soon as I could. How can this be? My brother Mark may die? Our family can't be our family without Mark. My roommate drove me to the airport so I could buy a ticket for the next day. Between crying and praying and thinking about losing Mark I didn't sleep that night.

As a Registered Nurse I did have an idea of what to expect when I walked into ICU. But it's so different when it's your brother lying on the table. All my nursing knowledge told me the severity of his injuries had him at death's door but my heart cried out to God "please save him!" Days passed as he battled to stay with us. Medical crises arose, new therapies were tried, and Mark stayed with us. One day, at the nurses' command, Mark squeezed his hand and then mom's. Oh what joy flooded our hearts! But it's not like the movies when the eyes flutter open and the person asks "what happened." It has proved to be a very long and difficult road. During Mark's recovery he had a flat affect for sometime, we all missed his smile and personality. Jeff one day said "I wish Mark would laugh" to which Mark, who overheard Jeff, responded very dryly "ha, ha, ha." The Mark we knew and expected to "wake up" had a long recovery ahead of him.

At the time of Mark's accident people were just beginning to survive severe closed head injuries. The therapies were basic as if caring for a stroke patient. The information available to families was practically nonexistent and of course most of it was very negative. So our family did what we could and what families do best. We stayed at his side, encouraged him, supported him, and of course prayed.

The time was drawing close for his discharge from the hospital. His therapies—speech, physical, and occupational, would need to continue. My parents lived 600 miles from the hospital in a very tiny community with no supportive therapies available. Mom called, burdened with what to do, and I said "I'll move to Lansing and Mark can live with me." I packed up my apartment in Minneapolis and moved to Lansing, Michigan.

I may be a nurse but I had zero practice being a therapist or a motivator. There wasn't anyone to explain what a broken brain did to a person. I worked with Mark with his exercises, speech, and activities of daily living. It was hard to keep pushing him. It was hard to have patience when he kept pushing back on me. The day came when the therapist said his therapy was nearing completion. Today I wish I would have known to insist that they continue for months or years. I suppose they felt they had done all that was possible but I knew there was more healing and growth needed before Mark could live independently.

Mark moved in with his friends and I moved in with my new friends in Lansing. Years have passed and most amazingly Mark continues to heal. The human body is miraculous! If that makes it sound easy to any degree— it is not! The recovery process is frustrating, hard, and even depressing, but joyful, amazing and miraculous at the same time. People faced with a traumatic brain injury need so much more support than is given them. Therapies, life coaches, job coaches, and someone needs to tell the story of recovery. That person could well be my brother Mark, the ultimate survivor!! Love you, brother, so glad God answered our prayers!!

Dorothy Condon, Mark's mother, remembers the night of Mark's accident:

It was 9:00 p.m. and we just finished feeding 100 people in the restaurant when my husband Tom came back to the kitchen crying. The State Police just called and said that our son Mark, a senior at Michigan State University, had just been in a car accident, was critically injured and was not expected to survive through the night. In a few minutes we were on our way driving 9 hours through the dark night. I didn't want him to die without us—or his brothers Tom and Jeff by his side. The police were trying to reach them but were not successful. There weren't any cell phones at that time so we kept stopping at gas stations using their pay phones to call Tom's dorm room. Finally we reached him at midnight and were comforted to know that Tom and Jeff were on their way to be with Mark.

We prayed and cried for the whole 9-hour drive and thanked God he was still alive when we walked into the ICU. It was such a shock to see our healthy son in a coma, hooked up to the respirator, IV's, etc. The doctors said if he survives he would probably have to be institutionalized. They wanted to give me some Valium but I said, "No, I have faith he will survive." It broke my heart to see him lying on a cooling mattress almost naked, just shaking and shivering. They were attempting to keep his body temperature down to keep his brain from swelling more. I stayed with him every day and didn't want to leave the hospital for several weeks—for I was afraid he might die without me there. We reluctantly signed a permit for a treatment that would either kill him or save him, what choice did we have, if we did not sign he would surely die. Thank God it was the right decision.

Through the years I shed many tears. The pain I encountered led me to a deeper spirituality. After many years of recovery, Mark graduating with a Master's Degree in Rehabilitation Counseling was nothing short of a miracle, especially when the doctors told us he will never be able to live independently or maintain a job. Granted, life for Mark with a brain injury was never easy: He breaks through medical barriers, solves big problems, then gets stuck in procrastination or self-doubt, makes a poor decision and takes a step backwards. It is like two steps forward, one step back, sometimes two steps back, or no steps at all, then forward again. However over the years he keeps steadily moving forward and the insights on life he has acquired have helped many people, including his father, his siblings and myself. Everything Mark has experienced and endured over the years since his accident prepared him for what he has become—a hope and help to other brain injury survivors. God prepared him for this.

Mark's father, Thomas, is a remarkable man in his own way, for his father, Joseph Condon, was an alcoholic who sometimes missed work and "forgot to come home," causing the family to always be short on money. Tom remembers having to hide many times as a young boy when the landlord came for the rent because his parents didn't have it. Because Tom loved his father and his family, he started working in eighth grade on a soda pop delivery truck to be able to give money to his mother. Like many children of alcoholics, Tom himself started drinking when he was in high school, and it became, for a significant part of his life, a problem. Later as a married man with two kids, he went to college on the GI Bill, but the money from that did not go far enough; so in addition to being a full-time student and a full-time dad, Tom worked for twenty-five to thirty hours a week. He told Mark, "Most of the time we didn't have two nickels to rub together, but we made it. I worked harder than the next guy on every job, leaving it in better condition than when I came on board, and I was always promoted. By the time we had five kids, I used to fear that I wouldn't make it, but all I could do was keep trying my best. I still am trying my best, and things keep working out. I believe the saying 'The only thing to fear is fear itself.'"

Tom began working for Central Michigan University in 1965, and he left ten years later in 1975 as the associate director of auxiliary services. He then, for thirty-five years, owned and operated, together with his family, Paul's Supper Club and Bar in Silver City, Michigan. Tom and the family expanded that business in 1995, building a forty-room Best Western Hotel and adding thirty employees. Over the years they were in business, Tom and Dorothy helped many people develop job skills, and they continued to help out various people with various kinds of problems even after they sold the business in 2010.

Today Tom, who is retired, has been clean and sober for over twenty-five years. Mark credits his own work ethic to that of his father and believes he would neither have survived his accident nor have been able to rehabilitate himself without his father's love and spirit. Tom Condon says his biggest achievement in life is "love for my loving, beautiful wife, our five amazing healthy children, our eleven wonderful grandchildren and thirteen great grandchildren."

Regarding Mark's accident, his father wrote:

> The crushing news from the State Police that my son was in a very bad accident that left his life hanging by a thread was hard to grasp. One day our family was living life to the fullest and then with a phone call, we were facing the hard fact that one of our sons may not

live through the night. Mark was a student at Michigan State University and was in his senior year in packaging design engineering.

We had a restaurant and bar to run in Upper Michigan, but thankfully our good employees took over and we started the long nine-hour drive to Lansing. No word yet that Mark would live. It was the longest night and we prayed, cried and asked God to spare him. We didn't want Mark to be alone, to die alone (which was too hard to accept) but Dorothy got through to Tom and Jeff around midnight. They went right over to the hospital and greeted us when we arrived and we all went to ICU. Mark was critical but thank God he had good doctors. Dr. Nieberg stayed all night monitoring Mark's vitals and figuring out how to save his life.

Mark was in a coma 32 days and survived. I was back in Silver City taking care of business when Dot called and said he was going to make it. I knelt down and thanked God with tears of joy. Mark's accident brought the whole family closer together. Not understanding how to rehabilitate a damaged brain was very hard on the whole family. We all learned patience and persistence and worked very hard to be a good support team. Through it all, Mark worked the hardest of any of us and set his goal on full recovery, he made great progress and surpassed all the limits the professionals said he would not be able to. With all the rejections and setbacks over the years he has never given up. With SSDI and part-time employment, Mark is self-sufficient, lives on his own in a 2-bedroom apartment with his daughter Lia who is 16 years old, and is still working hard on his recovery. I am the one who is inspired by *his* tenacity and spirit.

♦

Mark graduated from the University of Northern Colorado in December of 1998 surrounded by his own immediate family and his cousins Rob, Cathy, Erica, and Ethan Saffer as well as by Tom Higley, John Colvin, Mark Roe, and others. It was a great day for all involved. Mark rightly attributes his accomplishments to the family and friends who stood by him and believed in him when he was finding it difficult to believe in himself. When he thinks about how things *might* have turned out and about the love he has received from so many people, Mark says, "I'm not 'the luckiest man in the world,' but I'm pretty darn close." Mark's seventeen-year-old daughter, Lia Salomé, has been and is the joy of his life. He proudly put it this way: "She is so beautiful, so perceptive, so smart, so fun, and so loving that when things are good in her life, they are good in my life as well."

Clearly, Mark's faith, family, and friends have been the wind beneath his wings, yet it has been Mark himself who has angled his "disabled wings" to get him over the mountains of obstacles that lie before a brain injury survivor. As Mark has succeeded in climbing each new mountain, his family and friends have been encouraged to believe that now life for him will return to normal; but no, the lifelong complications of brain injury are such that there will always be another mountain and another after that—life goes on, but brain injury never really goes away. Mark's life has become more normal but only by degrees and to a certain extent so that, depending on what he (like any other survivor) chooses to focus on, he may feel either depression and defeat or encouragement and strength.

In recent years, Mark has found himself in demand as a public speaker on the topic of brain injury and its consequences. This phase of his life began with a big step forward when he was asked by Paul Herzog to speak at a fundraiser for his wife, Cathleen Schmidt-Herzog. While at home in Denver, Cathleen—a type 1 diabetic—lost consciousness in early January 2012, fell in her own kitchen, hit her head, and suffered a very severe traumatic brain injury. After spending four months at

Denver Health in various critical care units, she was referred to Craig Rehabilitation Hospital for the beginning of a journey and discovery process. What kind of progress could Cathleen make in an environment with dedicated therapists and specialists? The answer was some progress and some medical stability, but Cathleen still could not stand, walk, talk, or eat when she left Craig Hospital on August 1, 2013. She still required twenty-four-seven skilled nursing care. Cathleen's parents, Volk and Sharen Schmidt, together with her husband, Paul, and aided by family and friends, organized a gala fundraiser event to cover a year's worth of the $15,000 monthly cost for a night nurse and medications. Paul writes:

> When we contacted the Brain Injury Alliance of Colorado for a knowledgeable keynote speaker to help everyone understand what Cathleen and her family was going through, after thinking a couple of minutes, they said, "Why don't you contact Mark Condon? He works here at BIAC and is also a traumatic brain injury survivor." I called Mark and quickly established a good connection. The next week Mark joined Cathleen, our daughter Emma, Volk, and Sharen and me for dinner, and we agreed on the outline of what turned out to be an amazing speech about his experience as a brain injury survivor and the many challenges he has overcome. Initially what really impressed us about Mark were his caring questions and observations of where Cathleen was in her recovery. He told us we had a long and difficult road ahead of us, but offered a lot of hope as well, because Cathleen was aware and alert and showed a strong desire to recover—plus we had a strong support network. When Sharen asked Mark at dinner that night, "How long did it take for your recovery?"

Mark responded, "I still am recovering, every day."

At the November 2012 Gala Event, with Mark's help, his inspirational, heartfelt speech, and the generosity of our community, we were able to raise nearly $200,000, enough to cover 14 months of nighttime private pay nursing care for Cathleen. Mark has been so supportive of Cathleen and we her family—he has spoken at each subsequent Cathleen's Cause Annual Gala Fund Raiser. When he speaks the audience is captivated by his words. I think that is not only because of the brilliant ways he has of explaining what a brain injury is like, but also because of genuine authenticity that is a part of him, you feel what he is saying—you don't just hear it.

Mark's speech at the first annual Cathleen's Cause made such an impression on the audience and BIAC staff that he was also asked to speak at BIAC's 2013 breakfast with the board fundraiser. Again, Mark's speech was, at times, fraught with tears as various experiences flooded his memory and overwhelmed him emotionally. Again, the audience as well was heart struck, and many of those present were in tears. Colorado state representative Dianne Primavera was in the audience, and after the standing ovation at the end had subsided, she asked Mark if he would speak at the state capitol to other state legislators. He was glad to accept the offer. Mark, again, gave an emotional speech to those Colorado state legislators who are responsible for human services and related government affairs. BIAC has since asked Mark to be a national speaker and help educate the public about the far-reaching implications of brain injury. Their goal is to increase awareness, promote initiatives to prevent brain injuries, and encourage the development of rehabilitation facilities. Mark has entered into a speaking contract with BIAC that he feels is a win-win for all concerned, and he is even now working on his next speech.

In 2012, Travelers Life and Casualty, Mark's insurance company, stopped payment on his Bosick chiropractic and Lixin acupuncture as well as on Roann Riedel's massage therapies—the very therapies that had helped Mark reach his highest percent of muscle recruitment through Brucker biofeedback therapy and enabled him to reach his highest level of independence since his accident. Fortunately, Mark's friend Dan Sloane is a personal injury attorney and was the former president of the board of directors of the Brain Injury Alliance of Colorado. Sloane immediately got involved pro bono and contested Travelers' stopping payment for this combination of therapies (which had been identified as "medically necessary" by Dr. McIntosh).

Dan Sloane writes:

> I have been fortunate enough to know Mark Condon for over ten years. In that time, Mark has impressed, inspired and motivated me in more ways than I can count. Beginning with his accident Mark's story starts out as one of misfortune and adversity, but quickly becomes a story of survival, hard work, success and inspiration. I feel very confident that Mark's story going into the future will be equally inspiring.

> While Mark has been my friend, and lunch companion, for many years, it was not until 2012 that Mark needed my assistance as a lawyer. It was then that the insurance company that had been paying for Mark's rehabilitation tried to stop his benefits, potentially undoing much of the progress he had made over the years. When Mark called and told me about the decision, randomly made by a new insurance adjuster evidently trying to score a few meaningless points with the home office, by stopping many of his rehabilitation therapy benefits, I was incensed but not surprised. Unfortunately, as a lawyer who represents injured people every day, I see this happening all the time and the motivation is always the same—saving money. As is natural for Mark, he tried for quite some time to

deal with the adjuster himself and brought tremendous evidence to the table. Of course, it was to no avail. The insurance adjuster was not out to discover the truth about Mark and the treatments that had helped over the years. He was out to "paper" his file and then unjustly deny Mark treatment.

In an effort to help my friend, I spent several months communicating with the insurance company. No longer satisfied with the answers I was getting from the adjuster I sought out his supervisor. Unfortunately, it did not make a difference. After months of getting nowhere, Mark and I decided our only option was to bring a lawsuit against the company. For good or bad, the insurance policy that provided Mark coverage was a policy governed under the laws of Michigan, the state where Mark lived at the time of the accident. Being licensed only in Colorado, and having no knowledge of Michigan insurance law, I contacted a respected attorney in Michigan who I had worked with several years before on a large, nationwide product liability case, Bill Lamping. Thankfully Bill took the case.

William (Bill) Lamping felt certain Mark had a good case, and although he could not undertake it pro bono, he was able to begin work in Mark's behalf since Michigan's legal statute allows attorneys to collect their fees from the defendant if they win the case. Six months after becoming Mark's legal counsel, Mr. Lamping spoke with Travelers' attorney, who was of the opinion that the only way that Mark, who in the preceding years had been without an attorney, was able to get his case reopened twice after Travelers had closed it (something both Travelers' attorney and Mr. Lamping had never seen before) was through his legal-minded, documenting skills and the well-reasoned lengthy letters he had written—"he simply wore them out with the facts." A year later, the case was settled. Mark forfeited on some matters, but he won on others, a crucial one being coverage for continued biannual therapy at the Brucker biofeedback center, plus monthly physical therapy for the remainder of his life and the purchase of new therapies yet to be discovered that prove to restore functional abilities after brain injury.

Of Mark, Bill Lamping writes, "Mr. Condon is my most unique client. He has overcome travails that would overwhelm most people, and he has triumphed in circumstances that would make many succumb to despair. Mark's resiliency is an inspiration. He works every day to maximize his recovery. I hold him up as an example to other injured clients that they too can build a new life even after tragedy has changed everything for them."

It is a matter of public record that there comes a time, some twenty years or so after a brain injury, when survivors decline in their functional abilities, both physical and mental. That happens because of the secondary consequences of brain injury. Mark beat the average onset of decline, but thirty-three years after his TBI, decreased microcirculation on his hemiplegic left side resulted in a small posterior superior labral tear extending to the inferior posterior quadrant, resulting in a large paravertebral cyst, early denervation, glenohumeral osteoarthrosis, and mild subscapularis tendinopathy without discrete tear on his left shoulder. He had orthoscopic shoulder surgery in 2014 and was in rehabilitation for a year and a half before he regained much of his left shoulder function. Mark saw this as an opportunity to find a method, a therapy, a way to increase the microcirculation in his and other survivors' bodies and brains, for such a therapy is critically needed to prevent/heal such injuries and thwart the decline in function that most survivors experience twenty-plus years post-injury. When the PEMF microcirculation device came into his life, it was the way to increase microcirculation and the answer he was looking for. Today his company, Transforming Techniques Incorporated, has a franchise and is working to bring the PEMF microcirculation device into the homes of other survivors across the nation.

Mark does not know what the future holds for him, but he remains passionately committed to doing whatever he can to reduce the incident of brain injuries and to improve the outcomes of brain injury survivors. Mark quotes something humorous he once saw posted on an office wall—"What I need is a list of all the specific unknown problems we will encounter"—to acknowledge the fact that no matter how much a person may want to know the unknown future, it simply is beyond our grasp. The best anyone can do is prepare for the unexpected with education and training.

This is the end of Mark's first book. I would like to see him continue to write, for he seems to have an innate gift for writing in such a way that it is hard to forget what he has to say. Mark does not even remember a detail of his history I am about to mention, but his mother has shown me the clipping of a 1974 newspaper story from when he was only fourteen years old. He won that year the statewide Police Officers Association of Michigan (POAM) essay contest on prevention of juvenile delinquency. Mark's entry was chosen from among more than three hundred others, and he was among several other winners who won saving bonds totaling $2,575. His and the other contestants' thoughts and ideas about ways to prevent delinquency were incorporated in a booklet published by the POAM for distribution to law enforcement agencies throughout Michigan.

The text of Mark's present book, *The Silent Epidemic: What Everyone Should Know about Brain Injury*, does not exemplify either of two standard plot lines. David McRaney notes in his book *You Are Now Less Dumb* (*an in-depth analysis of psychological foibles*) that people generally prefer tales with the structure they've come to understand as the backbone of good storytelling: three to five acts, an opening with the main character forced to face adversity, a turning point where that character chooses to embark on an adventure in an unfamiliar world, and a journey in which the character grows as a person and eventually wins against great odds, thanks to that growth. That, according to mythologist Joseph Campbell and other students of literature, is the pattern of nearly every story ever written.

Tragedies, however—in which the leading character makes some mistake in judgment, refuses to change, chooses poorly, or is betrayed by some character flaw and as a result suffers great loss—represent a major exception and an alternative pattern. We are fascinated by both kinds of narrative because they reflect the ways in which we see real life played out for ourselves and those around us. People even tend to make use of both kinds of plot in shaping mentally their own narratives of what has happened to them, what they've accomplished, and what their futures may look like.

Mark's story reflects both these models in some ways. He did undertake a journey through an unfamiliar world, and through it, he has grown—against great odds. Certain things that he has lost, however—precious things—have not been restored or compensated for and never can be, not even by any amount of growth, yet his losses were not caused by any mistake or weakness of his own. Rather, in Mark's story, the tragic flaws were those of a drunk driver who, as far as Mark knows, has never faced any repercussions—neither been held responsible in any way nor even reached enough of an epiphany to stop drinking and driving. That lack of consequences is not common in stories; it may be unsettling for readers who expect justice and an "end."

What Mark wants people to understand is that living with a brain injury is also not typical and that it too has no end. Life remains for each survivor and his or her family a constant, continuing struggle, with ever-recurring highs and lows of varying degrees. However, as Charles Krauthammer wrote in the *Washington Post* on August 17, 2007, reflecting on the catastrophe that may, in an ordinary instant, befall any one of us from a single false move, wrong turn, or fatal encounter, "Every life has such a moment. What distinguishes us is whether—and how—we ever come back." Mark has made a most remarkable comeback from a severe traumatic brain injury. His indomitable search for and participation in rehabilitation therapies stands as an inspiring example to all of us in our own journeys over obstacles on the way to our own life goals.

Mark has written to me:

> I suffered some irreversible brain damage. I have been painted with a *mysterious otherness*, and I will remain painted with that for the rest of my life. My family and I have come to accept my brain-injury loss—our family's loss—but because of the ambiguous, incomplete nature of that loss, we have never really been able to navigate all the five stages of grieving as they were outlined by Kubler & Ross: denial, anger, bargaining, depression, and acceptance. It is as if we buried parts of me but not all of me, so we are partly thankful, partly mournful. We have had to find our own way to a different kind of acceptance. Someday someone will have to outline the stages for grieving "brain health loss." Those stages will not follow a straight line, and I am not sure how many stages there should be.

> In June of 2017 as I worked to complete this "Fourth Edition" of my book, I started my car one morning and the gas gauge read below empty. That was odd because I had recently filled the tank. I kept staring at the gas gauge and it slowly began to rise: "Oh good," I thought, "the gauge is old. It is just taking a little longer than usual to read correctly. But the needle did not go much above quarter of a tank, and it looked as if it wasn't going to go any higher. Perplexed, I looked around the instrument panel, only to realize I had been looking by mistake at the temperature gauge right across from the gas gauge! The gas gauge itself showed a near full tank—all was explained.

> I had to laugh because the whole incident reflected perfectly how a brain injury can deceive your perception/ your discernment in many ways when myopic vision

misses the whole picture. My client Andy reminds me often that, "We have to laugh at ourselves or else we will cry." I agree with Andy: A good sense of humor has served me and many other survivors well. Winston Churchill is said to have defined success as "the ability to move from one failure to another without loss of enthusiasm." I have had more than my share of failures. Staying positive, with a smile on my face, and looking to learn a lesson from each has helped me greatly.

Knowing what I have come through and how drastically worse things could have been if any one of my many supports or therapies had been taken away, I am *almost* proud of who I am today. I have been climbing one of life's "highest mountains," and I am nearing the summit! Even though I am not fully recovered and I accept I never will be; still, I keep trying to get closer to "100%"—1% at a time—because that goal, that beacon of hope, motivates me to continue with the rehabilitation systems I have in place. Some have suggested that in some ways I may already have surpassed what would have been my "pre-injury normal" and grown in ways that would not have been possible without such an obstacle as my severe TBI to "push against," such a bucket of cream to "struggle in," such a "suck" to embrace. Although I will never reach 100%, the goal and effort to do so will help me maintain my abilities longer than if I had not tried, and it will make me a better person than I was 10, 20, or 30 years ago.

You may be asking what good is a goal that can never be reached (being 100% my pre-BI self for instance)? The primary benefit of a goal is to serve as a beacon that marks a direction. The lifestyle we fashion, the habits we galvanize, the protocols and systems we employ daily, become the path we follow on our journey: Those daily habits are absolutely responsible for our rehabilitation progress or lack thereof. Being fixated on the goal of being the pre-injury "normal" Mark Condon (my missing tile) would undermine my whole program— for failing to attain that *impossible* goal would sap my energy and eventually crush me with despair and defeat. However, if instead I let the goal of being my normal self serve me *directionally* as the true North on my compass, to continually refocus my attention and to encourage my efforts with the CHAMP BRANDISE protocol: to follow, refine and develop its systems— then that goal—together with those effective programs and habits can sustain me in making further significant improvement 40 plus years post injury. According to the author James Clear,[106] "Ultimately, it is your commitment to the process that will determine your progress. Having a system is what matters. Committing to the process is what makes the difference. . . . I believe *Atomic Habits* is the most comprehensive and practical guide on how to create good habits, break bad ones, and get 1 percent better every day. I do not believe you will find a more actionable book on the subject of habits and improvement." Clear's amazing book *Atomic Habits*[50] is one more book you will want to own and refer to— again and again.

Abraham Lincoln failed in two businesses. When he was engaged, his fiancée died; he lost twice as many elections as he won, and he even wrote in his diary, "I am now the most miserable man living . . . Whether I shall ever be better I cannot tell." The first woman to swim across the English Channel failed on her first

---

[106] www.jamesclear.com/introducing-atomic-habits.

attempt because of the fog. Even though she had boats on either side of her she stopped one mile from the shore! Later in an interview she said that if she could only have seen the finish line she could have made it, but it had just seemed like she was swimming in circles. With the same strength but clear sight of the finish line, her second attempt was successful and record setting.

Of course ordinary people, unaware of brain injury, do not see me as normal, and they certainly do not want to be like me: Why would they want to be anything less than normal? Family members of the brain injury survivors I work with, however, tell me they want their survivor to be "just like me." If that is not possible, they want them to be at least "more like" me. This highlights again the ambiguous, incomplete nature of brain injury: I have not fully recovered, but I have progressed beyond what the medical community said was possible, and along the way I have been transformed. My whole family has been transformed as well. They continue to encourage and support me, and they help others in their communities as well as foreign refugees. My family does not take things for granted. They are all great people, humble people, and I am very proud to call them my family.

I am thankful for all the positive words people have said and written of me, but I know if they were to write about my negative qualities they could easily fill just as many or more pages. It is my prayer that at the end of my life when I am laid to rest and a tombstone is inscribed to mark my grave, instead of just putting a dash between 1958 and the year of my death, my family will instead put a dash between 1958 and 1981, the year of my brain injury, and then inscribe a three-dot ellipsis between 1981 and whatever year turns out to be my last (i.e., "1958–1981 . . . 20XX"). People will look at that and ask themselves, "Well, it looks as if he died in 1981, but there *somehow* must have been *something* more afterwards. I wonder what happened?"

An ellipsis indicates an intentional omission of words from a speech or text without altering its original meaning—because the communication can be understood from contextual clues. Truly, a dash before and an ellipsis after 1981 on my tombstone would be fitting because much of me did die in that car crash, yet that was not the end of my life or my story. In a real way it was the beginning. As a result of my brain injury and the rehabilitation protocol I have subsequently been able to put together in the course of more than 39 years, I will perhaps be able to significantly improve the lives of more people than I ever could have if I had not been brain injured. My family and friends would certainly understand an ellipsis on my tombstone: It might actually help them remember me both before and after the brain injury. This book may help all the other dear family and friends who have known me only with a brain injury put my "few cards short of a full deck" life in perspective.

Those of us who know Mark only through this book, may we never forget his story. Even more important, I would say, may we take to heart forever and widely share all that Mark has written about what can be done to prevent brain injury (so that our families, friends and neighbors may be spared from the brain injury epidemic) and to fully rehabilitate as many of the over ten million citizen survivors living among us as possible.

Mark's final commentary is:

A brain injury, mild to severe, can be a transformation unlike any other in the life of the survivor and his or her family. A severe brain injury is an unexpected one-way-door that, once you pass through, is closed with force and such finality that there is no going back. Your life and your family's life are divided in two: before the brain injury and after it.

In normal life a 'transformation' is generally a good thing: It often involves a spiritual epiphany, a wake-up call, or an 'aha moment.' (William James, the early 20th-century Harvard University psychologist and philosopher, writes about such moments of clarity in his book, *Varieties of Religious Experience: A Study in Human Nature*[51].) The revelations associated with such moments are deeply personal—even existential—and often give a purposeful new direction to life that was never felt before. The negative transformation involved in brain injury, however, confuses personal identity, bewilders life-purpose, dumbfounds communication skills, and perplexes relationships. A brain injury is an "*ugh* moment." However, I have worked, and continue working, to transform my *ugh moment* and the many subsequent gaffs into a purpose driven life full of meaning, quality relationships and joy.

Dr. David Walsh and Nat Bennett explain in their highly recommended 2004 book, *Why Do They Act That Way? A Survival Guide to the Adolescent Brain for You and Your Teen,*[52] that a baby's brain in his or her mother's womb, just before birth, is "knitted together" with about one hundred billion neurons, each having approximately ten thousand branches. Ten thousand branches coming off each and every one of the hundred billion neurons makes possible about a quadrillion connections. It is impossible to determine the number of different ways to arrange that many connections. Walsh wrote, "We cannot even calculate how many possible songs could be composed by arranging in different combinations and different sequences the eighty-eight keys on a piano keyboard" (p. 29). Francis Crick[107], who won the 1962 Nobel Prize in Medicine, calculated the viable number of neural arrangements in one human brain to inconceivably exceed the entire number of atoms in the universe. Given a quadrillion possible neural configurations, I can only believe there must be a way to recruit and reprogram a portion of them—to use this awe-inspiring, unfathomable abundance of brain capacity to our advantage—and see to it that significant progress, great progress, post brain injury—is the usual outcome—not the rare exception.

A newborn baby has about 17 percent of his or her neurons "linked." However, in the weeks and decades that follow birth, the remaining billions of neurons are connected and programed together. Walsh reported genetics and experience are the two forces "driving" the wiring, networking and development of the brain. Genetics provides the "hard drive," "guts" or capacity of the brain as well as the foundational programing that connects one neuron to another—allowing for continued neuronal branching and networking over a lifetime through experience. Walsh clarifies, "This wiring process driven by genetics is a kind of hard

---

[107] Francis Harry Compton Crick OM FRS (8 June 1916 – 28 July 2004) was a British molecular biologist, biophysicist, and neuroscientist. In 1953, he co-authored with James Watson the academic paper proposing the double helix structure of the DNA molecule.

wiring, complemented by the soft wiring shaped by life experiences" (p. 30). Our interpretation of experience programs the "software" that generates the commentaries played and replayed in our minds—for as long as allowed.[108]* Once in place, our "mindset" independently continues to write the programs that direct who we are, who we love, the decision-making/problem-solving process we employ, how we communicate and who we will become. After a brain injury we may not be able to affect the damaged "hard drive," but I believe through "experience" in therapy and through relationships—we can rewrite our mindset's software and positively shape our long-term outcomes.

Robert Love, Editor In Chief of *Health 2020,* said, "Only a few decades ago, doctors defined health as the absence of disease. Today we are much wiser, we know that without a strong mind, good relationships and a body that's prepped for the long haul, it's hard to say someone is fully well."[109] Love went on to explore how we can better maintain the honest and loving relationships that are foundational to health. After brain injury positive relationships become more important than ever, yet relationships often become the most difficult aspect of life post- injury: Survivors by and large migrate or are pushed towards isolation.

Victor Frankl who wrote the seminal book, *Man's Search For Meaning,* (*a book that the smartest people in my life recommend everyone should read*) said, "Everything can be taken from a man but one thing: the last of the

---

[108] * "for as long as allowed" – Clearly we can change our mindset if we so choose to replace the commentaries/programs played/written in our minds.

[109] "Stay Sharp Be Healthy Get Happy," *Health 2020* magazine April/May p31

human freedoms—to choose one's attitude in any given set of circumstances, to choose one's own way." Frankl said also, "Between stimulus and response there is a space. In that space is our power to choose our response. In our response lies our growth and our freedom." His opinion was formulated, however, without taking into account brain injury. Brain injury can take that "one thing"— the last of our freedoms—our ability to choose our attitude in any given circumstance, and steal it away. Inability to choose appropriate attitudes and responses, in turn, can cause survivors to be ostracized from others indefinitely.

Fortunately, most survivors do retain a degree of the ability to choose their attitude. They are aware of and able to make use of the "space" between a stimulus and their response. It is a fact, though, that many of us need more "space" or time to decide than normal—I implore every survivor to give him or herself that necessary accommodation, that needed space, to consciously formulate each response and how to communicate it – before in fact responding.

According to the AARP 2015 survey of Americans ages 34 to 75, nearly everyone (93%) understands the importance of brain health[110] (a drastic improvement from when I was brain injured in 1981). Absent from this understanding, however, is knowledge of how one can in fact maintain brain health. In AARP's April 1, 2020 Brain Health & Wellness article, "Sanjay Gupta's Prescription for Brain Health"[111] Dr. Gupta wrote, "I

---

[110] https://press.aarp.org/2015-01-20-Brain-Health-Important-to-93-of-Americans-But-Few-Know-the-5-Ways-to-Help-Maintain-or-Improve-It

[111] https://www.aarp.org/health/brain-health/info-2020/sanjay-gupta-brain-health.html

am more convinced than ever that the brain can be constructively changed – continually enhanced and fine tuned – no matter what your age or access to resources is." Since turning fifty Dr. Gupta has been working on building his brain's resiliency. Whereas he used to think of socializing as a "fun diversion," he now is certain it is a "healthy brain-building activity." Reflecting on the plethora of evidence that significant positive relationships with family and friends strengthen the prefrontal cortex and pave "the way for a more resilient brain," Dr. Gupta maintains socially engaged survivors are flexible in the face of change and less likely to see crises as "insurmountable problems." Such survivors demonstrate resiliency in action and can be an example to all of us. People who promptly address problems with confidence develop more resilient brains as they steadily move toward their goals. They habitually acknowledge and take note of the small accomplishments along the way while refining and expanding the magnitude of future goals. They are thankful people who express sincere gratitude to everyone that has been a part of his or her success. Such people routinely foster a positive view of themselves. Dr. Gupta reminds us, "It is very hard to cripple a brain that is decisive and views itself favorably."

It can be difficult after a moderate or severe brain injury to view oneself favorably or know where to turn. The CHAMP BRANDISE protocol may well be a way for survivors (no matter the degree of injury: mild – moderate – severe) to call upon and recruit many of those quadrillion neuronal configurations with which they can optimize rehabilitation success and fashion a satisfactory life. Employ the protocol daily with discipline and see where it takes you in two to ten years.

However, the CHAMP BRANDISE protocol certainly is not a panacea nor is it perfect. What I strongly encourage each survivor and every member of his or her family to do also is turn with all their hearts to their Higher Power, bring the Divine into the picture and never give up. The Hispano-Roman Stoic philosopher, statesman and dramatist Seneca said to all of mankind, "As long as you live, keep learning how to live." His words especially ring true for brain injury survivors who have to relearn, and keep relearning, how to live—for as long as they live.

I have named my company Transforming Techniques Incorporated to represent my journey through brain injury (more accurately my difficult, transforming journey with brain injury). This name reflects both my company's mission—namely, to positively transform the lives of brain injury survivors and their families—and its vision, bringing effective therapeutic methodologies and equipment into the homes of survivors, opening rehabilitation clinics/campuses, encouraging the expansion of BI support groups, advancing state brain injury alliances/associations, and educating the general public about the Silent Epidemic. Transforming Techniques Incorporated will prioritize helping survivors and their families maximize their *independence*. We will do so by teaching practical accommodation strategies, skills for adapting to post-brain-injury limitations and also developing social/communication skills for expanding participation in life—improving quality of life. Perhaps one day insurance companies, doctors and politicians interested in better outcomes and saving money will think of me as prescient when it comes to brain injury and invite me to work with them to improve the rehabilitation outcomes for the more than ten million survivors among us?

If I may adapt some words from our country's Declaration of Independence:

> When in the course of human events, it becomes necessary for people to dissolve the political and financial bonds that have connected them to a medical paradigm—acknowledged as inadequate—and to assume among their powers the right to confront the enormous forces arrayed against sensible reforms, they are both compelled and entitled to declare the medical and economical causes that impel them to dissolve these restrictive bonds. Prudence, indeed, will dictate that medical paradigms, long established and to which we are accustomed, should not be changed unless human suffering and financially prohibitive costs make it obvious that abolishing such paradigms is warranted. Further, when the long train of abuses and usurpations associated with the for-now standard brain injury rehabilitation medical paradigm evinces a design that reduces survivors and their families to a dark, restrictive dependence, it is their right and their duty to throw off such a failed medical paradigm and institute a bright alternative paradigm that provides new rehabilitation protocols for their well-being and future security.

If you feel compelled, please join me in this Transforming Techniques Incorporated venture. Initially it may look like a crazy circus, but over time it will become a more well-organized, medically effective, and cost-efficient operation. Thank you for helping me in any way that you can.

50   James Clear, *Atomic Habits: An Easy and Proven Way to Build Good Habits and Break Bad Ones* (New York: Avery, Penguin Random House, 2018).

51   James, W, *Varieties of Religious Experience: A Study in Human Nature,* Seven Treasures Publications, SevenTreasuresPublications@gmail.com Fax: 413-653-8797, ISBN 9781439297278, Copyright © 2009 by Seven Treasures Publications

52   Walsh, D, Bennett, N, *Why Do They Act That Way? A Survival Guide to the Adolescent Brain for You and Your Teen* FREE PRESS: A Division of Simon & Schuster Inc. 1230 Avenue of the Americas, New York, NY 10020 ISBN 0-7432-6071-6, Copyright © 2004 by David Walsh, Ph.D.

53   Frankl, V, *Man's Search For Meaning*, BEACON PRESS, 25 Beacon Street, Boston Massachusette 02108-2892, www.beacon.org ISBN 978-0-8070-1429-5 (pbk), Copyright © 1959, 1962, 1984, 2006 by Victor E. Frankl

REFERENCES

1. G. Whiteneck et al., "Prevalence of Self-Reported Lifetime History of Traumatic Brain Injury and Associated Disability: A Statewide Population-Based Survey," *Journal of Head Trauma Rehabilitation* (April 29, 2015), http://journals.lww.com/headtraumarehab/pages/results.aspx?txtkeywords=Prevalence+of+Self-Reported+Lifetime+History+of+Traumatic+Brain+Injury+and+Associated+Disability%3a+A+Statewide+Population-Based+Survey.

2. M. Faul et al., *Traumatic Brain Injury in the United States: Emergency Department Visits, Hospitalizations and Deaths 2002–2006* (Atlanta, GA: Centers for Disease Control and Prevention, National Center for Injury Prevention and Control, 2010).

3. D. Ludden, *The Psychology of Language: An Integrated Approach* (Thousand Oaks, California: SAGE Publications, 2016), https://books.google.com/books?hl=en&lr=&id=60YoBgAAQBAJ&oi=fnd&pg=PP1&dq=Dr.+Ludden+The+Psychology+of+Language:+An+Integrated+Approach.

4. P. Daniels, "Your Brain: A User's Guide, 100 Things You Never Knew" (Washington, DC: National Geographic Partners, LLC, 2018), https://www.amazon.com/National-Geographic-Your-Brain-Things/dp/B00AO70YGO.

5. D. McRaney, *You Are Now Less Dumb: How to Conquer Mob Mentality, How to Buy Happiness, and All the Other Ways to Outsmart Yourself* (New York: Gotham Books, 2013), https://www.amazon.com/You-are-Now-Less-Dumb/dp/1592408796.

6. M. Mehl et al., "Eavesdropping on Happiness: Well-Being Is Related to Having Less Small Talk and More Substantive Conversations," *Psychological Science* 21, no. 4 (2010): 539–541, https://www.ncbi.nlm.nih.gov/pmc/articles/PMC2861779/?TBiframe=true&width=921.6&height=921.6&mod=article_inline.

For more information about this study, please contact Matthias R. Mehl at mehl@email.arizona.edu.

7. N. Gibbs, "The EQ Factor," *Time* 146, no. 14 (June 24, 2001): 60–68, http://content.time.com/time/magazine/article/0,9171,133181,00.html.

8. A. Damasio, *The Feeling of What Happens* (New York, San Diego, London: Antonio Damasio, 1999), https://www.amazon.com/Feeling-What-Happens-Emotion-Consciousness/dp/0156010755.

9. J. Twenge et al., "Social Exclusion Decreases Prosocial Behavior," *Journal of Personality and Social Psychology* 92, no. 1 (2007): 56–66, http://www.uky.edu/~njdewa2/RejProsocJPSP.pdf.

10. D. Umberson and J. Karas Montez, "Social Relationships and Health: A Flashpoint for Health Policy," *Journal of Health and Social Behavior* 51(Suppl., 2010): S54–S66, doi: 10.1177/0022146510383501, https://www.ncbi.nlm.nih.gov/pmc/articles/PMC3150158/.

11. C. Elliott C, *The Ghost in My Brain: How a Concussion Stole My Life and How the New Science of Brain Plasticity Helped Me Get It Back* (New York: Penguin Publishing Group, 2015), https://www.thriftbooks.com/w/the-ghost-in-my-brain-how-a-concussion-stole-my-life-and-how-the-new-science-of-brain-plasticity-helped-me-get-it-back/9388336/item/9371439/.

12. J. Garbarino, *Lost Boys: Why Our Sons Turn Violent and How We Can Save Them* (New York: Anchor Books, 1999), https://www.ncbi.nlm.nih.gov/pmc/articles/PMC2722594/.

13. J. Didion, *The Year of Magical Thinking* (Knopf, October 2005), https://www.penguinrandomhouse.com/books/40771/the-year-of-magical-thinking-by-joan-didion/.

14. V. Murthy, *Together: The Healing Power of Human Connection in a Sometimes Lonely World* (April 21, 2020).

15. R. Manor, "Firestone Settles Tire Suit in Texas: Paralyzed Woman Gets $7.5 Million," *Chicago Tribune* (August 25, 2001), https://www.chicagotribune.com/news/ct-xpm-2001-08-25-0108250169-story.html.

16. H. Gravitz, "The Binds That Tie—and Heal: How Families Cope with Mental Illness," *Psychology Today* 34, no. 2 (March/April 2001): 70–76, https://www.psychologytoday.com/us/articles/200103/the-binds-tie-and-heal.

17. REAP Project can be accessed by calling Karen McAvoy, PsyD, coordinator of Mental Health Services, coordinator of the Cherry Creek School District brain injury team, at 720-554-4252 (phone), 720-554-4272 (fax), or kmcavoy@cherrycreekschools.org(email).

18. M. Lynch and P. Stretesky, *Exploring Green Criminology* (Farnham, England; Burlington, VT: Ashgate Publishing, 2014), https://core.ac.uk/download/pdf/41071488.pdf.

19. M. J. Lavery, *Whole Brain Power: The Fountain of Youth for the Mind and Body* (Blaine, WA: Lulu.com), www.wholebrainpowercoaching.com, https://www.amazon.com/Whole-Brain-Power-Fountain-Youth/dp/0557005140.

20. A. Sigman, *Remotely Controlled: How Television Is Damaging Our Lives*, new ed. (Vermilion, February 1, 2007), https://www.amazon.com/Remotely-Controlled-Television-Damaging-Lives/dp/0091906903.

21. W. Mackey and N. Coney, "The Enigma of Father Presence in Relationship to Son's Violence," *Journal of Men's Studies* 8, no. 3 (Spring 2000): 349–73, https://www.questia.com/library/journal/1P3-650097751/the-presence-of-the-social-father-in-inhibiting-young.

22. B. E. Weinstein, PhD, "Preventing Cognitive Decline: Hearing Interventions Promising," *Hearing Journal* 68, no. 9 (September 2015): 22–24, 26, https://journals.lww.com/thehearingjournal/Fulltext/2015/09000/Article.4.aspx.

23. N. Zasler, D. Katz, and R. Zafonte, *Brain Injury Medicine: Principles and Practice*, 2d ed. (Demos Medical Publishing, 2013), www.demosmedpub.com.

24. M. D. Wald, S. R. Helgeson, and J. A. Langlois, "Traumatic Brain Injury among Prisoners," *Brain Injury Professional, NABIS,*

216.97.226.57/node/66, https://www.brainline.org/article/traumatic-brain-injury-among-prisoners.

25. A. Chen, "Adolescents' Drinking Takes Lasting Toll on Memory: Even Moderate Drinking by Adolescents on a Regular Basis Can Cause Potentially Lasting Changes to the Brain," *Wall Street Journal* (April 27, 2015), https://www.wsj.com/articles/adolescents-drinking-takes-lasting-toll-on-memory-1430173521.

26. T. Tomlinson, "The Greatest Sports Moment I Ever Saw," *Reader's Digest* 100 (September 2012).

27. W. Nack, "The Wrecking Yard," *Sports Illustrated* 94, no. 19 (May 7, 2001): 60–75, https://vault.si.com/vault/2001/05/07/the-wrecking-yard-as-they-limp-into-the-sunset-retired-nfl-players-struggle-with-the-games-grim-legacy-a-lifetime-of-disability-and-pain.

28. M. Fainaru-Wada and S. Fainaru, *League of Denial* (New York: Crown Archetype, 2013), https://www.penguinrandomhouse.com/books/221286/league-of-denial-by-mark-fainaru-wada-and-steve-fainaru/.

29. J. Torg et al., "The National Football Head and Neck Injury Registry14-Year Report on Cervical Quadriplegia, 1971 through 1984," Journal of the American Medical Association 254, no. 24 (December 27, 1985): 3439–43, doi:10.1001/jama.1985.03360240051033, https://jamanetwork.com/journals/jama/article-abstract/402289.

30. F. Abreau, "Neuropsychological Assessment of Attention and Concentration in Soccer Players" (dissertation, California School of Professional Psychology, 1989; reproduction: photocopy, Ann Arbor, Mich.: University Microfilms International, 2000), viii, 63 p.; 28 cm, https://psycnet.apa.org/buy/1991-26117-001.

31. J. Matser, A. Kessels, and J. Troost, "Chronic Traumatic Brain Injury in Professional Soccer Players," Neurology 51, no. 3 (September 1, 1998): 791, https://n.neurology.org/content/51/3/791.abstract.

32. G. Voss, "Women and Concussions," Dr. Oz the Good Life 2, no. 5 (June 2015): 44–49.

33. M. Esiri and D. Perl, Oppenheimer's Diagnostic Neuropathology: A Practical Manual (London: Hodder Arnold, Hodder Headline Group, 2006), http://www.hoddereducation.com.

34. S. B. Shively et al., "Characterization of Interface Astroglial Scarring in the Human Brain after Blast Exposure: A Post-Mortem Case Series" Lancet Neurology 15, no. 9 (August 1, 2016): 944–53, https://www.ncbi.nlm.nih.gov/pubmed/27291520.

35. R. Kelley, "The Writing on the Wall," Newsweek 150 no. 20 (November, 12, 2007): 69, https://www.questia.com/magazine/1G1-170830860/the-writing-on-the-wall.

36. D. Snowdon, Aging with Grace: What the Nun Study Teaches Us about Leading Longer, Healthier, and More Meaningful Lives, unabridged (April 30, 2002), https://www.amazon.com/Aging-Grace-Teaches-Healthier-Meaningful/dp/0553380923.

37. S. Anderson, J. Cryan, PhD, and T. Dinan, MD, PhD, Psychobiotic Revolution: Mood, Food, and the New Science of the Gut-Brain Connection (Washington, DC: National Geographic Partners, 2017), https://www.amazon.com/Psychobiotic-Revolution-Science-Gut-Brain-Connection/dp/142621846X.

38. G. Bussiere, The Concussion Healing Solution: Clarity amid the Confusion (2017), https://www.amazon.com/Concussion-Healing-Solution-Clarity-Confusion-ebook/dp/B06XCDFGVD.

39. K. Kosik, Outsmarting Alzheimer's: What You Can Do to Reduce Your Risk (Reader's Digest Association, Inc., 2015), https://boulder.flatironslibrary.org/GroupedWork/fccb67bb-99d7-3567-6eec-747fc779d869/Home.

40. K. Eakin et al., "Efficacy of N-Acetyl Cysteine in Traumatic Brain Injury," PLOS One 9, no. 4 (April 2014): e90617, www.journals.plos.org/plosone/article/file?id=10.1371/journal.pone.0090617&type=printable.

41. B. Hoffer et al., "Repositioning Drugs for Traumatic Brain Injury—N-acetylcysteine and Phenserine" J Biomed Sci. 24, no. 1 (September 9, 2017): 71, doi: 10.1186/s12929-017-0377-1,

https://www.ncbi.nlm.nih.gov/pubmed/28886718, email: barry.
hoffer@case.edu.

42.   P. D. Harch and V. McCullough, The Oxygen Revolution:
      Hyperbaric Oxygen Therapy: The New Treatment for Post
      Traumatic Stress Disorder (PTSD), Traumatic Brain Injury,
      Stroke, Autism and More (Hatherleigh Press, 2016), https://www.
      amazon.com/Oxygen-Revolution-Third-Hyperbaric-Definitive/
      dp/1578266270/.

43.   N. Ortner, The Tapping Solution: A Revolutionary System for
      Stress-Free Living (Hay House, Inc., 2013), https://www.amazon.
      com/Tapping-Solution-Weight-Loss-Confidence/dp/1401945139.

44.   Brain Injury Professional 16, no. 3, North American Brain
      Injury Society, and HDI Publishers, PO box 1804, Alexandria,
      VA 22313, tel.: 703-960-6500, www.nabis.org, 2019, https://
      braininjuryprofessional.com.

45.   T. Meili, I Am the Central Park Jogger: A Story of Hope and
      Possibility (2003), www.shape.com/lifestyle/mind-and-body/
      trisha-meili-central-park-jogger-how-running-helped-heal-
      interview.

46.   A. MacNeill Horton Jr. and L. Hartlage, Handbook of
      Forensic Neuropsychology, 2d ed. (New York: Springer
      Publishing Company, 2003), https://www.amazon.com/
      Handbook-Forensic-Neuropsychology-Second-MacNeill/
      dp/0826118852.

47.   S. Aamodt and S. Wang, Welcome to Your Brain: Why You
      Lose Your Car Keys but Never Forget How to Drive and
      Other Puzzles of Everyday Life (New York, London, New
      Delhi, Sydney, 2008), https://www.bloomsbury.com/us/
      welcome-to-your-brain-9781596912830/.

48.   C. Symonds, "Concussion and Its Sequelae," Lancet 279,
      no. 7219 (1962): 1–5, http://www.oalib.com/references/
      14262809.

49.   C. Vash, Psychology of Disability (New York:
      Springer, 1981), https://www.amazon.com/Psychology-

Disability-Second-SPRINGER-REHABILITATION/
dp/0826133428.

50.   J. Clear, Atomic Habits: An Easy and Proven Way to
      Build Good Habits and Break Bad Ones (Hudson,
      New York: Avery, Penguin Random House LLC, 2018),
      https://www.penguinrandomhouse.com/books/
      543993/atomic-habits-by-james-clear/.

◆

Alexander, M. P. "Mild Traumatic Brain Injury: Pathophysiology,
      Natural History, and Clinical Management." *Neurology* no. 7
      (1995): 1253–60., 45

American Speech-Language-Hearing Association (ASHA). "TBI
      Recovery Hampered by Inadequate Health Insurance Coverage—
      On Eve of Capitol Hill Event, Group Urges Expanded Coverage
      of Services for Communication Needs." March 2011. http://www.
      asha.org., 15

Angell, M. "Handicapped Children: Baby Doe and Uncle Sam." *New
      England Journal of Medicine* no. 11 (September 15, 1983): 659–
      61., 309

Arras, J. "Toward an Ethic of Ambiguity." *Hastings Center Report* no. 2
      (April 1984): 25–33., 14

Betz, J., J. Zhuo, A. Roy, K. Shanmuganathan, and R. P. Gullapalli.
      "Prognostic Value of Diffusion Tensor Imaging Parameters in
      Severe Traumatic Brain Injury. *Journal of Neurotrauma* no. 7 (2012):
      1292–1305., 29

Brain Injury Professional no. 3. (Brain *Injury Professional is a* membership
      benefit of the North American Brain Injury Society and the
      International Brain Injury Association.), 16

Brooks, J. C., D. J. Strauss, R. M. Shavelle, D. R. Paculdo, F. M. Hammond, and C. L. Harrison-Felix. "Long-Term Disability and Survival in Traumatic Brain Injury: Results from the National Institute on Disability and Rehabilitation Research Model Systems." *Archives of Physical Medicine and Rehabilitation* no. 11 (November 2013): 2203–9, doi:10.1016/j.apmr.2013.07.005., 94

Brown, D. "Employment Considerations for Learning Disabled Adults." *Journal of Rehabilitation* no. 2 (April–June 1984): 74–77, 88., 59

Bullard, J., and R. Cutshaw. "Vocational Evaluation of the Closed Head Injury Population: A Challenge of the 1990s." *Vocational Evaluation and Work Adjustment Bulletin* (Spring 1991): 15–19.

Chandler, S., T. Czerlinsky, M. Moore, L. Starr Rutman, and A. Schumacher. "The Relationship between Vocational Decision-Making and Vocational Status of Individuals with Traumatic Brain Injury." *Vocational Evaluation and Work Adjustment Bulletin* (Winter 1993): 161–70.

Corrigan, J. D., J. P. Cuthbert, C. Harrison-Felix, G. G. Whiteneck, J. M. Bell, A. C. Miller, . . . and C. R. Pretz. "US Population Estimates of Health and Social Outcomes Five Years after Rehabilitation for Traumatic Brain Injury." *Journal of Head Trauma Rehabilitation* no. 6 (2014): E1–E9., 29

Corrigan, J. D., S. D. Horn, R. S. Barrett, R. J. Smout, J. Bogner, F. M. Hammond, . . . and S. Majercik. "Effects of Patient Pre-injury and Injury Characteristics on Acute Rehabilitation Outcomes for Traumatic Brain Injury." *Archives of Physical Medicine and Rehabilitation* no. 8 (2015): S209–S221, e206., 96

Crimmins, C. *Where Is the Mango Princess? A Journey Back from Brain Injury.* Vintage Books, 2000.

Daniels, P. *National Geographic Mind: A Scientific Guide to Who You Are, How You Got That Way, and How to Make the Most of It.* National Geographic Washington DC, September 15, 2017

Davis, L. C., M. Sherer, A. M. Sander, J. A. Bogner, J. D. Corrigan, M. P. Dijkers, . . . and R. T. Seel. "Pre-injury Predictors of Life Satisfaction at One Year after Traumatic Brain Injury." *Archives of Physical Medicine and Rehabilitation* no. 8 (2012): 1324–30., 93

Forslund, M., C. Roe, S. Sigurdardottir, and N. Andelic. "Predicting Health-Related Quality of Life Two Years after Moderate-to-Severe Traumatic Brain Injury. *Acta Neurologica Scandinavica* no. 4 (2013): 220–27., 128

Harrison-Felix, C., C. Pretz, F. M. Hammond, J. P. Cuthbert, J. Bell, J. Corrigan ... and J. Haarbauer-Krupa. "Life Expectancy after Inpatient Rehabilitation for Traumatic Brain Injury in the United States. *Journal of Neurotrauma* no. 23 (2015), 1893–901., 32

Hart, T., L. Brenner, A. N. Clark, J. A. Bogner, T. A. Novack, I. Chervoneva, . . . J. C. Arango-Lasprilla. "Major and Minor Depression after Traumatic Brain Injury." *Archives of Physical Medicine and Rehabilitation* no. 8 (2011): 1211–19., 92

Hart, T, J. M. Hoffman, C. Pretz, R. Kennedy, A. N. Clark, and L. A. Brenner. "A Longitudinal Study of Major and Minor Depression following Traumatic Brain Injury. *Archives of Physical Medicine and Rehabilitation* no. 8 (2012): 1343–49., 93

Hartlage, L. *Neuropsychological Evaluation of Head Injury.* Sarasota, FL: Professional Resource Exchange, 1990.

Hawley, L. *A Family Guide to the Rehabilitation of the Severely Head-Injured Patient.* Austin: Healthcare Rehabilitation Center, 1987.

Iverson, G. Outcome from Mild Traumatic Brain Injury. *Curr. Opin. Psychiatry* no. 3 (2005): 301–317., 18

James, W. *Varieties of Religious Experience: A Study in Human Nature.* Seven Treasures Publications, 2009.

Karp, D. *The Burden of Sympathy: How Families Cope with Mental Illness.* Oxford University Press, 2001.

Kartal, A., B. Yldran, A. Enköylü, and F. Korkusuz. "Soccer Causes Degenerative Changes in the Cervical Spine." *European Spine Journal* no. 1 (February 2004): 76–82., 13

Langlois, J., W. Rutland-Brown, M. Wald. "The Epidemiology and Impact of Traumatic Brain Injury: A Brief Overview." *Journal of Head Trauma Rehabilitation* no. 2 (2006): 375–78., 21

Lezak, M. *Neuropsychological Assessment.* New York: Oxford University Press, 1983.

Lippincott Williams & Wilkins, Inc. *Journal of Head Trauma Rehabilitation* no. 4 (July–August 2010): 225, www. headtraumarehab.com., 25

Marwitz, J. H., A. P. Sima, J. S. Kreutzer, L. E. Dreer, T. F. Bergquist, R. Zafonte, . . . and E. R. Felix. "Longitudinal Examination of Resilience after Traumatic Brain Injury: A Traumatic Brain Injury Model Systems Study." *Archives of Physical Medicine and Rehabilitation* no. 2 (2018), 264–71., 99

Masel, B. E., and D. S. DeWitt. "Traumatic Brain Injury: A Disease Process, Not an Event." *Journal of Neurotrauma* no. 8 (2010): 1529–40, https://www.liebertpub.com/doi/abs/10.1089/neu.2010.1358., 27

Mathias, J. L., and P. K. Alvaro. "Prevalence of Sleep Disturbances, Disorders, and Problems following Traumatic Brain Injury: A Meta-Analysis." *Sleep Medicine* no. 7 (2012): 898–905., 13

National Commission against Drunk Driving, 3D Prevention Month Coalition. 1900 L Street, NW, Suite Washington DC 20036. Ph.: 202-452-6004, fax: 202-223-7012., 705

NCAA Football Rule Book. Rule , 2

Omalu, B. I., S. T. DeKosky, R. L. Minster, M. I. Kamboh, R. L. Hamilton, and C. H. Wecht. "Chronic Traumatic Encephalopathy in a National Football League Player." *Neurosurgery* no. 1 (2005): 128–134, https://doi.org/10.1227/01.NEU.0000163407. 92769. ED., 57

Parker, R. *Traumatic Brain Injury and Neuropsychological Impairment*. New York: Springer-Verlag, 1990.

Rabinowitz, A. R. and P. A. Arnett. "Positive Psychology Perspective on Traumatic Brain Injury Recovery and Rehabilitation." *Applied Neuropsychology: Adult* no. 4 (2018): 295–303., 25

Sacks, O. *The Man Who Mistook His Wife for a Hat and Other Clinical Tales*. New York: Touchstone Book Simon & Schuster, 1985.

Silver, J., R. Kramer, S. Greenwald, M. Weissman. "The Association between Head Injuries and Psychiatric Disorders: Findings from the New Haven NIMH Epidemiologic Catchment Area Study." *Brain Injury* 11 (2001): 935–45.

Slaughter, B., J. Fann, and D. Ehde. "Traumatic Brain Injury in a County Jail Population: Prevalence, Neuropsychological Functioning and Psychiatric Disorders." *Brain Injury* 17 (2003): 731–41.

Thornhill, S., G. M. Teasdale, G. D. Murray, J. McEwen, C. W. Roy, and K. I. Penny. "Disability in Young People and Adults One Year after Head Injury: Prospective Cohort Study." *BMJ* no. 7250 (2000): 1631–35., 320

S. Vanost Wulz. "Acquired Traumatic Brain Injury." In *Medical, Psychosocial and Vocational Aspects of Disability*, edited by M. Brodwin, F. Tellez, and S. Brodwin, 473–89. Athens, GA: Elliot & Fitzpatrick, 1993.

Wardlaw, C., A. J. Hicks, M. Sherer, and J. L. Ponsford. "Psychological Resilience Is Associated with Participation Outcomes following Mild to Severe Traumatic Brain Injury. *Frontiers in Neurology* 9 (2018).

Wendell, S., and S. Tremain. "The Rejected Body: Feminist Philosophical Reflections on Disability." *Hypatia* no. 2: 219–24, 1997., 12

What America Thinks—MetLife Foundation Alzheimer's Survey, February 2011, Harris Interactive for MetLife Foundation, December 27, 1985.

APPENDIX

CHAMP BRANDISE PROTOCOL COST ESTIMATES

C   Cold therapy (therapeutic hypothermia) – $400
          CereScan – $4,500 for two scans
          qSPECT – $3,700
          QEEG – $700
          PET – $3,500
          Communication game coaching – $2,500

H   Hyperbaric oxygen therapy – 40 dives within the first 6 months – $12,000

A   Anti-inflammatory N-acetylcysteine (NAC) – $30

M   Microcirculation and anti-inflammation with European PEMF device – $6,000
          MojoFeet orthotics – $400

P   Prayer, power, pace, and penmanship – Whole Brain Power program – $40
          Perfect Penmanship – $40

B   Brucker biofeedback therapy – $4,000 per year
          FocusBand – $1,100

R   Reduce and rest

A   Activate – Muscle Activation Technique therapy – $7,500 per year

N   Neuro-optometric – Dr. Deborah Zelinsky's mind-eye evaluation and therapeutic lenses – $3,000
          Nutrition – organic diet including superfoods, unsweetened cocoa, and supplements – dietary budget shift

D	Designs for Strong Minds – Dr. Donalee Markus's brain injury apps: Strong Mind Puzzles and Strong Mind Treasure Hunt for iOS (iPhone, iPad) and Android – $60
I	Infrared light therapy – Vigen far-infrared light equipment – $5,000
S	Tapping solution – $300
	Integrated Listen System – $2,100
E	Educate

TOTAL CHAMP BRANDISE costs/year
First 20 years – $47,590
Subsequent 40 years – $15,990
60 years of CHAMP BRANDISE therapies – $991,000

The cost savings between the CHAMP BRANDISE functional medical protocol and the traditional AMA medical approach for a lifetime with a severe brain injury (sixty years) would be $1,446,500 for one person (based on averaging the estimated lifetime costs of a severe brain injury $3,000,000 - $1,875,000), $289,300,000,000 for the annual two hundred thousand people severely brain injured, and $1.7358e+13 for all severe survivors over a sixty-year period—which is nearly impossible to grasp. (I have never seen a number that big and do not know how to say it.)

The calculation/estimation above, if correct (I am not a mathematician but had the numbers verified at Westerra Credit Union in Denver, Colorado), does not include the majority of BI survivors— not the 1.8 million new moderate survivors hospitalized each year nor the 5.0 million people who were brain-injured but never hospitalized. Nor does it include any of the indirect costs to society or to families, such as the costs of social services; worker's comp, reduced work time, lowered productivity, or unemployment; marriage counseling; cognitive therapy; or the costs associated with suicide and violence. Further, the three calculations/estimations do not include the emotional and physical debts that arise in a survivor family and community as a result of brain injury because it is impossible to put a dollar figure on the ripple effect of brain injury consequences. However, the cost estimation is over a lifetime (sixty years) for the number of United States severe survivor citizens in a single year; if expanded for sixty years (close to a lifetime after a brain injury) to collect the new survivors from each of those sixty years, the lifetime cost savings from following the CHAMP BRANDISE protocol versus conventional medicine for severe brain injury adds up to a number so large that it dwarfs the United States national debt ($18.96 trillion). Had we followed the CHAMP BRANDISE protocol, we would have saved $289 trillion each year and been able to do much more than just pay off our national debt. I recognize that my calculations may not be exactly correct—and if they are a bit off—but that is no reason to dismiss this monumental medical paradigm shift. For there will certainly be a heretofore unimaginable cost savings associated with this new medical protocol.

INDEX

Corbett, Shaun. *See under* Brucker, Bernard S.

Cousteau, Jacques, 53

Covassin, Tracey, 116

COVID-19, 200, 202, 223–25

Craig Hospital, 27, 214–16, 310

Creole languages. *See* Bickerton, Derek, Creole languages

CTE (chronic traumatic encephalopathy), xix, 40, 96, 98–100, 102–7, 119, 198, 222, 232, 238, 247

D

Dahlia Campus for Health and Well-Being. *See* Prado, Lydia, Dahlia Campus for Health and Well-Being

Damasio, Antonio
Descartes' Error, 29

Daniels, Patricia S., 19, 24, 135
Your Brain, 18–19

degrees of disability, 19, 230

DeLay, Dave, 196

depleted ego. *See* ego depletion

depression, 29, 37, 43, 47, 51–53, 67, 83, 91, 96, 119–20, 145, 147–48, 164, 168, 199, 227, 239, 243, 309, 317

Designs for Strong Minds. *See* Markus, Donalee, Designs for Strong Minds

DeWall, C. Nathan, 40

Diaz, Diana. *See under* Brucker, Bernard S.

disinhibition, 28

distractibility, 20–21, 33, 44, 53, 58, 233

Domitrovich, Dorothy. *See* Condon, Dorothy (née Domitrovich)

Domitrovich, Martin, 197, 210
Equestrian Connection, 197, 210

Dr. Seuss, 255

drunk drivers, xv, 207–8, 222–23, 225–26, 293, 316

E

education, xi, xvii–xviii, 37–39, 42, 64, 76, 82, 104, 119, 181, 205, 208, 227–28, 249, 254, 279, 315

"Effective Concussion Treatment Remains Frustratingly Elusive, Despite a Booming Industry" (Meier and Ivory), 159, 164

ego depletion, 40, 43–44, 53

Einstein Soccer Study, 115, 124

elderly, xvi

emotional, 19–20, 27, 30, 32–33, 36, 43, 45–46, 51, 64, 66, 73, 81, 109, 129, 137–38, 142, 163, 186, 243, 258, 298, 300, 311

emotional bankruptcy, 32

empathy, xviii, 33, 136–37, 272, 274

Equestrian Connection. *See* Domitrovich, Martin, Equestrian Connection

Esmond family, 209

eye contact. *See* Parente, Frederick, eye contact

eye gaze, 135

F

face recognition memory, 23

Fainaru, Steve, 96–97

Fainaru-Wada, Mark, 96

far-infrared (FIR) light therapy, 129–30, 168–69, 175–76, 229
Vigen, 130, 168, 176–77, 229

fatigue, 13, 20–21, 33, 44, 49, 53, 69, 105, 119, 233, 239, 243, 285, 290

Faul, M., xvi

Feldman Barrett, Lisa, 33

Firestone tire failure. *See* Rodriguez, Marisa, Firestone tire failure

microcirculation, 148–49, 152–54, 166–67, 170, 184, 204, 216, 229, 253, 314

mild brain injury, xvi, 27–28, 38, 58–59, 110–11, 115–16, 119, 147, 214, 220, 235, 243, 273, 322

Mild dementia, 36

Minson, Ron, 84–85

Mirra, Lauren, 105–6

MMI (maximum medical improvement), 6, 170, 211, 229

mnemonics for cognitive skills, 139

moderate brain injury, 13, 20, 28–29, 38, 51, 159, 169, 182, 214, 220, 235, 240

MojoFeet Custom Orthotics, 130

"More Than 40 Percent of Retired NFL Players Had Brain Injury." *See under* Conidi, Francis X.

Murthy, Vivek H., 52

mysterious otherness, xvii, 236, 249, 317

N

N-acetyl cysteine, 159–60

National Center for Health Statistics, xv

National Research Council, 90

Nembutal drip, 1

Neuroeducator II Electromyography Biofeedback System, 76

neurologist, 2, 10, 108, 156, 242

"Neurometabolic Cascade of Concussion, The" (Giza and Hovda), 147, 182

"NFL's Concussion Priorities". *See* Jenkins, Sally, "NFL's Concussion Priorities"

Nicomachean Ethics. See Aristotle, *Nicomachean Ethics*

nonalkalyzed cocoa. *See* White, William, nonalkalyzed cocoa

normalcy bias, 38–39, 235

Null, Gary, 65

O

Occipital lobe, 19

Oldsmobile of General Motors, 269

Omalu, Bennet, 96, 104, 247

Oppenheimer's Diagnostic Neuropathology (Esiri and Pearl), 121, 158

Outsmarting Alzheimer's (Kosik), 151

overload, 45, 47

oxidative stress, 147–48

oxytocin, 136–38

P

Parente, Frederick, 138–39, 141–42, 204
  eye contact, 138, 140, 235
  listening skills, 139–40
  rhymes and mnemonics, 139, 141–42
  controlling anger, 142, 235

Parietal lobe, 18

Parker, Kevin "Kit," 118, 267–68

Pascrell, Bill, 214

PBA (pseudobulbar affect), 34

PEMF device, 153–54, 168, 184, 195

Perfect Penmanship. *See* Lavery, Michael, Perfect Penmanship

perplexity, 20, 33, 44, 53, 233

Pettibon System for spine rehabilitation, 130–31

Plutarch, 258

Prado, Lydia, 191, 205
  Dahlia Campus for Health and Well-Being, 205

prefrontal cortex, 19, 33

"Preventing Cognitive Decline" (Weinstein), 88, 94

prevention, xvi, xx, 58, 61, 80, 91, 100, 104, 115, 192, 225, 315

Price, Niki, 146

probiotics, 145–46

"Women and Concussions" (Voss), 116, 242
working memory, 22
Work of Christ Community, 268, 275
World Health Organization (WHO). *See* WHO (World Health Organization)

Z

Zhang, Li Xin, 129, 174–75